Chronic Disease and Disability

A Contemporary Rehabilitation Approach
to Medical Practice

Chronic Disease and Disability

A Contemporary Rehabilitation Approach to Medical Practice

Ross M. Hays, M.D.
George H. Kraft, M.D.
Walter C. Stolov, M.D.

Department of Rehabilitation Medicine
University of Washington School of Medicine
Seattle, Washington

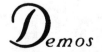

Demos Publications, 386 Park Avenue South, New York, NY 10016

Made in the United States of America.

ISBN: 0-939957-46-9
Library of Congress Cataloging-in-Publication Data

Chronic disease and disability: contemporary rehabilitation approach
  to medical practice / [edited by] Ross M. Hays, George H. Kraft,
  Walter C. Stolov.
      p.   cm.
    Includes index.
    ISBN 0-939957-46-9 (pbk.): $29.95
    1. Chronic diseases.   2. Medical rehabilitation.   3. Physically
  handicapped—Medical care.   I. Hays, Ross M.   II. Kraft, George H.
  III. Stolov, Walter H., 1928–
    [DNLM: 1. Chronic Diseases.   2. Disabled—rehabilitation.   WT 500
  C5555 1994]
  RC108.C455   1994
  616—dc20
  DNLM/DLC
  for Library of Congress   94-38226
                                                                         CIP

Preface

Medical students and physicians in training experience a standard of health care characterized by an unprecedented ability to overcome disease and the effects of injury. The explosion of knowledge and medical technology that began with the last generation of physicians includes an under-appreciated corollary: the ever-increasing number of patients surviving acute crisis, but living with chronic disease and disability. It has been estimated that over 14 percent, or 27 million individuals in the adult population, are suffering from one or more chronic diseases and that 70 percent of the population will suffer disability at some point in their lives. Impressive numbers of disabled people who are effectively and appropriately demanding that the health care establishment provide them with a reasonable quality of life. Therefore it is imperative that physicians and health-care practitioners in all specialties have a general understanding of the basic concepts of chronic disease and disability.

The University of Washington School of Medicine has mandated that all students have clinical experience in the area of chronic disease and disability. In order to provide students with a very general knowledge base from which to operate, the faculty of the Department of Rehabilitation Medicine, under the direction of Dr. Walter C. Stolov, developed its first syllabus on this topic. This text evolved as a refinement of that syllabus. It is intended to provide a brief basic foundation of information about chronic disease and disability. The first sections of the book describe general principles of assessment and treatment of the patient with disability. This is followed by descriptions of the commonly encountered disease syndromes that result in chronic impairment and by a discussion of the psychological and vocational aspects of disability management.

This book is designed to be used by health-care professionals who are being exposed to the concepts of chronic disease and disability for the first time. It provides the clinician with a basic understanding of the more common aspects of disability and the terminology used in rehabilitation. This text will be especially useful for medical students. It will also be useful for those who practice medicine in an acute care context but need an introductory reference to the more common disabling conditions.

Ross M. Hays, M.D.
George H. Kraft, M.D.
Walter C. Stolov, M.D.
Seattle 1994

This book is dedicated to the students at the University of Washington School of Medicine, to their intellectual curiosity, their industry, and their infectious enthusiasm. These are the students who challenge us, keep us accountable for quality in medical education, and who in their hearts and minds embody no less than the future of medical practice.

Acknowledgments

The editors gratefully acknowledge Diana M. Schneider, Ph.D., of Demos Publications for the insight that enabled her to see a useful textbook within the early syllabus and for her encouragement and patience, which were, more than anything else, responsible for the final production of this book. We thank Kim Klassen, who provided the sheer dogged determination necessary to get the job done.

Contributors

Elissa Barron, M.S.W.
Department of Rehabilitation Medicine
University of Washington Medical
  Center
Seattle, Washington

Rosemarian Berni, R.N., M.N.
Department of Rehabilitation Medicine
University of Washington School of
  Medicine
Seattle, Washington

Catherine Britell, M.D.
Clinical Assistant Professor
Department of Rehabilitation Medicine
University of Washington School of
  Medicine
Seattle, Washington

Jo Ann Brockway, Ph.D.
Clinical Associate Professor
Department of Rehabilitation Medicine
University of Washington School of
  Medicine
  and
Rehabilitation Psychologist
Providence Medical Center
Department of Rehabilitation Services
Seattle, Washington

Marvin M. Brooke, M.D.
Associate Professor and Chairman
Department of Rehabilitation Medicine
Tufts University School of Medicine
Boston, Massachusetts
  and
Physiatrist in Chief
Department of Physical Medicine and
  Rehabilitation
New England Medical Center
Boston, Massachusetts
New England Sinai Hospital and
  Rehabilitation Center
Stoughton, Massachusetts

Diana D. Cardenas, M.D.
Professor, Department of
  Rehabilitation Medicine
University of Washington School of
  Medicine
  and
Principal Investigator, Northwest
  Regional Spinal Cord Injury System
Seattle, Washington

Norma Cole, M.S.W.
Department of Rehabilitation Medicine
University of Washington Medical
  Center
Seattle, Washington

Joseph Michael Czerniecki, M.D.
Professor, Department of
  Rehabilitation Medicine
University of Washington School of
  Medicine
  and
Associate Director, Amputation
  Program
Seattle Veteran's Affairs Medical Center
Seattle, Washington

Barbara J. de Lateur, M.D.
Professor and Director
Department of Rehabilitation Medicine
The Johns Hopkins University School
  of Medicine
Baltimore, Maryland

Sureyya Dikmen, Ph.D.
Professor, Department of
  Rehabilitation Medicine
Adjunct Professor, Departments of
  Neurological Surgery and
  Psychiatry and Behavioral Sciences
University of Washington School of
  Medicine
Seattle, Washington

Brian Dudgeon, M.S., O.T.R.
Lecturer
Division of Occupational Therapy
Department of Rehabilitation Medicine
University of Washington School of
    Medicine
Seattle, Washington

Wilbert E. Fordyce, Ph.D.
Professor (Emeritus)
Department of Rehabilitation Medicine
    and Pain Services
University of Washington School of
    Medicine
Seattle, Washington

Andrew Gitter, M.D.
Assistant Professor
Department of Rehabilitation Medicine
University of Washington School of
    Medicine
    and
Physical Medicine and Rehabilitation
    Services
Seattle Veteran's Administration
    Medical Center
Seattle, Washington

Barry Goldstein, M.D., Ph.D.
Assistant Professor
Department of Rehabilitation Medicine
University of Washington School of
    Medicine
    and
Spinal Cord Injury Service
Seattle Veteran's Affairs Medical Center
Seattle, Washington

Mark R. Guthrie, Ph.D., P.T.
Assistant Professor, Division of
    Physical Therapy
Department of Rehabilitation Medicine
University of Washington School of
    Medicine
Seattle, Washington

Rochelle V. Habeck, Ph.D.
Professor, College of Education
Michigan State University
East Lansing, Michigan

Eugen Halar, M.D.
Professor
Department of Rehabilitation Medicine
University of Washington School of
    Medicine
    and
Chief, Physical Medicine and
    Rehabilitation Service
Seattle Veteran's Affairs Medical Center
Seattle, Washington

Margaret C. Hammond, M.D.
Associate Professor
Department of Rehabilitation Medicine
University of Washington School of
    Medicine
    and
Spinal Cord Injury Service
Seattle Veteran's Administration
    Medical Center
Seattle, Washington

Ross M. Hays, M.D.
Associate Professor, Departments of
    Rehabilitation Medicine and
    Pediatrics
University of Washington School of
    Medicine
    and
Associate Director, Department of
    Rehabilitation Medicine
Children's Hospital and Medical Center
Seattle, Washington

Kenneth M. Jaffe, M.D.
Professor, Department of
    Rehabilitation Medicine
Adjunct Professor, Departments of
    Pediatrics and Neurological Surgery
University of Washington School of
    Medicine
    and
Director, Department of
    Rehabilitation Medicine
Children's Hospital and Medical Center
Seattle, Washington

**D. Kiko Kimura-Van Zandt, R.N.,
    B.S.N., C.R.R.N.**
Department of Rehabilitation Medicine
Children's Hospital and Medical Center
Seattle, Washington

George Kraft, M.D.
Professor, Department of
    Rehabilitation Medicine
Director, Electrodiagnostic Medicine
Chief of Staff, University of
        Washington School of Medicine
Seattle, Washington

Michael J. Leahy, Ph.D.
Associate Professor, College of
    Education
Michigan State University
East Lansing, Michigan

Linda J. Michaud, M.D.
Assistant Professor
Departments of Rehabilitation
    Medicine and Pediatrics
University of Pennsylvania School of
    Medicine
Philadelphia, Pennsylvania
    and
Director, Department of
    Rehabilitation Medicine
Children's Seashore House
Children's Hospital of Philadelphia
Philadelphia, Pennsylvania

Charles P. Moore, M.D.
Clinical Associate Professor
Department of Rehabilitation Medicine
University of Washington School of
    Medicine
Seattle, Washington
    and
Department of Physical Medicine and
    Rehabilitation
Salem Hospital
Salem, Oregon

David R. Patterson, Ph.D.
Associate Professor
Department of Rehabilitation Medicine
University of Washington School of
    Medicine
    and
Department of Rehabilitation,
    Burn Unit
Seattle, Washington

Walter C. Stolov, M.D.
Professor and Chairman
Department of Rehabilitation Medicine
University of Washington School of
    Medicine
Seattle, Washington

Jay Uomoto, Ph.D.
Associate Professor
Department of Rehabilitation Medicine
University of Washington School of
    Medicine
    and
Brain Injury Rehabilitation Clinic
University of Washington Medical
    Center
Seattle, Washington

Stuart Weinstein, M.D.
Clinical Assistant Professor
Department of Rehabilitation Medicine
University of Washington School of
    Medicine
    and
Puget Sound Sports & Spine Physicians,
    P.S.
Seattle, Washington

Kathryn Yorkston, Ph.D.
Professor and Head
Division of Speech Pathology
Department of Rehabilitation Medicine
University of Washington School of
    Medicine
Seattle, Washington

Contents

Common Disabilities Requiring Chronic Care

The Rehabilitation of Children and the Elderly

Psychosocial and Vocational Aspects of Disability

Principles in the Diagnosis and Management of Chronic Disease and Disability

1 History and Physical Examination in Chronic Disease and Disability

Walter C. Stolov, M.D., and Ross M. Hays, M.D.

The "classical" history and physical examination is unchanged when dealing with a patient with chronic disease. Details can be found in standard texts, and will not be repeated here. The workup presented here elaborates on features that are essential to reaching a diagnosis of disability in addition to that of disease. As a framework for conducting an adequate history and physical examination in a person with chronic disease or disability (see Table 1.1), the examiner must have a clear understanding of the terms *disease, impairment, disability,* and *handicap.*

===== Definitions

A disease is best described as an interruption, cessation or disorder of bodily functions, systems or organs, characterized by at least two of the following:

1. a recognizable etiologic agent or agents;
2. an identifiable set of signs and symptoms (i.e., a syndrome); and/or
3. consistent anatomical alterations.

Most diseases result in some form of impairment—either permanent or transient. The World Health Organization (WHO) defines impairment as "Any loss or abnormality of psychological, physical, or anatomical structure or function." When an impairment interferes with tasks required for physical independence, it produces a disability. WHO defines disability as "Any restriction or lack (resulting from an impairment) of ability to perform an activity in the manner or within the range considered normal for a human being."

TABLE 1.1.

History and Physical Exam Outline

Problem List

Include functional, social, psychological, and vocational deficiencies as separate problems.

Patient Profile

1. Social Function
   a. Current: architectural layout of the home; the persons in it, and their responsibilities
   b. Past social history
2. Vocational Functions
   a. Most recent job, either within or without the home
   b. Job history
   c. Avocational activities
3. Psychological Function
   a. Lifestyle
   b. Response to stress—past and current
   c. Motivational factors

Present Illness and Problems

After developing historical specifics of the problems on your list, add a paragraph that describes current state and the evolution of impairment in the following categories:

1. Ambulation
2. Transfers
3. Dressing
4. Personal hygiene
5. Eating
6. Communication

Describe patient performance of these functions as: independent; requires standby assistance for safety or cues; requires partial physical assistance; or totally dependent.

Physical Exam

Include a thorough physical exam. Additionally, divide the neuromusculoskeletal examination into three parts.

1. Musculoskeletal
   Use the screening exam described in this chapter.
   Explore any abnormalities with a more detailed exam.
2. Neurologic
   Use a basic screening exam with the additions mentioned in this chapter.
   Include the expanded mental status exam.
3. Functional Neuromuscular Exam
   Observe patient performance in ambulation, transfers, dressing, personal hygiene, and eating.

This one-page form is designed for use at the bedside. The points outlined are additions to consider in examination of a patient with chronic disease or physical disability.

Diseases may be controlled, impairments may or may not be reversible, and disability can be reversed even if impairment can not. A handicap is that which remains after disability is reversed or improved. It is societal in origin. Its reversal is a societal responsibility. Diseases produce disability when part or all of the pathologic processes (e.g., impairments) are irreversible, or when a significant period of time must elapse before the impairments can be reversed. In both cases, acute resolution of the disease process is not possible; therefore these disorders fall into the category of chronic disease.

Chronic diseases and their impairments result in some degree of dependence on others for activities of basic physical function (i.e., the disability), and may result in problems in vocational function and in the ability to engage in avocational pursuits. Finally, chronic disease with loss of function and independence frequently results in emotional stress and the need for significant psychological adjustment not only by the patient, but also by the family. *The central process of comprehensive rehabilitation may thus be defined as the reversal of disability by restoration of functional losses.*

A host of conditions exists for which a diagnosis of disease alone—without the identification of disability—will lead to insufficient treatment. The disability must first be identified. The spectrum of disability problems that occurs depends on the interaction of the patient with his or her environment. This interaction is shown schematically in Figure 1.1. It indicates that the total disability (i.e., the disability diagnosis) as well as the total list of disability problems depends on factors specific to the patient and to the environment.

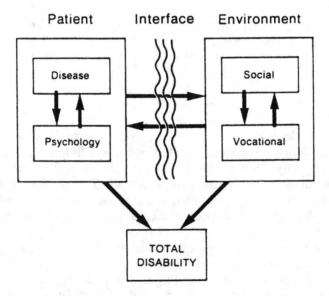

FIGURE 1.1. Schematic representation of the interaction of the patient with his or her environment. On the left, disease factors are reciprocally influenced by psychological factors. On the right, social factors are mutually influenced by vocational factors. The patient and his or her environment mutually influence each other through their interface. Total Disability is fed by all areas.

The database that will characterize the disability needed to determine the total disability extends beyond that needed for the determination of the diagnosis of the disease. The "Problem List" will include the problems (i.e., deficiencies) in self-care skills and problems in the social, vocational, and psychological areas. These functional issues may be a direct result of the physiological illness or may be concurrent problems that are affected by the disorder. The individual identification of these functional problems will lead to a plan for their solution and thus remediation of the disability.

History

Historical data of prime importance for the diagnosis of disability are obtained from the "chief complaint," "present illness," and "social and vocational history." The nature of the chief complaint may provide a hint to the existence of disability; the present illness data can determine the extent of lost function in basic self–care activities; the social and vocational history evaluates the environment, the family, and the social milieu and provides insight into the psychological background of the patient. The review of systems and past medical history contribute to the assessment of residual capacity.

CHIEF COMPLAINT

Chief complaints generally result from changes in health or well-being that create fear or anxiety, discomfort, or an inability to function. These unwelcome consequences lead the patient to seek medical attention. The chief complaints most likely to clarify areas of disability have to do with changes in the patient's function. The class of diseases most likely to produce complaints of loss of function are those that involve the musculoskeletal, nervous, or cardiovascular systems.

PRESENT ILLNESS

One of the hallmarks of disability is loss of independence. Historical information regarding dependence on others for activities of daily living (ADL) is best included under the category "Present Illness." Such data are really part of a symptom complex of the disease and describe the disability to be addressed in rehabilitation. For example, a patient concerned about reduced ambulation may actually be providing a description of muscle weakness; or a patient who has developed a tremor may describe the abnormality historically as onset of difficulty holding a cup of coffee. Similarly, it is not a reduction in shoulder and elbow range of motion that a patient wishes to correct but rather the loss of a functional ability, such as combing hair or attending to perineal hygiene.

The activities for which inquiries should be made can be divided into six categories:

1. Ambulation (movement from place to place);
2. Transfer activities (changes of position in place);
3. Dressing;

4. Eating;
5. Personal hygiene including use of the toilet and bathing; and
6. Communication.

The quantification of dependence in any of these activities of daily living is achieved by asking the patient: What type of assistance is needed? and Who provides it? Assistance may take several forms.

- *Stand–by Assistance.* When the activity is performed by the patient, there may be concerns about safety or correct execution of the activity. The assistant then is "standing–by" to guard against the occurrence of accidents and to ensure completeness of performance by noting errors and omissions.
- *Partial Physical Assistance.* The patient is able to do a good part of the activity independently but an assistant is needed to provide partial help. For example, the assistant may buckle the patient's belt after the patient has donned pants unaided; or the assistant may hold the wheelchair stationary while the patient transfers into bed.
- *Total Physical Assistance.* The patient contributes little or nothing toward performance of an activity. In these situations the patient is described as totally dependent. For the activity to occur, others must do it.

Ambulation History

In the broadest sense ambulation may be defined as travel from one place to another over a finite distance. It thus includes not only walking but also wheelchair travel, or even crawling. In order to assess the extent of disability with regard to ambulation, the patient's capacity for moving in different environments must be obtained.

The environments of significance are the home, its immediate vicinity, and the community at large. A patient may, for example, be totally independent in walking around the house but not out in the community. The environments found in theaters, restaurants, subways, or downtown stores may require partial physical assistance in order to negotiate safely. The disability diagnosis for such a patient will therefore include the problem of "decreased ambulation in the community."

If a patient uses a wheelchair, the extent of independence in its use needs to be known. For example, the examiner should determine whether the patient is able to maneuver it independently in the home, whether he or she is also independent in its use outside the home, and if he or she can use it successfully out in the community unaided. Sample questions in an exploration of ambulation skills are as follows:

- Are you able to walk without help from anyone?
- Do you use assistive equipment (canes, crutches, braces)?
- Do you use a wheelchair?
- Is there a limit to how far you can walk or use your wheelchair outside your home?
- Do you go out visiting friends or to restaurants or to theaters or stores?
- Do you fall very often?
- Do you drive?
- Can you climb stairs?

Transfer History

Transfers are movements that involve changes of position in place. They include such activities as turning over, moving from a bed to a wheelchair or a regular chair; going from a wheelchair to a toilet, bathtub, shower or car; and going from a wheelchair, regular chair, or toilet to a standing position. These activities are more basic than ambulation. For example, while a person may be independent in walking, he or she may need to depend on others for help to rise from a chair into the standing position. Independent ambulation therefore is not always available if assistance for the transfer into the upright posture is not always present.

Sample questions to begin an assessment of disability in transfers include the following.

- Can you get in and out of bed unaided?
- Can you get on and off a toilet unaided?
- Can you get in and out of the bathtub without help?

Dressing History

A disabled patient's ability to don and remove clothing must be carefully assessed. If the person is not independent in dressing, he or she is less likely to engage in community activities outside the home and less likely to receive guests. Dressing therefore has a significant impact on social adaptation after the onset of disability.

In obtaining a history of performance in dressing skills, it is not sufficient merely to ask: Do you dress yourself? An untrained, disabled patient may have, for some time, abandoned the use of garments that are more difficult to don. Typically abandoned are shoes, socks, pants, clothes with buttons, and close-fitting undergarments. The patient therefore may answer "Yes" to such a question without realizing how few clothes he or she actually wears. A complete probe into dressing history is necessary to gain insight into performance and function. Sample questions to explore dressing abilities include the following.

- Do you dress in street clothes daily?
- Can you put on, with assistance, your shirt, pants, dress, undergarments, etc.?
- Do you need help with shoes and socks?
- When you must go out, how much of your dressing do you do by yourself?
- How long does it take you to completely dress before school, work, etc.?

Eating History

The loss of independence in a person's ability to feed himself or herself can be devastating to self-esteem. Unlike the activities previously discussed, it is the one activity that must still persist even if total physical assistance is required. The association of passive feeding with dependence is exceedingly strong in our society, and such individuals often isolate themselves socially. Eating skills include the use of fork, spoon, and knife, and the handling of cups and glasses. Sample questions in exploration of this area include the following.

- Can you feed yourself without assistance?
- Are your able to cut meat?
- How do you handle messier foods, such as soup and cereal?
- Do you have trouble holding glasses and cups?

Personal Hygiene History

Personal hygiene activities include the spectrum of skills concerned with cleaning and grooming: toothbrushing, hair combing, shaving, the use of the tub and shower, perineal care, and the successful handling of bowel and bladder elimination. Loss of independence in the performance of these skills is severely disabling. This is particularly true when a patient cannot handle bowel and bladder elimination in a socially acceptable manner. If he or she is concerned with the possibility of becoming soiled with feces or urine, the emotional stress will be quite severe. Vocational rehabilitation efforts and improvements in social functioning will be unsuccessful until the person can develop a system for elimination that is consistent and successful.

It is more important to be continent socially than to restore elimination patterns that are anatomically and physiologically identical to those of the nondisabled population. Socially acceptable elimination can be achieved by the majority of disabled patients. Patients with catheters can develop a successful system if they can handle the emptying of collecting bags and can satisfactorily incorporate the necessary devices within their clothing. Sample questions to explore the personal hygiene area include the following.

- Can you shave (use makeup) and comb your hair without assistance?
- Can you shower or bathe without help?
- Are you able to use the toilet unaided?
- Do you need help with any aspect of using the toilet?
- Are bladder and bowel accidents a problem for you? If so, how often?

Communication

The term *communication* includes a broad range of skills associated with listening, speaking, reading, and writing. Communication encompasses the breadth and depth of language, and therefore reflects the patient's intellectual capabilities and educability. Listening and reading skills that form the receptive component of language function depend on the intact use of auditory and visual organs. Speaking and writing—the more expressive forms of language—depend on the integrity of motor functions associated with articulation and hand dexterity.

To obtain an accurate history of communication skills in patients with expressive communication deficits, the examiner will direct the inquiry to family members or others who have had a recent and long-standing relationship with the patient. To put the present level of disability into context, a clear idea of the patient's premorbid language skills must be obtained. For communication deficits that are changing, the time course of deterioration should also be ascertained. The communication history will sometimes be self-explanatory. Recognition of expressive aphasia, dysarthric speech, and so on are logical components of the physical exam and are often elicited during the mental status examination or incidentally noted during the general history. Frequently, specific questions regarding expressive verbal language are unnecessary. Sample questions that may augment the examiner's understanding of receptive language difficulty or deficits in written communication include the following.

- Do people often appear to mean something other than what you thought you heard them say?
- Do you have difficulty reading and understanding newspapers or magazines?
- Is writing possible for you?
- Do you have, or use, any special tools or methods to improve your ability to communicate either in speech or in writing?

General Principles in Determining Disability in Basic Functions

Several principles must be kept in mind when exploring disability in the basic functions of ambulation, transfers, dressing, eating, and personal hygiene:

1. When the patient reports that he or she is not independent, determine the extent of assistance required for the particular skill in question.
2. If assistance is being supplied, determine who is assisting the patient.
3. Separately interview the persons (usually family members) who are supplying the assistance. Assistant(s) may report a greater degree of dependence than that reported by the patient. The two may interpret differently what is occurring. A significant difference in their remarks may indicate that one or both are dissatisfied with the situation.
4. When it is expected or anticipated that the patient will be dependent, questions such as "can you" or "do you" should be rephrased. It may be more helpful to use questions beginning with "Who helps you . . ." Questions asked in this manner may yield more useful functional information because patients may initially wish to appear more independent than they actually are.
5. When the disability is one of acute onset, the inquiry should also include the premorbid level of independence. This is particularly important in the older patient or a person suffering an acute exacerbation of a long-term disability. Earlier disease or trauma may have left the patient with some residual dependence. An accurate understanding of the person's prior skills will obviate the possible error of expecting rehabilitation to improve the patient's functional status beyond that which was present in the premorbid state.
6. If there has been a loss of independence and the disease is of a progressive nature, determine the time course of this loss. Efforts to intervene in these situations are much more likely to be effective if the function was lost recently. Long-standing disability is likely to have already created some adaptive strategies.
7. In many cases the answers to the preceding sample questions may be obvious from observation and physical examination. It is best, however, to assume less and inquire more, to prevent omitting significant data.

When inquiry into the self–care functions of mobility (ambulation and transfers), dressing, eating, personal hygiene, and communication is complete, specific disability problems should be identified and documented separately in the patient's list of problems, even though they may be interdependent. The patho-logic condition underlying the functional disability may be irreversible in part or in whole, or the decreased function may not be eliminated by reversal of the disease process. Therefore disability problems may be more appropriately addressed individually with their own set of predisposing conditions, so that strategies may be designed to restore function when none are available to cure the disease and its impairments.

PAST MEDICAL HISTORY

Like the review of systems, the Past Medical History provides information regarding the patient's residual capacity. Concurrent disease or previous trauma and surgery may have produced residual impairment which, although it no longer produces disability itself, may compound the disability of the present illness.

A careful review of Past Medical History is therefore an essential component when evaluating the patient with disability. A simple recitation of past or concurrent disease or trauma may not be sufficient. The inquiry requires an understanding of the impact that past illness has had on the present disability, regardless how minor.

PATIENT PROFILE

The patient's social and vocational history will provide the database necessary for understanding the interaction between the patient and his or her environment. A careful review of these issues will identify environmental factors that are either secondary to or concurrent with the disease, and will also provide insight into the personality of the patient and his or her ability to adjust to the stress of chronic disability. A careful understanding of the complexities of adaptation to disability should be obtained as a foundation for further rehabilitation intervention. It is convenient to divide the personal history data into three categories: (1) social, (2) vocational, and (3) psychological.

Social History

The family unit may be compromised when a person becomes dependent on others for the performance of self–care skills, or when vocation is disrupted secondary to disease. Other family members' plans may alter significantly due to the need to assist the disabled person in performing the activities of daily living, as well as by the loss of income incurred by chronic disability. A major disability of one member of a family unit will create problems of adjustment for all and may even threaten the integrity of the unit. The superimposition of major disability on a family unit already beset with social difficulties is particularly threatening. Identification and inclusion of secondary and concurrent social issues into the patient's history and problem list will allow the physician to begin to understand the environmental factors that influence the patient's physiologic and medical problems.

The assessment of social impairment is obtained with inquiries into the stability of the family. Its history, the resources available to its members, and the responsibility of the patient within his or her family should all be ascertained, as should a clear understanding of the physical environment of the patient's home and community. In this context the word *family* must be broadly interpreted to mean "all interested parties with whom the patient interacts in an interdependent manner."

The physical environment is important because dependence or independence in the performance of activities of self-care is directly related to the location in which that activity is performed. Sample questions that begin the search for problems in social functioning include the following.

- Do you live in the city? a rural community? the suburbs?
- Do you rent or own your residence?
- Are the bedroom, bathroom, kitchen all on the same floor?
- Are there entrance stairs or stairs within your residence?
- Do others live with you? If so, do any of them go to work? to school? Do they have any health problems of their own?
- Do your parents, brothers, and/or sisters live in your immediate vicinity? Do you maintain contact with them?
- Are you married? If so, for how long?
- What activities and functions did you perform for your family that you no longer are able to do (e.g., parental discipline, financial management, chores, sexual activity, avocational activities)? How are these functions now being handled?
- Where were you born and where else have you lived?
- What did (or do) your parents and siblings do for a living?
- At what age did you leave your parents' home?

The answers to these questions will provide the necessary information on social background and current resources, as well as some insight into current or potential problems. "Abnormal" responses to these questions should be pursued. For example, if the patient has experienced major disruptions within the family unit, further questioning regarding the roles of individual family members may yield important clues regarding additional social stressors and past coping strategies.

Vocational History

A patient's disease may also lead to unemployment. Whether there is, or will be, a significant disability in this area depends on the physical, intellectual, and interpersonal requirements of the patient's job. Sample questions that will elucidate the interconnection between disease, lost function, activities of daily living, and employment are as follows.

- When did you last work?
- For whom did (do) you work?
- How long have you worked for them?
- Describe what you do (did) on the job. Be specific. Start with what you do (did) when you first arrive(d) at work and give a brief outline of your day.
- Was (is) your income sufficient to support your family or do you have other resources? Do you have significant debt?

Answers to these questions should provide information about the patient's premorbid vocational pattern. If the description given by the patient of current or last job seems incompatible with present illness, even with rehabilitation management, further inquiries may be necessary.

- What type of work do you plan to do in the future?
- What type of work have you performed in the past? How long ago did you do this type of work? Would you be interested in returning to it?
- What qualifications do you have (education, memberships, licenses, special skills)?
- What is your educational background?

This additional information will indicate whether the patient has had work adjustment problems. The strengths in the person's vocational background, which may be successfully exploited in the process of vocational adaptation, will become more clear in this portion of the history. If the patient has been unemployed, it is important to understand his or her current sources of financial support and their likely sufficiency for the future.

When working with persons who are not employed outside the home, or for those who live alone, it is important to inquire about household tasks and skills. Sample questions would include the following.

- When did you last do the cooking, shopping, light/heavy housekeeping?
- Who does these things now?
- Is this arrangement satisfactory for you and your family?

Avocational activities are also an important aspect of a patient's function. Many people derive more of their enjoyment of life from their avocational pursuits than from their vocational activities. To understand the impact of the disability in this area, the following sample questions are useful.

- What do you do with your leisure time (by yourself, with your family) after work and on weekends?
- What organizations or religious groups are important to you?
- When did you last participate in these activities?

Psychological History

Psychological function must be assessed in patients with chronic illness or physical disability for several reasons. Since the organic, pathologic changes may be incompletely reversible, the stress of the disease is often persistent. This stress may be of great magnitude. For example, a patient who loses a limb has to adjust not only to this loss but also to the secondary stress of loss of employment if the physical requirements of the job are incompatible with activity limits of an artificial limb. The patient and his or her family may then have to relinquish established goals and patterns of activity. The patient may have to learn to be more active in protecting his or her health than when premorbid. These new modes of behavior are likely not the patient's prior preferred way of doing things. Thus the patient's psychological background needs to be assessed and understood in order for new learning and adaptation to take place. A clear understanding of the reinforcers most likely to be successful in motivating a given patient will also be necessary to change behavior. For patients with brain damage from trauma or disease, an understanding of intellectual function will be required in order to successfully devise treatment strategies to reduce the disability.

Psychological problems should be included in the patient's problem list when reaction to the stress of the disease interferes with adaptation to the disability, and when new learning is potentially impaired. While the mental status examination can provide some assessment of current function, the social and vocational data will yield a great deal of valuable information about the person's personality. The same social and vocational data that identify the person's lifestyle will also identify the types of activities that can be used as goals toward which the person will work to remove dependence during treatment. The likelihood of success in an activity, consistent with premorbid lifestyle, will serve as a motivational factor, even if the work the patient must perform to achieve his or her goals includes activities that are, in themselves, alien to his or her usual style. For example, an interpersonally oriented individual may be motivated to perform certain heavy exercises important for health if increased social contact with others will be possible when a required level of strength is achieved. Similarly, an intellectually oriented individual may be motivated to develop independence in transfer skills if successful transfers will afford opportunities to attend lectures or concerts.

Social and vocational data provide information that allows the clinician to build upon the patient's strengths in planning for the removal of disability. Interpreting social and vocational data to yield psychological characteristics is a relativity simple matter when organized into four categories: (1) the patient's previous lifestyle; (2) the patient's past history or response to ordinary life stresses; (3) the patient's current response to the stress of his or her disease; and (4) the activities likely to motivate the patient to adapt to his or her disability.

The Physical Examination

The information obtained from the physical examination of a person with a disability serves three functions:

- The examination searches for the signs that signify deviations from normal structure and function. Correlation of these signs with the patient's history and laboratory data will yield the disease diagnosis.
- In examining a disabled patient, the physician searches for signs of secondary problems that are not necessarily a direct consequence of the disease. Such secondary problems are physical complications that result from the loss of ability to initiate preventive health habits, or as a consequence of the medical treatment of the disease.
- The physical examination assesses the residual strength in the body systems that are unaffected by disease. These strengths provide the foundation upon which the patient and his or her physician will build a strategy to reverse or minimize the disability and reestablish lost functional skills.

The importance of secondary problems, whether unavoidable, treatment-induced, or due to omission of prevention measures, is that these add to the patient's disability and may lengthen the treatment time necessary to remove the disability associated with the primary disease.

All patients with chronic disease and disability require a complete physical exam. The interaction between health-care professionals who provide rehabilitation or management of chronic disease and disability with professionals who provide acute care suggests that primary diagnostic issues have usually been addressed by the acute care providers. Frequently, new and important clues to previously unrecognized or underappreciated acute medical concerns will become apparent in the process of carefully evaluating a patient for chronic disability; it is therefore always necessary to evaluate a patient from a fresh point of view with a complete physical exam.

In the thorough general physical exam, special attention should be paid to the cardiovascular and the respiratory systems to determine if there will be any cardiorespiratory limitations to retraining in self-care and activities of daily living. Because chronic disability frequently includes alterations in bowel and bladder function, special attention should be paid to the genital and rectal exam, especially in the evaluation of sacral mediated reflexes. Evaluation of loss of skin integrity or the incidence of skin breakdown is another essential aspect of the general physical exam, which may have significant implications for the disabled patient.

In addition to the thorough general physical exam, the examination of the patient with disability must include an expanded examination of the nervous system, the musculoskeletal system, and the interaction between the two in functional activities; this is sometimes referred to as the functional neuromuscular examination.

NERVOUS SYSTEM

The neurologic exam should be performed with the same care exercised by neurologists in searching for signs in a difficult diagnostic problem. All twelve cranial nerves should be carefully evaluated. The screening neurologic exam should be expanded with the addition of a careful sensory exam. The use of a standardized patient map illustrating spinal cord level dermatomes and the distribution of peripheral nerves is helpful in sorting out observed abnormalities and sensation. In addition to the sensation of superficial touch and pain, the examiner should test position sense, vibration sense, stereognosis and two-point discrimination, as well as hot and cold perception. Cerebellar and coordination functions should be tested in both gross and fine motor movements.

The general neurologic exam of deep tendon reflexes should be expanded to include the bulbocavernous reflex, in order to evaluate the S2 through S4 reflex arc. This is tested by noting involuntary contraction of the external anal sphincter in response to brief stimulation of the glans of the penis or clitoris, or to a tugging applied to an indwelling urinary catheter. The exam should include the evaluation of abnormal reflexes, including the Babinski reflex in the lower extremity, Hoffman's reflex in the upper extremity, and careful evaluation of primitive reflexes in the brain-injured patient.

CARDIOVASCULAR SYSTEM

Retraining to restore basic self-care skills that are lost as a result of musculoskeletal and neurologic disease usually requires specific therapeutic exercise regimens. An adequate cardiovascular reserve and optimized cardiovascular function are therefore essential.

Examination should therefore include the blood pressure (supine, sitting, standing), liver size, peripheral pulses, carotid pulses, venous return systems, peripheral skin temperatures, peripheral skin hair, and peripheral edema. Cardiac size, cardiac rhythms, and cardiac sounds will need correct interpretations. All treatable abnormalities will need identification.

RESPIRATORY SYSTEM

Much like the cardiovascular system, the respiratory reserve must be assessed to evaluate exercise tolerance.

Examination should include the respiratory rate and rhythm, the chest shape, the fingers for clubbing, the facies for cyanosis, and the lungs for congestion and obstruction. Supplementary pulmonary function laboratory tests may also be required.

GENITALIA AND RECTUM

Particularly critical for patients with diseases that affect the functions of micturition and defecation are examination for cystocele and rectocele, prostate size, sphincter tone, anal wink reflexes, perineal sensation, the presence of orchitis and epididymitis, and the presence of the bulbocavernous reflex.

If present, the bulbocavernous reflex signifies that the sacral conus of the spinal cord at the level of S2 and S4 is intact. The afferent sensory stimulus is elicited by pressure on the clitoris or glans. For patients with catheters, a tug on the catheter will stimulate the response. The efferent response is contraction of the external sphincter. It can be detected by a finger in the anus; visualization of the anal opening may suffice.

MUSCULOSKELETAL SYSTEM

The functional unit of the musculoskeletal exam is the joint and its associated structures: the synovial membrane, capsule, ligaments and the muscles that cross the joint. Examination of this complex anywhere in the body cannot be completed unless the underlying anatomy is well understood. The screening examination is useful for localizing abnormalities when the disability problems are minor. However, examination of individual joints is necessary for conditions that result in major disability. Such examinations include inspection, palpation, passive range of motion, stability, active range of motion, and muscle strength.

Inspection

The two sides of the body should be observed for symmetry in contour and size, and any differences measured. Atrophy, masses, swelling, and skin color changes should be noted.

Palpation

The origin of a pain symptom may be localized by palpation of the various anatomic structures about the joint. Palpation of the bones may determine their discontinuity in fracture assessment. Palpation of masses and swelling for consistency can distinguish between bony masses, edema, and joint effusion. To determine the presence of a muscle spasm, muscle palpation with the patient at rest will identify sustained involuntary reflex contraction resulting from pain.

Passive Range of Motion

These tests are performed by the examiner while the patient is relaxed. When range of motion is limited, the examiner must determine if the limitation is due to joint surface incongruities, joint fluid excess or loose bodies, or to capsule, ligament, or muscle contracture.

Stability

To assess whether a pathologic condition of the bone, capsule, or ligament is causing abnormal movement (subluxations or dislocations), the joint should be moved under stress in the direction its contour ligaments and capsule do not normally permit it to move, with the patient at rest. Tears in a ligament or laxity of the capsule will result in abnormal mobility. During movement, joint stability is also supported by active muscle contraction.

Active Range of Motion

These tests should be performed prior to strength tests in the event that pain is a problem. Muscle tension and joint compressions induced by an active movement are less than those in a strength test. If pain is minimal in the active range of motion, the examiner can more easily proceed with the strength test. When active range of motion is less than the passive range of motion, the examiner must decide between true weakness, hysterical weakness, joint stability, pain, or malingering as possible causes.

Muscle Strength

Muscle strength can be tested if its prime action is known. The body part can be positioned to allow this prime action to occur. Grading systems are based on the ability of the muscle to move the part of the body to which it is attached against the force of gravity.

GRADE 5: Normal Strength. The muscle is able to move the joint it crosses through a full range of motion against gravity and against "full" resistance applied by the examiner.

GRADE 4: Good Strength. The muscle can move the joint it crosses through a full range of motion against gravity with only "moderate" resistance applied by the examiner.

GRADE 3: Fair Strength. The muscle can move the joint it crosses through a full range of motion against gravity only.

GRADE 2: Poor Strength. The muscle can move the joint it crosses through a full range of motion only if the part is positioned so that the force of gravity does not act to resist the motion.

GRADE 1: Trace Strength. Muscle contraction can be seen or palpated but strength is not sufficient to produce motion—even with gravity eliminated.

GRADE 0: Zero Strength. Complete paralysis; no visible or palpable voluntary muscle contraction.

Grade 3 is the key muscle grade with regard to disability assessment. Determination of grade 3 is objective and independent of the examiner's strength. Since any activity a patient may perform is done in a gravity field, muscles with grade 3 strength will allow the involved body part to be used. For grades less than 3, external support may be necessary to allow the involved part to be useful to the patient. Additionally, joints having muscles across them with less than grade 3 strength are prone to develop contractures.

Different examiners should concur about whether a muscle should be graded 0, 1, 2, or 3. For grades 4 and 5, ratings may vary among examiners depending on the expectations of different age groups and the amount of resistance that different examiners are able to apply. With experience the examiner's accuracy will likely increase. In patients where motor strength deficits are asymmetrical, grades 4 and 5 are more readily appreciated because the unaffected body part can be used as a control.

This grading system is not as useful for the prediction of motor strength in conditions where weakness is associated with spasticity.

A useful abbreviated musculoskeletal exam is outlined in Table 1.2. It may be used as a framework for quickly evaluating the patient for gross impairments. When abnormalities are noted on the screening exam, a more detailed examination must be performed in order to clearly understand the nature of the impairment. The outline is a helpful guide to assist in the accurate assessment of the musculoskeletal system. It was developed at the University of Washington as a physical exam screening tool. Although this brief outline will not detect subtle pathophysiology, it will indicate areas of gross impairment that can then be further evaluated with a more detailed examination. This method is easy to learn and especially appealing because the entire exam can be completed within a few minutes.

FUNCTIONAL NEUROMUSCULAR EXAMINATION

A functional examination translates the objective neurologic and musculoskeletal exams into performance. It defines at a given time the skill of the patient in the execution of activities of daily living. It is the starting point from which improvement may occur through treatment, even if the objective neurologic and musculoskeletal disorders are unalterable.

TABLE 1.2.

Musculoskeletal System Exam Outline

A. Essential Symptoms to Evaluate in the History
   1. Pain
   2. Weakness
   3. Deformity (deviations from normal posture, including limitation of movement)
   4. Stiffness
   5. Injury
   6. Functional limitations

B. Screening Musculoskeletal Exam to Localize Impairments
   1. Inspection of body in anatomical position
      a. From front, back, and side
      b. Symmetry, alignment
   2. Inspection of gait
      a. From front (or back) and side
      b. Look for:
         (1) abnormal truncal movement,
         (2) abnormal pelvic movement,
         (3) stride length,
         (4) base,
         (5) toe, heel walking.
   3. Cervical spine movements
      a. Flexion is normal when chin can touch the sternum
      b. Extension is normal if the occiput comes within one finger width from the C7 spinous process
      c. Rotation left and right should allow the plane of the head to make an angle of 70° to shoulder plane
   4. Elbows extended and arms are placed in front of the body with the shoulder at 90° of forward flexion
      a. Inspect for symmetry
      b. Test hand intrinsic strength by having the patient abduct his or her fingers and attempt to squeeze them together
      c. Shoulder flexion strength is tested by resisting upward motion of the arm
   5. Arms abducted overhead with external rotation
      a. Inspect rhythm of movement, symmetry of scapulae; smooth movement at the shoulder, sternoclavicular and acromioclavicular joints
      b. Can the upper arms touch the patient's ears?
      c. Test lateral deltoid strength by resisting horizontal abduction with resistance applied to the elbows
   6. Test internal and external rotation of the shoulder by having the patient touch the inferior border of the scapula at the back to demonstrate full internal rotation and elbow flexion (external rotation is indicated by the ability to touch the back of the head)
   7. Any limitation of elbow, wrist or finger range of motion will be apparent from careful observation of the previous manuevers; note any limitations.
   8. Upper extremity strength screen
      With elbows at side flexed at 90°, the patient grasps examiner's hands and holds himself or herself rigid while examiner tests finger flexors, wrist flexors, wrist extensors, forearm supinators and pronators, elbow flexors, elbow extensors, shoulder protractors and retractors by moving in the direction that is resisted by these motions

(cont'd.)

TABLE 1.2. (cont'd.)

B. Screening Musculoskeletal Exam to Localize Impairments (cont'd.)
   9. Examination of back
      a. With the patient's back bare, have him or her stand facing away from the examiner. Check for level shoulders and pelvis; is the head in midline, spine straight? Observe for symmetry of space between trunk and upper limbs.
      b. Have the patient flex his or her trunk forward with knees straight; observe for a paraspinal prominence in thorax, or lumbar area (i.e., fixed scoliosis).
      c. When the patient extends trunk check for flexibilty.
      d. Have the patient rotate his or her trunk to right and left while the examiner stabilizes pelvis; the plane of shoulders should rotate to a 45° angle with the plane of the pelvis.
      e. Ask the patient to laterally flex or her his trunk to right and left; the fingertips should touch head of fibula.
   10. Lower extremity hip and knee range of motion and extensor strength screen can be grossly evaluated by one manuever: The examiner holds patient's hands while he or she squats with heels remaining on floor and then returns to upright position. Limited extensor strength will result in loss of control of the smooth descent and extensor weakness will interfere with ascent. Any limitation in range of motion at the hips, knees, or ankles will be obvious during the manuever. Any abnormality observed during the brief screening exam should be evaluated more thoroughly. A useful system for more detailed evaluation follows.

C. Specific Regional Exam of the Various Joint–Muscle Complexes Found To Be Impaired on the History and Screening Exam
   1. Inspection
   2. Palpation of key anatomical structures in region (Consider percussion of muscles for myotonia)
   3. Passive range of motion, using goniometer for accurate assessment
      a. Joint evaluation for contracture
      b. Assessment of muscle tone
      c. Search for tightness in two-joint muscles (e.g., hamstrings)
   4. Stability tests (Stress joint in direction opposite to normal movement for ligament laxity or rupture)
   5. Active range of motion, using goniometer for accurate measurement (Examine if added compression force of muscle contraction induces pain)
   6. Muscle strength—use 0–5 grading system:
      0 = No visible or palpable voluntary contraction
      1 = Visible or palpable contraction present but insufficient to produce range of motion (ROM)
      2 = Sufficient strength to produce full ROM with gravity eliminated
      3 = Sufficient strength to produce full ROM against gravity
      4 = Strength can be overcome with moderate resistance
      5 = Normal, sustains against high resistance.

Once the musculosketal system is evaluated, the patient's actual ability can be more accurately assessed with the functional exam.

The functional examination confirms the status of skills reported by the patient and the history regarding ambulation, transfers, eating, dressing, and personal hygiene. The functions to be tested include the following.

Sitting Balance

Sitting is a necessary prerequisite for transfer skills. It is tested by placing the patient in the sitting posture, with the feet on the floor and back unsupported; the patient's hands are in his or her lap. If the patient can hold this position, then gently push him or her in various directions to observe the ability to use protective extension to recover from the tendency to fall (i.e., dynamic balance).

Transfers

Movements to be examined include turning from supine to prone and back, rising to a sitting position, rising from sitting to standing, and moving from a bed or a low examining table to a chair.

Standing Balance

This is a necessary prerequisite for safe ambulation. It should be assessed with support and, if adequate balance is present, the person should be gently pushed from side to side to assess the ability to use protective responses.

Eating Skills

Eating skills may be assessed by demonstrating hand-to-mouth abilities with various examining room objects or, for an inpatient, by means of actual observation at mealtime.

Dressing Skills

Range of motion and strength of the upper extremities, including grip and fine motor skills as well as the flexibility of the lower hips, knees, and spine, are required for independence in dressing. Patients should be independent in dressing skills if they have the ability to touch the tops of their heads, the small of their back, and their feet; have the ability to flex at the hips and knees; and have the manual dexterity to handle snaps and buttons. Isolated parts of dressing, such as manipulating buttons or managing a garment, frequently can be simulated in the examination setting to represent the patient's dressing skills.

Personal Hygiene Skills

Upper extremity strength and range of motion required for dressing are also required for personal hygiene skills. The motions necessary for face, perineal, and back care can usually be simulated by the patient in the examining room. Direct observation of a specific task when it is actually performed may be useful in clarifying some of the details of sequencing and organizing complex tasks.

Ambulation

Walking should be observed if the patient has standing balance. The person should wear minimal clothing so that major joints and the back may be observed as much as possible. Walking should be inspected with and without street shoes, and from the front and back as well as from the side. Abnormalities should be described in relation to the phase of gait in which they occur. If pain is present, it too should be related to phase of gait. The following format should be used in the systematic examination of gait.

- Observation and description should be systematically performed and recorded.
- Cadence should be observed for symmetry and consistency.
- Trunk position should be noted for flexibility or presence of abnormal posturing and especially for exaggerated movements in the anterior, posterior, or lateral planes.
- Arm swing—especially asymmetry—should be evaluated.
- The position of the pelvis should be observed for posture and placement. Abnormalities in anterior and posterior placement result in lumbar lordosis or kyphosis or obliquities associated with a lurching gait.
- The base should be observed to determine whether it is normal, narrow, or broad.
- Heel-strike and push-off should be carefully evaluated.
- Swing phase hip and knee flexion and circumduction should all be considered and noted when present.

If the person cannot walk, wheelchair mobility should be evaluated. The patient's ability to travel in a straight line and to negotiate turns should also be observed. Careful attention should be paid to the patient's seating and positioning in the wheelchair. If posture is not appropriate, recommendations should be made to improve positioning to allow the patient to have better use of the upper extremities for propulsion of the wheelchair. Seating and positioning may be critical for patients using a power wheelchair to allow them access to the electronic interface necessary to control its independent use.

MENTAL STATUS EXAMINATION

For a patient with chronic disease or disability, the screening neurologic evaluation should be expanded to include a comprehensive mental status exam. This examination and the psychological history provide the background for understanding the person's basic personality structure and current emotional reaction to the disability.

Removal of the disability is an educational process that involves retraining and relearning. The mental status examination becomes particularly important in patients for whom disease or trauma has produced brain damage. The orientation of the mental status examination for the patient with physical disability differs from that usually emphasized in a psychiatric evaluation. The general categories to evaluate in the disabled patient include recent memory, perception, affect, and judgment.

Recent Memory

It is important to evaluate recent memory function in order to ascertain the patient's ability to relearn skills and thus make progress in rehabilitation. The patient may, for example, need to learn a specific technique to execute a safe transfer, or to coordinate crutch-walking skills. Learning such new skills requires the patient to assimilate, retain, and reproduce new material, which may not have been previously learned, or which may have been learned and lost.

Recent memory function with regard to language information may be assessed by asking a patient to remember, for example, an address provided. Retention is evaluated when the patient later is asked to reproduce the address, perhaps on the next day. A simple new motor task, taught during the evaluation, can be used to assess motor learning. Retention of this motor skill can then be assessed at a later date. A clear understanding of strengths and weaknesses in the recent memory area will guide the rehabilitation team in their approach to training the patient to use new adaptive skills.

Perception

Perception includes the process by which the patient organizes sensory information about his or her environment. In this context the term *perception* is used to describe how the patient interprets his or her real environment because disturbances of this interpretation may have an organic or a psychiatric etiology. The disabled patient will frequently have subtle disturbances in perception, relating to the ability to process visual information of form, space, and distance. These visual representations of the environment require correct interpretation in order for the patient to make a correct motor response. Errors in visual perception may result in serious accidents if they are not appreciated and incorporated into the adaptive strategies designed for the patient. For example, a patient with monocular blindness may suffer deficits in depth perception that may result in an inability to judge the correct distance for transfer from bed to wheelchair; this will result in accidents. A patient with right parietal lobe injury may not be able to accurately interpret the difference between the inside and outside of a garment and thus will require adaptive strategies for dressing.

Disturbances in perception of this type are more likely to occur with damage to the right cerebral hemisphere. These can be assessed by asking the patient to copy figures such as a square, a triangle, and a Maltese cross. He or she can also be asked to reproduce a clock face from memory. When disturbances in perception of form exist, these reproductions are distorted. The finding of disturbed perception suggests that the teaching of basic self-care will be more successful by verbal instruction than by demonstration.

Affect

A reactive depression is common following the acute onset of a major disability, or after a relatively sudden additional functional loss in a person with long-standing disease. It is a realistic response, and indicates that the patient has enough insight to recognize his or her losses. This same insight will be useful to the patient in helping him or her to remove the disability. A reactive depression requires remedial action if it is associated with eating or sleep disturbances or if it interferes with the patient's ability to respond to treatment. The absence of a reactive depression may be considered abnormal in some cases. If the patient is unable to confront his or her physical or functional losses, the ability to overcome the disability created by the loss may be reduced.

Mood swings are another feature of affect to consider. Rapid transitions from laughter to tears and back can represent the lability associated with psychological disturbances or can be due to brain injury. Certain features may be helpful in delineating the emotional liability associated with organic brain disease from that associated with more traditionally psychiatric affective disorders. For example, vigorously changing the subject of the conversation or the simple immediate distraction of attention by snapping fingers will frequently alter the patient's mood if the lability is of organic origin. The presence of pseudobulbar neurologic signs will also suggest that the lability of mood is of organic origin.

Judgment

In brain damage judgment factors relate to difficulties that the patient may have in self-monitoring behavior. These may include the failure to detect errors, such as the omission of behaviors normally incorporated in eating or dressing. These problems must be distinguished from carelessness associated with apathy and depression. If such behavior is observed in the general assessment of the patient's appearance and the various activities performed during the course of the evaluation, judgment problems may exist. Insight into judgment can also be obtained during observation of the patient as he or she performs the various tasks given in the mental status exam. An organic origin is likely when such behaviors are associated with the onset of disease or trauma. When judgment errors are present, standby assistance and increased supervision may have to be provided as the person performs various functional activities.

═══ The Problem List

A person with a disability is described here to illustrate how a problem list may be constructed.

> A 19-year-old woman fractured her cervical spine in a small plane accident, resulting in quadriplegia. Her male companion, with whom she had been living for the previous year and a half, was killed in the crash. Their relationship had been close and family-oriented; she served as a "stepmother" for her companion's two small children from a prior marriage. Following the accident, responsibility for the children was legally assumed by the natural mother.
>
> The patient was hospitalized for a short period on an acute neurosurgical service and then transferred to a comprehensive rehabilitation center for inpatient care. Following a complete comprehensive evaluation shortly after admission her problem list included:
>
> 1. C7 fracture dislocation
> 2. C7 complete quadriplegia
> 3. ambulation dependent
> 4. transfer skill dependent
> 5. eating, dressing, personal hygiene skills dependent

    6. neurogenic bowel dysfunction
    7. neurogenic bladder dysfunction
    8. decreased respiratory function
    9. potential for pressure sores
  10. potential for thrombophlebitis
  11. history of impulsive behavior
  12. reactive depression
  13. home architecture incompatible with paralysis
  14. financial obligations without immediate resources
  15. diminished contact with her family of origin
  16. unemployment without prior work history
  17. absence of independent transportation

Seventeen problems create an impressive list. It may be argued that the list need not be this long because nearly all the problems are secondary to the first—C7 fracture dislocation—and that this one diagnosis should be sufficient. Such an approach might be valid if there were a therapeutic technique to reverse spinal cord damage and restore full nervous system function. Unfortunately, such a technique does not exist. There does exist, however, a set of techniques for each of the 17 individual problems. These can be used to minimize the severity of the problems and to fully resolve some of them.

Problems 1, 2, 6, 7, 8, 9, and 10 are examples of more "classic" medical problems. Problems 3, 4, 5, and 17, while also direct results of the trauma, relate to the patient's physical disabilities. Problems 11 and 12 relate to the patient's psychological condition and problems 13, 14, and 15, to the social sphere. Problem 16 succinctly identifies the vocational disability.

══════ Conclusions

The diagnosis of disease alone is insufficient for the planning of a comprehensive treatment program. The symptoms and signs required to diagnose disease are not synonymous with those required to diagnose disability. An understanding of disability—that is, specific losses in physical, social, vocational, and psychological function—requires investigation beyond the history and physical exam ordinarily required in the treatment of acute disease. The techniques described will also identify those medical problems secondary to but not natural consequences of a chronic impairment. To achieve a successful treatment program that removes disability, the clinician must also be prepared to assess and appreciate the patient's residual strengths.

Following an appropriate evaluation, the clinician will be able to list all of the patient's problems. This problem list will include disease, diagnosis, and secondary complications. It must also include the specific losses in physical, self-care, social, vocational, and psychological function. Once this problem list is established, the rehabilitation treatment process can begin. Successful strategies to remove disability can be planned for each of the problems on the list. Therapeutic techniques used will fall within one of six general areas:

    1. Methods to prevent or correct secondary complications;
    2. Methods to enhance the capability of systems unaffected by disease;
    3. Methods to improve the functional capacity of affected systems;

4. Methods to promote function through the use of adaptive equipment;
5. Methods to modify the social and vocational environment; and
6. Methods derived from psychological theory to improve the patient's performance.

═══ Annotated Suggested Reading List

Dinsdale SM, Gent M, Kline G, Milner R. Problem oriented medical records: Their impact on staff communication, attitudes and decision making. *Arch Phys Med Rehab* 56:269–274, 1975.

Grabois M. The problem–oriented medical records: Modifications and simplification for rehabilitation medicine. *South Med J* 70:1383–1385, 1977.
  Both of the above attempt to deal with the complexity of long problem lists.

Heimburger RD, Reitan RM. Easily administered written test for lateralizing brain lesions. *J Neurosurg* 18:301–312, 1961.
  A description of a useful bedside test of cerebral function.

Rosse C, Clawson DC. *The musculoskeletal system in health and disease.* New York, Harper & Row, 1980.
  A basic text on the musculoskeletal system. This text first introduced the screening musculoskeletal exam.

Stolov WC, Clowers MR (Eds.), *The handbook of severe disability.* Washington DC, U.S. Government Printing Office, 1981.
  A basic easy–to–read review of the disability problems and vocational implications of a host of impairments productive of disability.

Stolov WC, Hays RM. Evaluation of the patient. In Kottke FJ, Lehmann JF (Eds.), *Krusen's handbook of physical medicine and rehabilitation* (4th ed.) Philadelphia. W.B. Saunders, 1990, pp. 1–19.
  Further elaboration of the principles outlined in this chapter.

World Health Organization. *International classification of impairments, disabilities, and handicaps: A manual of classification relating to the consequences of disease.* Geneva, World Health Organization, 1980.
  The most widely accepted definition of the terms used to describe chronic disease and disability.

Erickson RP, McPhee MC. Clinical evalution. In DeLisa JA (Ed.), *Rehabilitation medicine: principles and practice.* Philadelphia, J.B. Lippincott, 1988, pp. 25–65.
  This chapter details the evaluation of the patient in much greater detail than is possible in this text. It is an excellent resource for those who wish to further pursue the basic principles of evaluation of the patient with disability.

2 Treatment Strategies in Chronic Disease

Walter C. Stolov, M.D., Ross M. Hays, M.D., and
George H. Kraft, M.D.

The history and physical examination of a patient with disability will identify the medical problems and the limitations of function that are in need of resolution, both of which constitute the problem list. A patient with chronic disease and disability will usually have a combination of both physiological and functional items on the list.

It is not unusual for such a patient to have an extensive problem list in which the physiologic and functional items are interdependent. The "classical" items on the problem list include pathologic and physiologic disorders that are frequently irreversible. The functional items, however, will be amenable to rehabilitation treatment as outlined in this book.

Many, and in some cases all, of the functional problems directly result from the classical medical problems. Notwithstanding, each needs a separate identification because they all have their own set of treatment techniques. Thus L2 paraplegia secondary to vertebral fracture causes an "ambulation dependency." Removal of this dependency through treatment to achieve bipedal or wheelchair ambulation involves techniques that have nothing to do with treatments which deal with the fracture and the damage to the cauda equina, and do not change the paraplegia itself.

Strategies have to be carefully planned in order for the patient to achieve resolution or improvement of these specific functional deficits. Six classes of treatment strategies have been identified for patients with chronic disease. Their purpose is not to reverse the pathological derangement but to remove disability, and include the following:

1. prevention or correction of additional (secondary) disability;
2. enhancement of systems unaffected by pathology;
3. improvement of the functional capacity of affected systems;

4. the use of adaptive equipment to promote function;
5. modification of social and vocational environments; and
6. psychological techniques to improve patient performance.

Prevention or Correction of Additional Disability

Perhaps the most important initial treatment for the patient with chronic disease and disability is the prevention of secondary complications that would increase disability. Anticipatory guidance, based on knowledge of the primary pathology, guides the team and the patient in the development of strategies that will prevent secondary disability. Examples of such strategies would include:

- medication to avoid congestive heart failure in patients with atherosclerotic cardiovascular disease;
- medication to maintain control of diabetes, to reduce the chance of peripheral neuropathy and peripheral vascular disease;
- anticoagulation to reduce the risk of cerebral thrombosis in patients with transient cerebral vascular insufficiency;
- passive range of motion exercises for joints where motor strength is less than grade 3 to avoid the development of soft tissue contracture;
- appropriate management of the neurogenic bladder to prevent infection and hydronephrosis and resultant renal damage;
- progressive resistive exercises (PRE) to reduce muscle weakness associated with bed rest;
- a system of periodic relief of pressure at insensate body surfaces to avoid loss of skin integrity and decubitus ulcers; and
- time-contingent medication to prevent addiction in the patient with chronic pain.

Enhancement of Systems Unaffected by Pathology

Impairments that result in disability are frequently not systemic in nature. Disability can often be reduced by either providing improvement beyond the previous level of function of body systems unaffected by the present disease, or by using those unaffected systems in novel ways to accommodate a loss of function elsewhere. Examples of the enhancement of systems unaffected by pathology include:

- exercises to strengthen muscles on the nonparalyzed side of a hemiplegic stroke patient or in the upper limbs of a paraplegic spinal-cord-injured patient;
- adaptive techniques using visual monitoring of hand function for patients with cutaneous sensory loss; and
- adaptive training using hearing and tactile sensation to improve mobility in a patient with low visual acuity.

Improvement of Functional Capacity of Systems Affected by the Disease

The disabled patient who suffers derangement of body function may be helped by directly addressing the deficits responsible for the disability. These strategies are most successful when the natural history of the impairment suggests that improvement will occur over time. In these cases the improvement initiated by the body's own healing capacity can be augmented by well-planned, adaptive strategies. Examples of enhancement of functional capacity of affected systems include the following:

- graded exercise programs to improve systemic conditioning after myocardial infarction;
- exercises to improve the strength of muscles weakened by prolonged bed rest; and
- the use of visual cues in brain-damaged patients to assist impaired memory function.

Use of Adaptive Equipment to Promote Function

Perhaps the most rapidly growing area of medical rehabilitation is the use of adaptive equipment. The advent of computer-assisted technology and the miniaturization of electrical circuitry has allowed the development of a new generation of technical adaptations for disability. In many cases such technical aides may restore function in a patient who otherwise would remain severely disabled. It would be erroneous to assume that all adaptive equipment is complicated and electronic. Frequently, simple approaches will also have great benefit for the patient with disability. Specific examples of the use of adaptive equipment include the following:

- shoe modifications to improve standing balance;
- mechanical equipment to extend hand function for dressing—long shoehorns, stocking pullers, and buttonhooks;
- canes, crutches, and braces to improve energy expenditure and safety in ambulation;
- wheelchair training for travel when walking is not possible;
- prostheses for amputee patients to allow independent ambulation or to replace upper extremity function.
- adaptive hand controls for patients unable to use an automobile in the conventional fashion.
- computer-assisted augmentative communication systems for patients with the cognitive potential for language but with severe oral motor impairment.

Modification of Social and Vocational Environments

Disability is frequently as much related to the patient's environment as it is to his or her impairment. Environmental barriers may combine with the individual's disability to produce a handicap. For example, the patient is not handicapped, the patient has a disability, but the lack of access to an elevator may be a handicap. Adaptations of the environment at home and in the workplace may restore function. In many cases modifications of a patient's environment must be made before the patient can be discharged from the medical facility. Examples of environmental modifications include the following:

- procurement of a one-level home for patients unable to climb stairs;
- alterations to hallways and doorways to allow easy wheelchair access;
- addition of rails and grab bars to promote safety and mobility within the home;
- provision of assistance in the home for physical and homemaking needs;
- employment to reduce physical or mental demands on patients who have reduced motor strength or ambulation, or cognitive problems due to head injury;
- redesign of the work area for patients who will be expected to use wheelchair mobility; and
- training of family members to adapt to changes in the disabled individual in order to reinforce constructive behavior and discourage unnecessary dependence.

Support from health professionals and the family can exert a potentially powerful influence over the patient's performance. Once a working relationship between the health-care team, the family, and the patient has been established, further work can progress to replace lost function. It is the responsibility of the health-care team to identify for the family which skills should be independently performed by the patient and which should be replaced, either by assistance from others or by technological adaptations. A clear differentiation of the tasks that can be expected from the patient will help prevent the frustration in the family caused by a mismatch of expectations after the patient returns to the community. As recovery continues, flexibility should be maintained to allow the patient greater independence as warranted by improved performance.

Psychological Techniques To Improve Patient Performance

Principles of behavior management can be extremely helpful in the recovery of function. Although certain behavior management strategies may be intuitive to the family, others may need to be pointed out by a more objective third party unemotionally tied to the patient. Examples of psychological techniques that can be used to improve patient performance include the following:

- the use of repetition in training self-care skills in patients with memory problems;
- adaptive strategies using demonstration for patients with receptive language deficits;
- the development of a consistent milieu to provide reorientation for the confused or agitated patient emerging from coma associated with traumatic brain injury; and

- the judicious use of operant conditioning techniques to improve performance and minimize unwanted or harmful behaviors.

Summary

In the presence of irreversible pathology, disability (i.e., functional problems) can be modified and reduced. The six treatment strategies emphasized in medical rehabilitation are not themselves directed at modifying the pathology. They are, however, effective means of reducing disability.

3 The Spectrum of Physical Treatment

Barbara J. de Lateur, M.D.

A number of so-called physical measures play a large role in the treatment of a disabled patient with chronic impairments. They serve to generate within the patient the capacity for progressive independence even though the extent of pathology may not be altered. These measures are also useful in a number of acute neuromusculoskeletal problems that are not associated with major disability.

This chapter will introduce most of those likely to be included by physicians of any specialty as part of a total treatment package.

The Physiologic Effects of Heat

Since the diathermies and superficial heat have their therapeutic effect through the production or transfer of heat, it would be well to begin with a statement of some of the general physiologic effects of heat that have therapeutic benefit as well as the general contraindications to its use.

- Heat alleviates pain by a direct effect on nerve and nerve endings, as well as indirectly by alleviating painful conditions, such as muscle spasms and joint stiffness (e.g., subjectively and by objective measurement, heat decreases the morning stiffness of rheumatoid arthritis).
- An important effect of heat is that it alters the viscoelastic properties of collagen tissues, making joint contractures more amenable to stretching exercises.
- Heat increases blood flow and may assist in the resolution of chronic inflammatory processes.

It is often desirable to distinguish between vigorous and mild heating. In vigorous heating the highest temperature in the distribution is applied at the site of pathology; relatively high temperatures are reached rapidly and maintained for relatively long periods of time. Vigorous heating is appropriate for chronic disorders. In acute disorders—particularly in acute inflammatory disorders—heat should either not be used at all or only mild heating should be used. In contrast to vigorous heating, with mild heating the highest temperature in the distribution is at some distance from the site of pathology, and relatively low temperatures are achieved at the site of pathology (for example, superficial heat may be used over a deeply placed, acutely inflamed joint).

The therapeutic temperature range for physiologic effect is 40°C–45°C (104°F–113°F), and the effective duration of treatment is generally 5–30 min. The therapeutic range is close to damage temperatures. These begin at 46°C (115°F) for long durations, but can be higher if exposure is shorter (e.g., damage is proportional to temperature × time).

General contraindications to heat include malignancy in the area to be treated, ischemia in the area to be treated, impairment of sensation or obtundation of consciousness, and hemorrhagic diathesis. In addition to these general contraindications, there are some specific contraindications with the specific diathermies.

Modalities

DIATHERMY

The term *diathermy* is taken from the Greek *dia* meaning "through" and *thermi* meaning "heat." The implication is that diathermy heats through tissues or at least deeply into tissues, rather than just heating the surface. The three forms of diathermy are shortwave, microwave, and ultrasound. These, as well as infrared radiation, are said to heat by conversion because a different form of energy is converted into heat energy.

Shortwave Diathermy

Shortwave diathermy (SWD) is the therapeutic application of high-frequency electrical currents, which are converted into heat as they pass through the tissues. This is perceived by the patient as warmth and not as a shock or the usual type of electrical stimulation. The equipment available for SWD varies, but all SWDs have in common the three basic components of the circuitry: a power supply, an oscillating circuit, and a patient circuit. These machines operate at a frequency of 27.33 megahertz (MHz), with a wavelength of 11 meters. The patient circuit is part of the total circuitry; therefore the equipment must be tuned so that the frequency of the patient circuit is made equal to that of the oscillating circuit of the machine (resonance frequency). This must be done at low output to avoid a surge of current, which might result in a burn. After the machine has been properly tuned to the patient circuit, the output can be increased, depending on the vigor of heating desired.

Accurate dosimetry is not available for SWD; therefore one must rely on intact sensation of warmth and pain to effectively and safely use this modality. Various types of applicators are available, which use either a condenser (Figure 3.1) or an induction coil (Figure 3.2). With condenser plates, spacing is provided by the space plates, which are part of the equipment. For the other types of application, spacing must be provided by several layers of terrycloth to avoid burns caused by too great current density in the superficial tissues. The various applicators permit heating of essentially all body surfaces, regardless of shape.

With SWD, heating is generally greatest in deep subcutaneous tissue and superficial musculature, depending to some extent on the technique of application and thickness of the subcutaneous fat. Internal vaginal and rectal electrodes are also available, which are used with an external belt and alcohol thermometer. These must be used with caution and may be contraindicated in borderline congestive heart failure because the great increase in pelvic blood flow resulting from SWD may strain a failing heart. SWD also has the potential for hazardous interference with cardiac pacemakers; the technique should not be used in patients with implanted pacemakers, and in particular should not be used to treat the area containing the device or electrode wires.

Precautions should be used to avoid accumulation of sweat beads as these may be selectively heated. The layers of terrycloth thus serve a dual function, in that they not only provide spacing but also prevent accumulation of sweat beads. General contraindications to heat should be observed. Additionally, SWD should be avoided where there are metal implants.

Microwave Diathermy

Microwave diathermy is the therapeutic application of electromagnetic radiation, identical to radar. Microwaves are propagated even in a vacuum; thus the patient is outside of the circuitry. As with light waves, microwaves can be reflected, scattered, refracted, or absorbed. The basic components of the apparatus for microwave consist of a power supply, a magnetron that produces the high-frequency oscillation, and the applicator. The applicator is an antenna, and is often

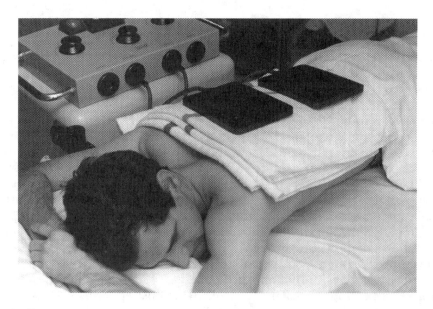

FIGURE 3.1.

referred to as a director. The commercially available directors are called A, B, C, and E. The field patterns they produce vary. Although there are some nonthermal effects of microwaves, all demonstrable therapeutic effects are due to heat. The pattern of relative heating varies with the frequency of the machine. Frequencies allowed by the FCC for use of microwave diathermy include 2456 MHz and 915 MHz. Unfortunately, at the time of this writing, only machines operating at 2456 MHz are commercially available. Machines operating at 915 MHz have a greater depth of penetration, particularly in the muscle, which may be more desirable than merely heating the fat. Further, the depth of penetration may be enhanced by using a contact applicator (instead of one of the standard directors) with preliminary superficial cooling. Ten min of superficial cooling before turning on the power of a 915 MHz microwave can induce, after subsequent 20 min of microwave heating, uniform heating of deep muscle. Depth of penetration with microwave, then, depends on the frequency at which the machine operates, the thickness of subcutaneous fat, the type of applicator, and the presence or absence of superficial cooling. The greatest depth of penetration and most uniform muscle heating occurs with a contact applicator and previous superficial cooling. At the time of this writing such applicators are not commercially available, but it is anticipated that they will be in the relatively near future.

As with SWD, caution should be taken to avoid selective heating in accumulations of fluid and with metal implants. Pacemaker inhibition may also occur and should be avoided. Care should be taken to avoid exposure to the eye as cataracts may occur from long-term exposure; experimentally, these have not been shown to occur at intensities below 100 milliwatts per square centimeter (mw/cm^2). Less stray radiation occurs with the contact applicator, an advantage of this technique when it becomes available commercially. An advantage of currently available directors is their great ease of application, which is about as simple as shining a light on a part to be heated.

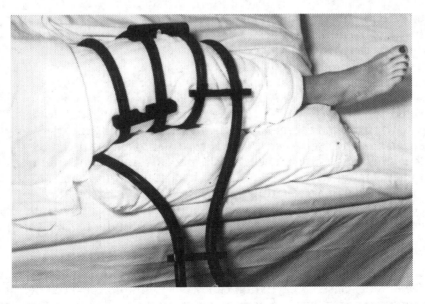

FIGURE 3.2.

Ultrasound

Ultrasound is an acoustic vibration characterized by compression and rarefaction of particles in a medium. It is similar to audible sound in all respects save its frequency. Somewhat arbitrarily, frequencies below 17,000 Hertz (Hz) are referred to as sound whereas higher frequencies are referred to as ultrasound. The propagation of ultrasound depends on a medium; in contrast to microwaves, ultrasound cannot be propagated in a vacuum. Because wavelength (λ) is inversely proportional to frequency (f) ($\lambda = c/f$, where c is the velocity of sound propagation in the medium), it follows that the wavelength of ultrasound is very much shorter than that of sound. Thus, anatomic structures in the body are large relative to the wavelength, and bones and joints represent a barrier to ultrasound. For this reason, multiple aspects (fields) of joints (like the shoulder) must be treated. For therapeutic purposes it is desirable to have an ultrasonic applicator with good beaming properties. Other things being equal, there will be less divergence with applicators of large diameter. However, contact with tissues, which is essential for propagation, may be lost when applicators are too large. Therefore the applicator size chosen is a compromise between these two factors. An applicator with a radiating surface of 7–13 cm^2 is a useful range.

Ultrasound is a very effective deep-heating agent, and has the deepest penetration of the three diathermy modalities. It can easily bring the temperature of the hip joint into the therapeutic range, whereas SWD and microwave have little or no effect when applied over the hip. Ultrasound can also be used safely in the presence of metal implants in the area to be treated, although the available data at this time suggest that it should not be used in the presence of methyl methacrylate, the "glue" used in total joint prostheses.

Accurate dosimetry is available for ultrasound. Therapeutic intensities range from 1–4 watts per square centimeter (w/cm^2). The appropriate amount depends upon the vigor of heating required as well as the volume (area × thickness) of tissue to be treated. If a deeply placed joint capsule is to be heated, an intensity should be chosen that will produce pain (temperature = 46°C) within approximately 11 or 12 min. The patient will not experience pain during the actual treatment because the treatment time will be, for example, 10 min, stopping short of the time required to elevate temperature to a level that will produce pain. If it is possible to treat an area for 20 min or more without ever producing pain, the intensity used is probably too low, and the structures intended to be heated will not be brought into the therapeutic temperature range. Taking the patient to the pain level and then slightly decreasing intensity until pain disappears may be used to ensure that treatment is being given in the therapeutic temperature range. In general, the benefits from ultrasound relate to its heating effect, but streaming of fluids may also result in a stirring effect that may be beneficial in accelerating the diffusion of injected medications.

General contraindications to heat should be observed. Under carefully controlled conditions, it is possible to heat an area of impaired sensation if the ultrasonic dosage is first standardized on the unaffected side and then, for safety, the wattage cut back slightly. So, for example, a stiff shoulder in a hemiplegic patient might safely be treated if the dosage were standardized in this way on the unaffected side. Gaseous cavitation can occur in fluids of low cell density, but does not occur clinically when proper equipment with full wave rectification and filtering is used along with adequate pressure of the applicator on the tissue and a stroking technique. Even with good equipment, the ultrasonic beam is not perfectly uniform in the so-called near field; therefore a stroking technique (e.g., applicator head not held stationary) must be used to mix or "average" the maxima and minima of intensity.

A good coupling medium must be used because of the mismatch of acoustic impedance between the applicator and air. Ultrasound is reflected at interfaces, which contributes to its utility for heating deeply placed structures, such as joint capsules. However, nerves may be heated selectively, and care must be taken to avoid their inadvertent heating; however, a low intensity application to nerves may be desirable and helpful in pain control in an area supplied by the nerve, or in the case of an amputation neuroma.

Ultrasound is most useful when combined with a therapeutic exercise program of stretching and active exercises of a contracted joint, such as the shoulder or hip. For maximum effectiveness, the stretching should be applied with low loads for relatively prolonged periods (20 min+) during the application of the ultrasound, or immediately thereafter if it is not possible to stretch during the application. For a patient with a flexion contracture of the right hip, a typical prescription might be as follows: "Place patient in Thomas position with prolonged low-load static stretch to the right hip flexors. Apply ultrasound to the anterior aspect of the hip joint; 2–2.5 w/cm^2 with stroking technique for 10 min."

SUPERFICIAL HEAT

Superficial heat can be applied utilizing a wide range of techniques and equipment. Virtually all methods of superficial heat application have the same depth penetration; that is, a few mm, and therefore the choice of modality is related to other factors. For example, with hydrotherapy the other factors include buoyancy cleansing. In a Hubbard tank, which allows full immersion, the shape of the tank allows the patient to exercise upper and lower extremities and also permits the therapist access to the patient to assist in range of motion or dressing changes.

Some facilities have deeper walk-in tanks that allow the patient to walk with less stress on the joints and with some support provided from the water, although additional external support from an overhead harness may be needed if the patient is unstable. Hydrotherapy is very useful in the management of burns and pressure sores, where the cleansing effect is desired. It is also useful in rheumatoid arthritis, when many joints are affected and a mild heating effect may be desired. The temperature of various forms of hydrotherapy baths depends on the extent of the body to be heated. For the Hubbard tank 39°C (102°F) is the upper limit, although I personally do not go beyond 38°C (100°F). Temperatures of 41°C (105°F)–43°C (110°F) may be used for the extremities, although if one is treating an ischemic ulcer the temperature should be kept in a more neutral range of 35°C–37°C (95°F–98°F) to obtain the cleansing effect of the agitated water without additional heating of an ischemic area.

Superficial heat is also conveniently applied in the form of hot water bottles, which are inexpensive and readily available, but are not thermostatically controlled; pads with circulating water thermostatically controlled at a safe level and often available in hospitals; heating pads which, if of good quality, are thermostatically controlled to prevent exceeding a safe level; and Hydrocollator™ packs (that are commercially available and contain a silica gel), which retain the heat of the water bath in which they are heated. These packs are heated in a thermostatically controlled water bath to a temperature of 140°F–160°F; burns are prevented by applying several layers of terrycloth towels between the Hydrocollator™ pack and the skin.

Noncontact dry heat may be applied using various types of heat lamps, either the powerful lamps available in a physical therapy department or the relatively inexpensive heat lamps (such as the Mazda lamp) available in most drug and hardware stores. Care should be taken that the patient does not obtain a sun lamp that emits ultraviolet radiation when only heat is desired. In addition to the benefit of the heat from infrared lamps, drying may be useful in treating some stages of pressure sores.

THERAPEUTIC COLD

The application of cold has some things in common with therapeutic heat. Both alleviate pain and muscle spasm, although some patients will have a definite preference for one over the other. When the "spasm" is muscle splinting protecting a painful structure, heat is appropriate. When true spasticity is present, 20 min cooling, sufficient to cool the muscle spindles, will notably decrease the clinical manifestations of spasticity for as long as 90 min. Cold is more appropriate in acute processes, particularly in acute inflammatory processes, which might be aggravated by heat. When treating acute trauma, such as sprains and strains, the application of cold plus compression immediately following the injury may lessen the development of swelling and hemorrhage. Cold may lessen the damage from a burn if it is superficial and if the cold is applied no later than 2 min after the burn occurs. If it is a full-thickness burn or if the application of cold is delayed beyond 2 min, cold may actually increase edema and delay healing. In contrast to heat, cold increases joint stiffness, although many patients with rheumatoid arthritis obtain relief of pain and stiffness by alternating heat and cold in the so-called contrast baths.

ULTRAVIOLET RADIATION

Ultraviolet radiation is a physical treatment modality, but is not a heating modality. Various portions of the spectrum of the ultraviolet have different effects, which may be either beneficial or harmful. The major divisions of the ultraviolet spectrum are referred to as UVA, UVB, and UVC. Normally all of the UVC is screened from the sun's rays by the ozone layer of the atmosphere. UVB, which has been dubbed the "sunburn spectrum," is present in sunlight but does not penetrate ordinary window glass, although it does penetrate quartz, from which the envelope of mercury vapor of arc lamps is made. UVA, which is closer to the visible spectrum of light, is available in abundance in sunlight but is very weak in producing sunburn or tanning. Thus, one cannot ordinarily get a sunburn through window glass, which permits UVA but screens out UVB. The skin, however, can be sensitized to UVA by drugs, such as methoxypsoralen, following which UVA may tan the skin; indeed, if patients are not careful they may even get a sunburn through ordinary window glass. This technique has gained some favor in the treatment of chronic psoriasis and is called the PUVA technique.

The standard physical treatment for psoriasis, the Goekerman technique, involves painting the affected area with coal tar to sensitize the skin, following which ultraviolet light is applied using a standard clinical unit. Because sensitivity to ultraviolet varies inversely with the thickness of stratum corneum and the amount of pigment in the skin, and is highly individual, the dosage must be determined individually. The dosage unit is a biologic one called the minimal erythema dose (MED). The MED is that amount of radiation which produces erythema within 4–6 hr and which disappears in 24 hr. After this is determined, the ultraviolet is prescribed in increasing multiples of the MED. This technique is highly effective, but is also quite messy for the patient and the therapist, which may be one of the reasons for the popularity of the PUVA technique. UVA can be applied by a lamp source after sensitization of the skin by oral administration of 8-methoxypsoralen. It may also be applied outdoors by screening out the UVB with a large sheet of Mylar™ plastic. This technique understandably has found greater favor in sunny climates.

Other uses of ultraviolet include its surface antibacterial effect, for example, in the elevators of hospitals; as an adjunct to the management of acne vulgaris; and particularly in the management of neonatal jaundice, using the blue portion of the visible spectrum. While some use ultraviolet in the management of pressure sores for its antibacterial effect, I believe cleansing several times a day and mechanical debridement is superior. For drying, an infrared lamp or ordinary light bulb are preferred.

IONTOPHORESIS

The technique of iontophoresis involves the transfer of ions into the body by electromotive force. Positive ions are driven in under the anode, negative ions at the cathode. This technique still has some utility as a research tool in the investigation of drugs. It has been almost completely abandoned as a therapeutic tool, however, because much better control of localization and dosage is obtained by injection. As with ultraviolet, iontophoresis is a physical treatment modality but not a heating modality.

Traction

Traction of the cervical and lumbar spine is used to provide an axial distracting force. Prolonged low-force traction may be applied with tongs in the distraction and realignment of cervical fractures. In the physical therapy department, however, relatively high-force traction, often with the patient in a seated position, is applied to the cervical spine to alleviate pressure on nerve roots. It is important that the traction pull the neck toward slight flexion to obtain the desired effect. Flexion alone will increase the vertical diameter of the intervertebral foramina. Traction added to the slightly flexed position will further increase this diameter and alleviate pressure on the nerve roots. After a series of treatments, the benefit obtained often far outlasts the treatment time. Sitting cervical traction at 10 lbs simply supports the weight of the head and unloads the neck muscles. At about 20–25 lbs actual distraction occurs. Maximal traction is likely not to exceed 50 lbs for 2 min. Patient response dictates how forceful the traction will be. Preheating with superficial heat or SWD usually helps patient relaxation.

It is assumed that the mechanism of this effect is to permit fluid to return to the intervertebral discs. It is also possible to produce demonstrable distraction in the lumbar spine, but special equipment with the application of relatively high forces is required. It is important here that traction be applied to the pelvis and not to the legs, as this will increase the lumbar lordosis, an undesired effect in patients with low back pain or an acutely herniated disc. Bed rest with the application of 10–30 lbs of pelvic traction is simply a form of enhanced bed rest; there is no additional benefit to this low level of traction.

Manipulation

Manipulation is a difficult treatment modality to study scientifically, but has its advocates, among them many patients who have obtained prompt and long-lasting relief. Theories differ regarding what is actually done by manipulation and how it produces relief. Perhaps the foremost proponent of manipulation in the United States is John Mennell (5). He theorizes that the most important effect of manipulation (as he describes it) is restoration of "joint play." By joint play he refers to the involuntary range of motion of a joint. An example of Mennell's manipulations would be long axis extension of the interphalangeal joints of the finger or a distracting force pulling the glenohumeral joint away from the body in the long axis of the arm. These movements should be short and sharp, not prolonged. They are referred to as nonvoluntary because none of the patient's own muscles can produce them; they must be performed passively by the therapist.

Therapeutic Exercise

STRENGTH

Even an apparently simple concept, such as "strength," must be defined in view of the various capabilities of muscle. Muscle can shorten actively by concentric contraction, and can lengthen actively by an eccentric contraction. Muscle can maintain an overall length against resistance, termed an *isometric* or *setting contraction*. The kinesiologic functions of each of these types of contractions are, respectively, acceleration, deceleration (shock absorption), and stabilization. Strength, then, can be defined as the maximal force one can exert either concentrically, eccentrically, or isometrically. The measured values for each of these will differ in any one individual. The highest value will be obtained with a fast lengthening contraction; lower values are seen with slow lengthening contractions, lower still with isometric, lower still with slow shortening contractions, and the lowest force or tension in the muscle developed with fast shortening contractions. These are referred to as the classic force–velocity relationships first described by A.V. Hill (3). Additionally, owing to length-tension relationships, the torque which a muscle can exert, even at constant velocity of contraction, varies throughout the joint range due to variations in angle of insertion of the muscle tendon. All of these considerations are important for angle-specific and rate-specific effects of muscle training.

Strength is determined by the physiologic cross-sectional area of the muscle combined with certain neural or skill elements, such as the ability to synchronize. In muscles with long parallel fibers, the physiologic cross-sectional area is simply the cross section of the main belly of the muscle. In pennate muscles, which have short fibers coming in at an angle to the tendon of insertion, the physiologic cross-sectional area is found by taking multiple sections at right angles to the fibers until all are included. Thus, for any given volume of muscle tissue, the pennate muscle will have a greater ability to exert force although it does so over a shorter range than the parallel muscles.

ENDURANCE

Endurance is defined as the ability to continue a specified task, either in terms of time or number of repetitions. Endurance is one factor in work capacity, defined as the product of force X distance X number of repetitions. Endurance is the converse of fatigue, which may be defined operationally as the inability or unwillingness of the subject to continue the prescribed task under conditions of reinforcement in effect and known to the subject. As a general rule, a subject can sustain 5–15 percent of maximum force "indefinitely."

AEROBIC CAPACITY: $\dot{V}O_2MAX$

This is the maximal ability of the subject to consume oxygen despite increasing performance of external work. The dot over a symbol ($\dot{V}O_2max$) always indicates a rate.

ENDURANCE EXERCISE

This term is used by exercise physiologists to describe an activity that requires the prolonged and reciprocal use of multiple groups of muscles (e.g., swimming, running).

OTHER ANATOMICAL ASPECTS OF THERAPEUTIC EXERCISE

Muscle is under neural control in its anatomic as well as physiologic aspects. Motor units, which consist of the nerve and the muscle fibers it innervates, fall into two basic types. The smaller units, described as type I, have slow-twitch characteristics, are recruited early (at low forces) in a voluntary contraction, fire regularly, exert low tensions, have high oxidative ability, and are fatigue-resistant. Type II units have fast-twitch characteristics, are larger, are recruited at high thresholds, fatigue rapidly, fire irregularly, and are low in oxidative ability. A subtype of type II units has an intermediate fatigue resistance and oxidative ability, but retains the fast-twitch characteristics. The twitch characteristics of a motor unit are highly stable and change only with cross innervation. Type I units are also referred to as slow oxidative (SO). The two subtypes of the type II are referred to as fast glycolytic (FG) and fast-oxidative glycolytic (FOG), respectively. Using histochemical techniques, type I and type II units can be distinguished by staining for myosin ATPase preincubated at pH 9.4 or 10.2. Thus identified, adjacent serial sections will also be identifiable and can be stained for other metabolic properties such as NADH-diaphorase, which reflects oxidative ability, and phosphofructokinase (PFK), reflecting glycolytic ability.

═══ Response to Training

Muscle may respond to training by an improvement in skill (neural factor), which generally includes an increased efficiency of contraction (lower metabolic demand for a given task). Muscle may also respond by an increase in strength (increase in physiologic cross-sectional area plus certain neural factors, such as the ability to synchronize), and by enhancement of metabolic capability, either the aerobic or the anaerobic capacity or both. Endurance at a given task is related to strength and metabolic capacity, which in turn is related to the metabolic apparatus (such as the cytochrome oxidase system) and the amount of glycogen contained in the muscle. Within rather wide limits, endurance is mathematically related to strength. These limits may be as wide as 20–100 percent of maximal voluntary contraction (MVC) capacity. The higher the force of contraction, the more closely is endurance related to strength. As force decreases, metabolic capacity becomes increasingly important. At an intensity that is sufficiently low to be maintained for 1–2 hr or more, endurance will be limited by the amount of glycogen contained in the muscle, assuming an adequate metabolic apparatus.

What type of exercise produces these results? Within wide limits, that is, between 40–100 percent MVC and perhaps as wide as 20–100 percent MVC, there is a high degree of positive transference from low-intensity training to high-intensity performance, and from high-intensity training to low-intensity performance, as long as the subjects go to fatigue in training. However, for extreme quantitative differences as well as for qualitative differences (e.g., isometric versus isotonic, i.e., static versus dynamic exercise), there will be little positive transference; there is some evidence—albeit limited—that there may be such a thing as negative transference, that is, interference. Thus it may be safely said that the best type of training for a given task is that task itself. The more that skill is involved in a particular activity, the more it is true that the best training for a task is the performance of that task itself. Available evidence suggests that an eccentric (lengthening contraction) component is necessary if hypertrophy is to result from isokinetic exercise.

PROGRAMS AND EQUIPMENT

A wide range of programs and equipment exist for therapeutic exercise but only a few can be mentioned here because of space limitations. Perhaps the most well-known strengthening programs are those described by DeLorme (2) and a modification of this technique by Zinovieff and coworkers (6), referred to as the "Oxford" technique. In either of these the 10 repetition maximum (10 RM), that is, the highest weight that can be lifted by a subject 10 times, is determined once a week for each muscle group to be trained. At each treatment session, 10 repetitions are done at 50 percent of the 10 RM, 75 percent of the 10 RM, and 100 percent of the 10 RM. In the DeLorme technique it is done by adding weights; in the Oxford technique it is done by removing weights. Although the Oxford technique is more widely used today, in this author's opinion the DeLorme technique is probably the superior of the two because contracting initially at the lower force provides a warm-up and working gradually to the higher forces results in fatigue, which has a long-term beneficial effect in training.

In addition to strengthening by increasing the load, strengthening may be achieved by increasing the rate of contraction at a constant weight, as described by Hellebrandt and Houtz (4). This is referred to as progressive rate training. It is not used widely, but has as an advantage the fact that training is efficient; a fixed number of repetitions takes slightly less time each day as the metronome setting is advanced.

Brief isometric exercises have been advocated by some. These are very effective and efficient in developing isometric strength. However, because most activities require some dynamic strength, and because transferability from isometric to dynamic contractions is limited, training for dynamic tasks should not be confined to isometric exercises. For joints painful on movement, isometrics are likely to be preferred.

Two of the newer types of equipment deserve mention (1). The Cybex isokinetic exerciser allows one to preset a rate of contraction, which cannot be exceeded no matter how hard the subject pushes against the resistance arm. It provides accommodating resistance to the concentric contractions throughout the range of motion, and thus provides rate-specific and angle-specific training. It has a write-out device that gives immediate feedback to the subject regarding his or her contraction ability. Another device or set of devices is available in Nautilus equipment which, through its nautilus-shaped cam, provides variable concentric and eccentric resistance to approximate the torque curves of the muscle as previously described. Because the resistance varies to match the torque curves, it subjectively feels uniform throughout the range, and provides uniform muscle training throughout the range.

RATE OF INCREASE AND LOSS WITH IMMOBILIZATION

The most rapid increases of strength with training and the most rapid losses of strength with immobilization occur early in the course, and therefore reported average figures will vary depending on the length of the training or immobilization. A good average figure for six weeks of immobilization is 8 percent loss per week and for a 6-month daily training program 5 percent gain per week. These figures must be taken only as a rough rule of thumb. Both figures will be higher for shorter training programs and shorter immobilization. Gains are less likely if training is less than three times per week, although the latter can usually sustain gains made on a daily program.

Electrical Stimulation

Innervated muscle has the property of responding to short duration stimuli, as can nerve. Denervated muscles can respond to stimuli only of long duration. With a relatively long duration of 100 msec, denervated muscles may be even more sensitive than innervated muscles to stimuli—that is, respond at a lower intensity in milliamperes. However, as one proceeds to relatively shorter durations, the intensity required to produce a contraction becomes for practical purposes "infinite." So-called faradic current is of necessity short duration current, while galvanic (direct) current may be of long or short duration. Innervated muscle might be stimulated, for example, as a reeducation technique in someone who has temporarily lost central control, as in stroke patients. Denervated muscle may be stimulated to maintain muscle bulk until expected reinnervation occurs. In order to have any significant effect, this stimulation of denervated muscle must be carried out several times a day with multiple contractions in each session.

Massage

Massage has both reflex and mechanical effects. The most important of the reflex effects is relaxation. Mechanical effects include improvement of circulation and intramuscular movements, which may assist in the removal of adhesions. The general types of massage are stroking (effleurage); compression (petrissage), which includes kneading, squeezing, and friction; and percussion (tapotement). The subtypes of compression or petrissage are useful in mobilizing adhesions. Stroking and well-done percussion are relaxing, and stroking is useful in assisting the circulation. Stroking must always be done in the direction as to assist return flow circulation—that is, toward the heart. Massage is contraindicated in infection, malignancy, deep-vein thrombosis, and in hemorrhagic diathesis. Massage does not provide muscle strengthening and is not a substitute for active exercise.

Orthotic Devices

An orthosis assists the function of or protects a painful or otherwise impaired part of the body. A prosthesis restores one or more functions of an absent part of the body. Orthoses or orthotic devices include spinal braces; collars; molded body jackets, such as the TLSO (thoraco-lumbar-sacral orthosis); corsets with stays; static and dynamic splints for the upper limb; and varying splints and braces for the lower limb. The latter might be an off-the-shelf or custom-molded shoe insert to prevent excessive pronation of an athlete's foot; or, more extensive bracing of the ankle(s), knee(s), and even the hip(s) with pelvic band and drop lock(s). In lower-limb braces, the anterior stop at the ankle, combined with a rigid sole plate in the shoe, partially substitutes for the function of the gastrocnemius and tibialis posterior muscles, respectively; the posterior stop substitutes for the function of the tibialis anterior muscle. Thus the former gives a measure of "pushoff" and the latter gives "toe pickup." Lower-limb braces are available which, when properly designed, give relief of weight-bearing of the skeletal system. In the upper limb, orthoses can give passive stability, maintenance of skeletal alignment, and even dynamic prehension (grasp and release).

References

1. de Lateur BJ, Lehmann JF. Therapeutic exercise to develop strength and endurance. In: Kottke FJ, Lehmann JF (Eds.), *Krusen's handbook of physical medicine and rehabilitation* (4th ed.). Philadelphia, W.B. Saunders, 1990.
2. DeLorme TL. Restoration of muscle power by heavy resistance exercises. *J Bone Joint Surg* 27:645–667, 1945.
3. Hill AV. The dynamic constants of human muscle. *Proc Roy Soc London Series B* 128:263–274, 1940.
4. Hellebrandt FA, Houtz SJ. Methods of muscle training: The influence of pacing. *Phys Ther Rev* 38:319–322, 1958.
5. Mennell JM. *Joint pain*. Boston, Little, Brown, 1964.
6. Zinovieff AN. Heavy-resistance exercises: The "Oxford technique." *Br J Phys Med* 14:129–132, 1951.

Annotated Suggested Reading List

Colachis SC Jr, Strohm BR. A study of tractive forces and angle of pull on vertebral interspaces in the cervical spine. *Arch Phys Med Rehab* 46:820-830, 1965.
  A study of the forces and flexion angles and intervertebral space separations produced in normal subjects.
de Lateur BJ. Exercise for strength and endurance. In: Basmajian JV (Ed.), *Therapeutic exercise* (4th ed.). Baltimore, Williams & Wilkins, 1984.
  An enlarged discussion of strength and endurance.
de Lateur BJ. The role of physical medicine in problems of pain. *Adv Neurol* 4:495-497, 1974.
  Clinically oriented application of the modalities in relation to pain.
de Lateur BJ, Lehmann JF, Stonebridge JB, Warren CG, Guy AW. Muscle heating in human subjects with 915 MHz microwave contact applicator. *Arch Phys Med Rehab* 51:147–151, 1970.
DeLorme TL. Restoration of muscle power by heavy resistance exercises. *J Bone Joint Surg* 27:645-667, 1945.
Hellebrandt FA, Houtz SJ. Methods of muscle training: The influence of pacing. *Phys Ther Rev* 38:319–322, 1958.
Henneman E. Peripheral mechanisms involved in the control of muscle. In: Mountcastle VB (Ed.), *Medical physiology* (13th ed.). St. Louis, C.V. Mosby, 1974.
  Includes a discussion of motor unit types.
Hill AV. The dynamic constants of human muscle. *Proc Roy Soc London Series B* 128:263–274, 1940.
  A discussion of force-velocity relationships.
Lehmann JF (Ed.). *Therapeutic heat and cold* (4th ed.). Baltimore, Williams & Wilkins, 1990.
  A major text covering the physics, physiology, and clinical applications of temperature elevation or depression.
Lehmann JF, de Lateur BJ. Diathermy and superficial heat, laser and cold therapy. In: Kottke FJ, Lehmann JF (Eds.), *Handbook of physical medicine and rehabilitation* (4th ed.). Philadelphia, W.B. Saunders, 1990.

Lehmann JF, McMillan JA, Brunner GD, Blumberg JB. Comparative study of the efficiency of shortwave, microwave and ultrasonic diathermy in heating the hip joint. *Arch Phys Med Rehab* 40:510–512, 1959.

Documentation of the penetration power of ultrasound.

Mennell JM. *Joint pain.* Boston, Little, Brown, 1964.

A text that discusses manipulation and "joint play."

Sloan JP, Giddings P, Hain R. Effects of cold and compression on edema. *Phys Sportsmed* 16:116–120, 1988.

Zinovieff AN: Heavy-resistance exercises: The "Oxford technique." *Br J Phys Med* 14:129–132, 1951.

4 Electromyography, Nerve Conduction Studies, and Somatosensory Evoked Potentials in the Evaluation of Motor Unit and CNS Diseases

George H. Kraft, M.D.

Electrodiagnostic techniques are powerful tools for assessment of the site, severity, and type of dysfunction of both peripheral and central nervous system (CNS) diseases. The basic functional unit of the neuromuscular system is the motor unit (MU). It includes an anterior horn cell (AHC), its motor nerve root, myelinated peripheral axon, neuromuscular junction, and all of the skeletal muscle fibers innervated by that motor neuron. There is a wide range in the number of muscle fibers in each motor unit. Weak muscles that are involved in fine movements (e.g., extraocular muscles) may have as few as 8–12 muscle fibers per motor unit, whereas large, strong postural muscles may have more than 1,000. The neural elements are referred to as a lower motor neuron (LMN) (See Figure 4.1).

The weakest contraction of which a muscle is capable consists of all of the muscle fibers in a single motor unit firing slowly at a rate of approximately 6 Hz. Because all muscle fibers in a MU must contract as the motor unit fires, a minimal contraction of a large postural muscle will generate more force than a minimal contraction of a facial muscle. The normal mechanism of gradually increasing force production in skeletal muscle consists both of increasing the

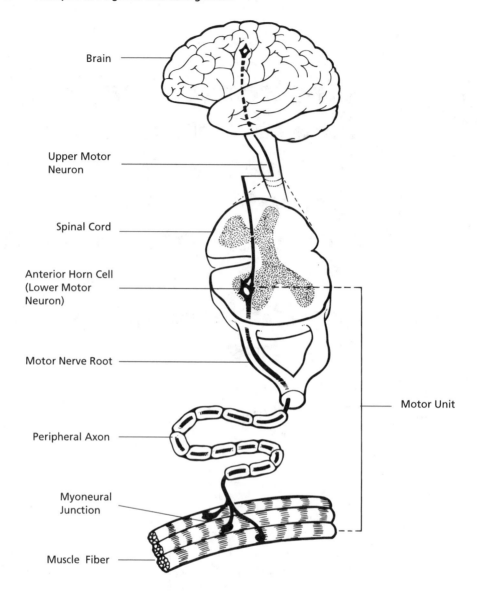

Brain

Upper Motor
Neuron

Spinal Cord

Anterior Horn Cell
(Lower Motor
Neuron)

Motor Nerve Root

Motor Unit

Peripheral Axon

Myoneural
Junction

Muscle Fiber

FIGURE 4.1. The upper motor neurons descend through the pyramidal tracts to synapse with cell bodies of the lower motor neurons in the anterior horns on the opposite side of the spinal cord. The motor unit consists of the anterior horn cell, motor nerve root, peripheral axon, myoneural junction, and the skeletal muscle fibers it innervates.

firing rate of MUs and recruiting more MUs to participate in the contraction. A normal motor unit will fire as rapidly as 20 Hz on maximal contraction. In a trained athlete, MU firing can be as great as 40 Hz.

When an anterior horn cell is stimulated above threshold by descending CNS impulses, a wave of depolarization is transmitted down the peripheral axon. As depolarization reaches the many myoneural junctions, acetylcholine (ACH) is released, and the individual muscle fiber membranes are depolarized. This electrical event produces chemical changes in the sarcoplasmic reticulum (SR), and contraction of all the muscle fibers of the MU then occurs.

The electrical activity of individual motor units—the composite activity of many synchronized muscle fibers—is called the motor unit action potential (MUAP) This action potential may be recorded by needle electrodes inserted into a muscle. In this technique, known as electromyography (EMG), the electrical potentials recorded are amplified and may be observed on an electromyographic display and heard over a loudspeaker system. By convention, positive potentials are downward going.

From the above, one can appreciate why MUAPs from the larger muscles have a greater voltage (amplitude) on the EMG display than MUAPs from facial muscles: it is because they contain a greater number of muscle fibers. One can also understand that as the strength of contraction increases, the number of MUAPs on the screen will increase.

Electromyography is performed with Teflon™-coated monopolar needle electrodes or with concentric needle electrodes. After identifying the muscle to be studied, the electrode is inserted into the muscle and the EMG display observed while both the needle and patient are at rest. In the normal state, no electrical potentials should be seen.

The insertional activity of the muscle is then studied by probing the muscle with the intramuscular electrode. Normally the electrical activity that accompanies these movements stops shortly after the needle motion terminates.

When the patient is asked to contract the muscle at low levels of force, individual MUAPs are easily identified, and their amplitude, duration, waveform, and firing rate can be evaluated. In normal individuals, the MUAP's peak-to-peak amplitude ranges from 300 microvolts to 3 millivolts, depending on the muscle studied and the MUAP evaluated. The total duration is from 3 to 16 milliseconds, and the typical minimal contraction firing rate is 6 Hz. The MUAP represents the summated electrical potentials of the muscle fibers innervated by a single lower motor neuron. The typical biphasic or triphasic waveform is the result of spatial and temporal summation of the electrical activity produced by the individual muscle fibers of the motor unit (Figure 4.2a).

With increasing muscle contraction, the recruitment pattern for motor units may be observed and an evaluation of the integrity of the total motor unit pool may be made at a maximum contraction. A full interference pattern is normally noted.

Fasciculation potentials are MUAPs of either normal or abnormal size and configuration, occurring sporadically. They represent the spontaneous firing of the motor unit, and can be seen in disease processes involving the anterior horn cell or more distal axons.

In acute MU diseases that produce axonal loss, some muscle fibers become denervated. Denervated muscle fibers are not under voluntary control and fire spontaneously. These spontaneously firing muscle fibers produce short duration potentials known as fibrillation potentials (Figure 4.2b). As the denervated muscle fibers undergo atrophy, the amplitude of the fibrillation potentials decays. Positive sharp waves are also seen in denervated muscles and represent discharges initiated by the mechanical stimulation at the needle tip (Figure 4.2c). Fibrillation potentials and positive sharp waves can also be seen in primary muscle diseases, such as muscular dystrophy and polymyositis.

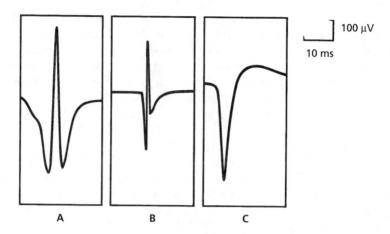

FIGURE 4.2. (a) Normal motor unit action potential. (b) Fibrillation potential from recently denervated muscle. (c) Positive sharp wave. In all traces, positive deflection is down.

Polyphasic, low-amplitude MU potentials of increased duration are observed in early stages of nerve reinnervation. These "nascent" potentials are produced by the electrical activity generated by only a few skeletal muscle fibers innervated by immature, slowly conducting, terminal nerve twigs. Thus there is little synchronization of the individual muscle fiber potentials. As regeneration occurs and the MU matures, more skeletal muscle fibers will be added to the motor unit, with greater synchronization resulting in large amplitude MUAPs.

Polyphasic MUAPs with five or more phases and an amplitude and duration greater than normal are seen in chronic neuropathic processes. They represent reorganization of the motor unit, with some muscle fibers from denervated MUs having been incorporated into existing or regenerating ones, along with spatial reorganization of the motor unit. In such conditions there are fewer than normal MUAPs to participate in a full recruitment, and a "decreased interference pattern" is noted.

Small amplitude MUAPs of short or normal duration result from fewer than normal skeletal muscle fibers participating in the motor unit discharge. These motor units are often polyphasic as well. Primary muscle disease is the usual source of these potentials.

Abnormalities of the interference pattern may also be observed in disease processes. When motor unit reorganization has occurred, large amplitude units will be recruited earlier and maximum recruitment effort will show a reduced number of MUAPs. Low amplitude but full recruitment patterns with maximum effort are seen in myopathic diseases.

In addition to needle electromyography, other techniques are available to the electromyographer. Peripheral nerves may be stimulated by electrical currents. Such a stimulus can be delivered to any mixed or motor nerve percutaneously, and the electrical activity of the muscle innervated measured. This synchronized muscle activity—known as the compound muscle action potential (CMAP) or "M wave"—can be recorded, and the time interval between the stimulus and response—known as the latency—can be measured. By stimulating the peripheral nerve at two different points along its course and determining the latency in each case, the nerve conduction velocity (NCV) may be calculated. This is achieved by subtracting the distal latency from the proximal latency (giving the time required to travel between the two points of stimulation), and dividing this time into the distance between the two points (Figure 4.3). NCV = M/sec.

All of these techniques can be used to provide the electromyographer with information about the motor unit. Additionally, information about sensory nerve fibers may also be determined and sensory latencies or sensory NCV may be measured. A sensory nerve action potential (SNAP) produced by electrical stimulation of an afferent nerve distally may be recorded over the sensory nerve proximally (Figure 4.4). This is known as "orthodromic" conduction. Conversely, the sensory nerve can be stimulated proximally and the action potential recorded distally, a technique known as "antidromic" conduction. The time interval between the onset of the stimulus to the negative peak of the response—the peak latency—is recorded. Alternatively, the latency to the onset may be recorded and a NCV calculated after the latency of activities has been subtracted from the measured latency.

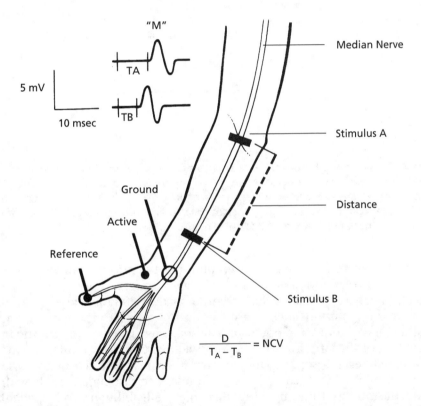

FIGURE 4.3. Motor NCV technique. In this example of median nerve recording, the reference and ground electrodes are placed over electrically inactive areas. The active electrode is placed over the abductor pollicis brevis. The median nerve is supramaximally stimulated with bipolar surface electrodes distally at the wrist and proximally at the antecubital fossa. The latencies from stimulus artifact to the initial negative deflection of the CMAP (TA and TB) are noted. The distance between the two sites of stimulation (D) is measured. The NCV in meters per second is calculated by dividing D by $(T_A - T_B)$, where D is measured in mm and T is measured in msec.

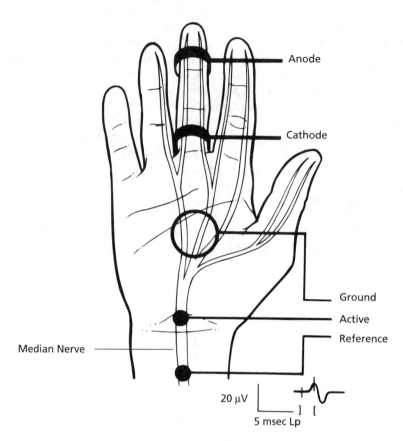

FIGURE 4.4. Sensory latency technique. In this example of median nerve orthodromic recording, stimulating ring electrodes are placed on the digit with the negative (cathode) electrode proximally. Recording electrodes are placed over the median nerve at a standard distance from the stimulating electrodes. The peak latency (Lp) from the stimulus artifact to the negative peak of the SNAP is recorded.

A modification of motor nerve conduction techniques can also be used to study the myoneural junction. Instead of single stimuli, motor nerves can be stimulated repeatedly at fixed rates. Such techniques are useful for studying disorders of the myoneural junction, such as are seen in myasthenia gravis, Eaton-Lambert (myasthenic) syndrome, and botulism. The characteristic electrodiagnostic finding is variability of the amplitude of the M wave to successive stimulation, in a pattern unique to each disorder. The most common myoneural junction disease is myasthenia gravis, in which M wave amplitudes decrease progressively with each subsequent stimulus, thus mirroring the clinical fatigability noted by patients.

In addition to the CMAP, action potentials can be recorded at long latencies when stimulating certain nerves, and are known as "late responses." The most common of these are the F waves (frequently studied in the ulnar nerve, with a latency of less than 30 msecs) and the H reflex (studied in the tibial nerve, having a latency of greater than 30 msec). H reflexes and F waves are useful for evaluating the function of the most proximal segments of the peripheral nerves. In the H reflex, the mixed peripheral nerve is stimulated at low voltage. This stimulates the afferent fibers and an impulse travels centrally through the dorsal roots, synapsing on the anterior horn cells, producing a depolarization of them and a subsequent response of the MU. This entire time period can be measured, giving information about nerve conduction in the roots. F waves are similar, except the centripetal impulses are transmitted along the efferent (motor) fibers, "bouncing back" from the anterior horn cells to produce a muscle response.

Another type of late response is a complex cranial nerve (CN) V and CN VII reflex known as the blink response. This reflex is useful in evaluating patients with Bell palsy, multiple sclerosis, and other brainstem and cranial nerve disorders. Such recordings require two EMG channels, and record late reflex responses from both ipsi- and contralateral facial muscles after stimulating one supraorbital nerve. These reflexes traverse polysynaptic brainstem regions and identify pathology of this area of the CNS as well as the PNS.

A more sophisticated EMG technique is the single-fiber EMG (SFEMG), which allows analysis of the irregularity of firing of different muscle fibers within the motor unit. It is useful primarily in the study of myoneural junction disorders.

A technique known as macro EMG has been developed to provide information about the entire motor unit. Macro EMG can be useful in assessing the size of the motor unit and, hence, information about its innervation.

Somatosensory evoked potentials (SEPs) are powerful techniques that can be applied in the clinical setting to measure conduction through the peripheral nervous system, nerve roots, spinal cord, and brain. In SEP recordings, mixed nerves, pure sensory nerves, and even dermatomes (known as DSEPs) can be stimulated. Sensory fibers are stimulated in the periphery, and electrical potentials are recorded over the spinal cord and somatosensory cortex of the contralateral brain. Because the cortical potentials are very small, hundreds of stimuli are given and the evoked potentials are averaged. An averager is an electronic system that "looks" at the electrical potentials recorded following a peripheral nerve stimulation. Many potentials may be recorded, including electronic or environmental "noise," unrelated biologic signals (such as EEG), and time-locked responses to the peripheral stimulus. The averager enhances the signals (which are time-locked) and averages out those which are unrelated to the stimulus. Recordings are generally made in several locations, with one recording made from the most proximal portion of the peripheral nerve studied before cord entry, with additional recordings made over various segments of the spinal cord and somatosensory cortex on the contralateral scalp.

The current areas of greatest practical use of SEPs are in multiple sclerosis, nerve root disorders, spinal cord trauma, nerve plexus trauma, and many other CNS and PNS disorders. DSEPs are especially useful in lumbosacral spinal stenosis.

A very new technique is magnetic evoked potentials (MEPs). A rapidly changing magnetic field is placed over neural tissue, causing the fibers to discharge. Impulses conducted down motor neurons cause muscle to contract; the latency can be measured. Although at the present time, MEPs are only FDA approved for stimulation of peripheral nerves, the technique looks most promising for motor cortex stimulation.

Using electrodiagnostic techniques, it is possible to delineate the segment of the motor unit or sensory nerve that is involved in a disease process. For example, in peripheral nerve diseases it is possible to discriminate between myelin and axon disorders. Demyelinating diseases generally show greater slowing of NCV because segmental loss or thinning of myelin can cause slowed conduction or a conduction block. Nerve root compression and peripheral nerve entrapment can be identified by the pattern of skeletal muscle found to be involved. In the former, muscles supplied by the same affected nerve root, including limb and paraspinal muscles, will show abnormalities; in the latter, only muscles supplied by a given peripheral nerve will show abnormalities. Additionally, NCV will be altered in regions of nerve abnormality.

The combination of EMG, NCV, and SEP techniques is useful in the diagnosis and evaluation of both peripheral and central nervous system diseases. The presence of disease of the motor unit or sensory system can be identified; muscle disease can be separated from nerve disease; and the severity, duration, and change in a disease can be determined. Electrodiagnostic techniques are thus powerful tools for the assessment of weakness and sensory loss.

═══ Annotated Suggested Reading List

1. AAEE glossary of terms in clinical electromyography. *Muscle & Nerve* G1–60: October 1987.
   The definitive "dictionary" for the field.
2. Brown WF, Bolton CF (Eds.), *Clinical electromyography* (2d ed.). Stoneham, MA, Butterworth-Heinemann, 1993.
3. Chiappa KH. *Evoked potentials in clinical medicine* (2d ed.). New York, Raven Press, 1990.
   The most authoritative source of evoked potential information.
4. Johnson EW (Ed.), *Practical electromyography* (2d ed.). Baltimore, Williams & Wilkins, 1988.
   A good general EMG text.
5. Kimura J. *Electrodiagnosis in diseases of nerve and muscle: Principle and Practice* (2d ed.). Philadelphia, F.A. Davis, 1988.
   A comprehensive, definitive EMG text.
6. Kraft GH. Doctors' questions answered. In: MacLean IC (Ed.), *EMG: A guide for the referring physician. Vol. 1: Physical medicine and rehabilitation clinics of North America.* Philadelphia, W.B. Saunders, 1990:1–15.
   A current, easy-to-read summary of electrodiagnostic medicine for general physicians.
7. Kraft GH. Fibrillation potential amplitude and muscle atrophy following peripheral nerve injury. Muscle & Nerve 13:814-21, 1990.
8. Slimp JC, Rubner DR, Snowden ML, Stolov WC. Dermatomal somatosensory evoked potentials: cervical, thoracic, and lumbosacral levels. Electroencephalography and clinical neurophysiology 84:55-70, 1992.
9. Snowden ML, Haselkorn JK, Kraft GH, Bronstein AD, Bigos SJ, Slimp JC. Stolov WC. Dermatomal somatosensory evoked potentials in the diagnosis of lumbosacral spinal stenosis: Comparison with imaging studies. *Muscle & Nerve* 15:1036-1044, 1992.
10. Stalberg E, Trontelj JV. *Single fiber electromyography*. Old Woking, Surrey, UK: The Miravile Press Limited, 1979.
    A detailed manual of SFEMG by the originator of the technique.

5 The Team Approach to Rehabilitation

Ross M. Hays, M.D., Rosemarian Berni, R.N.,
M.S.N., Mark Guthrie, Ph.D., Brian Dudgeon,
M.S., O.T.R., Kathryn Yorkston, Ph.D., and
Kiko Kimura–Van Zandt, R.N., B.S.N.

The process of rehabilitation is invariably wed to the concept of a team. While the rehabilitation team as a model of health care delivery is frequently written about and referred to, it is so rarely studied that it has no generally accepted definition. The use of a team in health care delivery was initially an attempt to deliver a more comprehensive form of medical treatment mandated by the knowledge explosion in medical and basic sciences technology that occurred during the middle twentieth century. It has evolved, according to Rothberg, "as a compromise between the benefits of specialization and the need for continuity and comprehensiveness of care" (10).

The small amount of research addressing the efficacy of a team approach to rehabilitation collected by Halstead (5) suggests that;

1. for persons with long-term illnesses a coordinated team is more effective at delivering services than is fragmented care;
2. the team approach is effective in maintaining restoration of function;
3. patients managed by a team are less likely to suffer status deterioration;
4. team care leads to increased use of health services; and
5. greater use of health services results in increased health care costs.

Like many other aspects of modern medicine, team delivered rehabilitation has the benefit of increased effectiveness but is accompanied by a larger expenditure of health care dollars.

Health care teams may be multidisciplinary or interdisciplinary. Frequently and erroneously, these descriptive terms are used interchangeably. The "multidisciplinary" model refers to activities provided by professionals from a variety of disciplines, with each team member remaining within his or her own area of expertise. The summation of benefits, and occasionally the disadvantages, of uncoordinated care are known only to the patient receiving the services because the health-care providers remain segregated with control over only their own activities. An "interdisciplinary" approach assumes that each professional provides a unique aspect of health care, but also has an understanding of the general principles of services provided by others. In this model, the responsibility for overall patient care is more clearly shared and team members have accountability to each other (4). In order for the best possible care to be provided, final responsibility should rest with one team member. Interdisciplinary team management affords the possibility of synergistic activity among the team to resolve potential conflicts, reduce redundancy of services, and coordinate the timely provision of interventions. In this system, where the whole is greater than the sum of the parts, the eventual outcome may have greater value to the patient (6).

Historically the health care team consisted of four disciplines: physicians, nurses, volunteers, and the chaplaincy. This aggregate of care providers could adequately handle the scope of existing medical expertise and provide state-of-the-art, humane care until the latter years of the last century. The dramatic expansion of health care knowledge and technology, often accelerated by the tragedy of war and epidemics, resulted in the development of a diverse group of health-care professionals, all of whom play an important role in the process of rehabilitation (7).

Rehabilitation Nursing

Nurses who specialize in rehabilitation possess the knowledge and clinical skills needed to deal with the profound impact of disability on individuals, their families, and significant others. The essence of rehabilitation nursing is the diagnosis and treatment of human responses to actual or potential health problems characterized by disability, altered function, and lifestyle. Practice settings vary widely from the acute-care hospital phase to home-based care and community programs (2). Nurses practicing in such settings are accountable for the knowledge and skills necessary in providing care to people with disabilities. Certification for specialty practice, which recognizes a level of expertise in rehabilitation nursing, began in 1984 (8). This certification is administered by the professional organization, the Association of Rehabilitation Nurses (ARN), which was established in 1974.

Believing that individuals have intrinsic worth that transcends disability, the goal of rehabilitation nursing is to assist patients in the restoration and maintenance of maximal physical, psychosocial, and spiritual health. This is accomplished through the diverse roles of the rehabilitation nurse, that of teacher, caregiver, patient advocate and care coordinator, counselor, consultant, and researcher (3).

As a teacher, the rehabilitation nurse shares information and assists the patient and family to develop the skills necessary to move toward future self-management, independence, and achievement. The nurse provides instruction to the patient and family regarding specific nursing procedures or patient needs, such as intermittent bladder catheterization, routine skin check techniques, or the side effects of medications. The rehabilitation nurse also reinforces the instruction of other members of the interdisciplinary team. The nurse provides educational information for other team members or community resources, such as the community public health nurse and other home health-care providers, school personnel, or primary care physicians.

The nursing staff provides 24-hour care to the patient. This direct contact provides opportunity for the assessment of efficacy of treatments and therapies provided by other disciplines. Skills such as transfers, ROM, ADLs, and communication strategies can be observed on the unit and supervised by a nurse. Direct daily care is done until the patient and family acquire the competence necessary for independence outside the medical facility. All care is aimed at the restoration and maintenance of function and at prevention of complications, which may result in further functional loss. The nurse is responsible for the provision of a therapeutic environment that is reality based, wellness-behavior oriented, optimistic, encouraging, and socially appropriate.

In the role of advocate, the nurse bridges communication gaps between patient and family and the remainder of the rehabilitation team. Because the relationship is developed by round-the-clock contact, the nurse may be in the unique position to convey the patient's needs and concerns to the team. Advocacy may also include interpretation of technical medical information for the family. This role results in the development of a relationship between patient, family, and nurse based on mutual confidence and trust.

The unique relationship forged by nurse and patient allows the exploration of issues that the newly disabled person experiences, such as changed self-concept and redefined personhood. The nurse encourages the maximal use of the patient's remaining abilities, assisting him or her to develop appropriate responses to new situations. The operating concepts in the rehabilitation nurse's counseling role are a pragmatic approach to problem solving and the insight that allows patients to recognize their own residual strengths. The nurse works with the family to maximize the disabled person's functional independence and to reintegrate him or her into the home and community. This process is acheived by encouraging the patient to reestablish and maintain control over as many aspects of his or her own life as possible.

As a consultant, the nurse promotes the concept of rehabilitation and the restoration of function. The rehabilitation nurse consultant is qualified to offer support and expertise to other nurses and team members. The nurse also advocates for the rights of the disabled, community accessibility, and primary prevention of disease and trauma. Some nurses in this role are employed by insurance companies to do case utilization review in order to influence appropriate allocation of resources.

The rehabilitation nurse uses medical and nursing research methods to improve the quality of care provided to patients. Nurses frequently participate in the design and implementation of clinical research in rehabilitation. In academic settings, rehabilitation nurses contribute to nursing and medical science by initiating and conducting independent research study.

By working to achieve realistic independence for patient and family, rehabilitation nurses encourage their clients to look beyond the disability. It is a responsibility of the nurse to promote quality of life for individuals with disability and to support activities that prevent disability and chronic illness.

Physical Therapy

Physical therapists are specialists in the conservative management of patients whose ability to move is impaired. For one patient that might mean designing a program to increase strength, flexibility, and endurance to achieve the goal of

Olympic competition. For another it could mean balance and coordination drills that allow that person to simply get from bed to wheelchair.

The training of physical therapists has evolved from certification to baccalaureate programs, and is now in the process of moving to the postbaccalaureate (masters) level(1). These programs include intensive study of musculoskeletal anatomy, kinesiology, exercise physiology, and therapeutic exercise. Many hours are spent in refining hands-on skills in joint mobilization, guided exercise, and the use of electrical modalities. Additionally, physical therapists become experts in physical examination, including assessment of strength, range of motion, coordination and balance, gait, and functional status.

Historically, physical therapists have been employed primarily in hospitals, treating patients with acute and chronic illness and disability. Therapists are, for example, actively involved in the design and implementation of programs to increase strength and range of motion, decrease pain, and adapt new techniques or devices to assist in movement of patients with degenerative joint disease, thus helping those patients avoid or postpone the need for corrective surgery. When surgery is indicated, physical therapists are critical in enhancing the patient's recovery via the use of intervention strategies designed to efficiently and effectively restore optimum function. Physical therapists are also involved in all stages of managing cardiac disease, designing and monitoring exercise programs for patients with coronary artery disease or postmyocardial infarction, and after coronary artery bypass graft surgery. Similarly, physical therapists work with cancer, AIDS, amputees, and burn victim patients. A large part of the profession is involved in the treatment of disabled children (9).

Within recent years, due to expansion of the practice of physical therapy and changes in reimbursement policies, the physical therapy service delivery areas have shifted to outpatient care. Outpatient settings are often part of a large medical center, but are just as likely to be independent, private physical therapy clinics. The types of patients seen in these settings are frequently those with common musculoskeletal disorders, such as neck and back pain. The success of physical therapists in this type of setting has been responsible for the development of such innovative practices as emergency room consultation by physical therapists, to more quickly and effectively rehabilitate victims of acute bouts of low back pain or joint sprains. In many settings, physical therapists include or limit their practice to the prevention and management of sports-related injuries.

It is in the areas of rehabilitation of patients with chronic disabilities, such as spinal cord injury and stroke, that the practice of physical therapy is perhaps best defined. The physical therapist has extensive daily contact with the patient and is therefore perhaps in the best position to monitor progress and report changes to the other members of the rehabilitation team. The physical therapist conducts complete initial and ongoing assessments, paying particular attention to strength, tone and deep tendon reflexes, sensation, position sense, range of motion, functional status, pain, and the integrity of skin and soft tissue.

The physical therapist initiates treatment as soon as the patient is medically stable. Following a completed stroke, for example, this typically begins within 24–36 hrs and is aimed at such goals as maintaining range of motion, preventing deconditioning, minimizing the effects of abnormal tone, mobilizing the patient, improving trunk control, promoting awareness, and initiating self-care activities. Physical therapy treatment progresses over weeks or months in response to the patient's improving status. The goal, of course, is optimal physical function. Most physical therapists tend to follow a developmental sequence in their approach to treatment: bed mobility, trunk control, sitting balance, and simple transfers are stressed before quadruped kneeling and standing activities are initiated. Gait training may be one of the last activities to be addressed. Techniques are often used to facilitate movement, which include brushing and tapping of skin, quick-stretching electrical stimulation of muscles, and biofeedback.

The physical therapist works closely with other members of the rehabilitation team, offering suggestions for reinforcement of gains in physical function and the incorporation into other aspects of rehabilitation. In the same manner, input from other team members is incorporated into the physical therapy treatment. For example, the speech therapist may offer suggestions for cuing a patient in performance of a wheelchair to bed transfer. Education of patients and their families is an important aspect of treatment. The nature and extent of contact with the patient allows the physical therapist to help patients and family achieve an understanding of principles of management and compliance in completion of home exercises and assignments.

Occupational Therapy

The major purpose of occupational therapy (OT) is to develop, maintain, and/or restore function in persons with disabilities through the use of activities. The occupational therapist assesses and trains individuals in living skills and works to clarify environmental and personal-care needs within the community setting to enhance functional independence and safety at home. Performance of activities, exercises, and play are used in goal-directed programs to promote independence in persons who are hampered by physical illness or injury, social and emotional difficulties, congenital or developmental problems, or the aging process. Functional outcome goals are influenced by age, gender, and sociocultural background. Particular tasks of self-care, work, and leisure function are addressed through collaboration with other rehabilitation team members.

Occupational therapy interventions may include physical techniques, such as sensorimotor stimulation, neurodevelopmental handling, or biomechanical methods that facilitate movement. OTs also design and fabricate orthotics and other devices to prevent deformity and improve function. Educational approaches are used by OTs to teach and supervise patients in the performance of exercises or activity routines in order to maintain or maximize range of motion or to improve strength endurance, coordination, and fitness. Self-care and home-living activities are addressed by training patients to perform modified self-help routines or by using adaptive devices and assistive technology. Consultation may be provided relative to strategies for overcoming architectural barriers, coping with social consequences of disability, or otherwise adjusting to handicaps.

The use of therapeutic activities to facilitate the development of physical, cognitive, and psychological skills has its origins in ancient civilizations. In more modern times the precursors of OT began in the eighteenth and nineteenth centuries in mental health facilities in Europe and the United States, where a more humanitarian approach toward persons with mental illnesses and retardation was evolving. In the early 1900s, and particularly during and after World

War I, allied health practitioners and educators were trained to use activities to help restore function to the physically impaired as well as to the emotionally disabled. During this period the modern practice of OT emerged. Schools developed and the profession was promoted by the establishment of an organization in 1917, known today as the American Occupational Therapy Association (AOTA). The practice of OT grew even more rapidly during World War II and expanded to civilian rehabilitation programs to respond to workmen's compensation rights and other social mandates for rights to public education, employment, and independent living.

Registered Occupational Therapists (OTRs) have completed a bachelor of arts or science degree or basic master's degree from a college or university program accredited by the AOTA. Six months of fieldwork training and successful completion of a national examination are required. Certified Occupational Therapy Assistants (COTAs) have an associate degree or certificate from an AOTA accredited community college program, have completed two months of fieldwork, and have also passed an examination. Both OTRs and COTAs are licensed in most states. In many practice settings, the OTR conducts and interprets evaluations to formulate a treatment plan with a patient. The OTR carries out the treatment or utilizes a COTA to conduct treatment while providing periodic supervision. Although there are nearly 50,000 practitioners today, a severe shortage of personnel is predicted during the next several decades.

Occupational therapists work with clients throughout the physical medicine and rehabilitation process. With injury, acute onset of disease, or the exacerbation of chronic disease, the occupational therapist's first concern is the prevention of further limitation, such as muscle or joint contractures, unnecessary deconditioning, or further injury due to falls or poor judgment. A second priority is to encourage the patient's family and other careproviders to allow as much return to normal independence as possible. Simple adaptation of routines may permit the patient partial or complete independence in self-help skills, which can often offset the development of overly dependent behaviors.

The OT then works with the patient, family, and community to restore function. Such efforts may involve improvement of performance skills: prerequisites to purposeful and functional activity. Performance skills include sensory and motor ability, perception, and cognition, as well as psychological and social skills. Evaluation and treatment through exercise and activity training includes motor skill development via techniques of reflex integration, range of motion, gross and fine coordination, and strength and endurance building. Activities to develop sensory skills may address awareness and integration, visuospatial skills, body integration, and motor planning. Cognitive skill training approaches include interventions to promote orientation, concentration, attention span, memory, generalization to new situations, and effective problem-solving strategies. Activities and training in self-expression and control, as well as dyadic and group interaction, may be used by a therapist to improve psychological and social skills.

Techniques are employed to restore the occupational skills of activities of daily living, work, and play necessary for independent living concurrently with efforts to improve skills that aid functional ability. Direct evaluation and training of independent living skills include the daily life activities of grooming and hygiene, feeding or eating, dressing, functional mobility, functional communication, and object manipulation. Work-skill development addresses homemaking, child care and parenting, employment preparation, and leisure skills. Psychological daily living skill training includes techniques to promote self-concept and identity, situational coping, and community involvement.

Both performance skills and functional task training are impacted by the use of therapeutic and prevention programs. Adaptive techniques include the selection and training in use of orthotics, prosthetics, self-help devices, and assistive technology. Prevention approaches include training patients in personal energy conservation, joint protection, positioning, and planning daily life activities.

Hallmarks of the OT training approach are activity analysis and the breakdown of tasks into achievable steps. Specific training may involve use of modified sequences and assistive devices. Training is often reinforced by repetition of functional tasks at normally occurring times and by use of training aids, such as cue cards or other self-prompting routines.

Simulation of independent living skills is another intervention used in OT. Community visits, home visits, and other means may be used to evaluate and train the patient in an environment that replicates the challenges they will face after discharge. In many cases, the patient cannot be expected to regain or maintain performance skills, and likewise will peak in his or her ability to function independently. In such cases, the OT works with family and other careproviders in the community to modify and reduce environmental barriers, and trains careproviders to appropriately assist the patient, on occasion by modifying behavioral expectations to better match the patient's level of function.

Occupational therapists practice in a variety of settings familiar to all rehabilitation practitioners. Hospitals, outpatient clinics, home-health agencies, skilled nursing facilities, community mental health centers, public schools, and independent living centers employ OTs. Therapists may provide direct patient care, serve as consultants, or as case coordinators.

Speech Pathology

The field of speech/language pathology seeks to understand the process of human communication and how this process may be disrupted by physical or neurologic disorder. Among the major goals of the field is remediation of problems that interfere with normal communication. Speech/language pathologists and audiologists hold either a master's or doctoral degree and are certified by the American Speech-Language-Hearing Association. Certification requires, in addition to a graduate degree, the completion of a supervised clinical fellowship year and satisfactory completion of a written examination. Speech/language pathologists practice in a number of settings, including hospitals, outpatient clinics, home-health agencies, residential or extended-care facilities, and educational settings.

In the medical rehabilitation team, the speech pathologist provides assessment, program planning, and treatment to patients with communication and swallowing disorders, including those with aphasia, apraxia of speech, dysarthria, laryngectomy, glossectomy, and voice disorders. Common medical etiologies include stroke, traumatic brain injury, degenerative neurological disorders, and cancers involving the speech production mechanism.

Assessment involves the establishment of baseline performance, the evaluation of strengths and weaknesses upon which to base a treatment program, and followup testing to determine the extent of change in performance. In terms of language assessment, a number of standardized tests are available to measure comprehension and expression of verbal and written material. When assessing motor speech production, the speech/language pathologist will evaluate respiratory support, phonation, velopharyngeal, and oral articulatory function. Treatment of motor speech disorders involves the maximization of residual physiologic capability and teaching the speaker techniques to maximize intelligibility and naturalness of speech. A variety of augmentative communication devices are available for patients who are unable to meet their communication needs via natural speech. These augmentative approaches range from gestures and signs, to simple alphabet/word board, to complex computer-based equipment. Speech/language pathologists are also involved in the rehabilitation of individuals after ablative surgical procedures, such as laryngectomies or glossectomies. In the case of the laryngectomized patient, a variety of alternative sound sources are available. Because the listener is such an integral part of the communication process, the members of a patient's family will frequently need considerable training to improve the effectiveness of communication. The speech/language pathologist frequently consults in the evaluation and treatment of patients with swallowing disorders. This approach may involve the selection of appropriate food, the evaluation of the efficiency of the swallowing mechanism, and training in specific techniques to enhance the safety and efficiency of the swallowing process.

══ REFERENCES

1.   APTA. Statement adopted by the House of Delegates, at the Annual Conference of the American Physical Therapy Association, 1983.
2.   ARN and ANA. *Standard of rehabilitation nursing practice.* ANA, Kansas City, MO, 1986.
3.   ARN and ANA. *Rehabilitation nursing: Scope of practice; process and outcome criteria for selected diagnoses.* ANA, Kansas City, MO, 1988.
4.   Gaston, EH. Developing a motivating organizational climate for effective team functioning. *Hospital Community Psychiatry* 31:407–412, 1980.
5.   Halstead LS. Team care chronic illness: A critical review of the literature of the past 25 years. *Arch Phys Med Rehab* 57:507–511, 1976.
6.   Keith RA. The comprehensive treatment team in rehabilitation. *Arch Phys Med Rehab* Vol 72, April 1991.
7.   Melvin JL. Interdisciplinary and multidisciplinary activities and the ACRM. *Arch Phys Med Rehab* 61:379–380, 1980.
8.   Mumma CM (Ed.). *Rehabilitation nursing: Concepts and practice.* Rehabilitation Nursing Foundation, Skokie, IL, 1989.
9.   O'Sullivan SB, Schmitz RJ. *Physical rehabilitation: Assessment and treatment.* Philadelphia, F.A. Davis, p. 351, 1988.
10. Rothberg JS. The rehabilitation team: Future direction. *Arch Phys Med Rehab* 62:407–410, 1981.

Management Problems of Disabling Diseases

6 Disuse Syndrome: Recognition and Prevention

Eugen M. Halar, M.D.

Disuse syndrome is the name that is used to describe the group of symptoms and signs caused by the limited use of body systems and which are not caused by any specific pathological condition. Disuse syndrome refers to complications that are caused by prolonged bed rest, immobility, immobilization, and physical inactivity. These may produce a wide range of problems and dysfunctions.

Lack of use of muscles as in immobilization of an extremity in a cast or physical inactivity may produce muscle weakness, atrophy, and parallel loss of endurance even in an absence of any neurological or musculoskeletal pathological conditions. The lack of mobility, with limited muscle pull on the bone and lack of gravity may produce profound calcium loss from the axial bones. The absence of simple stretch to the collagen tissue of the joint capsule or muscle may cause limited joint range of motion or muscle contractures. Prolonged bed rest, if associated with deprivation of social and environmental cues, may cause anxiety, irritability, depression, and decline in intellectual functioning. It has been well documented that bed rest, reduced mobility, and inactivity may produce a wide range of complications, which are commonly called the disuse syndrome.

Complications that accompany prolonged bed rest and inactivity are widespread and do not spare any age or gender. However, the chronically ill with associated functional impairments are particularly at high risk. Patients with any preexisting musculoskeletal, neurological, and/or cardiopulmonary conditions will develop adverse effects at an accelerated rate if bedridden. The compounded effect of the disease and inactivity creates a troublesome vicious cycle of side effects (Figure 6.1).

In some cases, complications of inactivity in chronically ill and disabled patients may become a greater problem than that of the primary disease, resulting in additional dysfunction and disability. It is important to realize that many of these problems either in healthy subjects or in patients with chronic diseases can be easily prevented or treated if recognized in time. Hence, one important

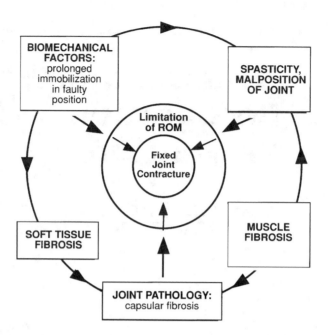

FIGURE 6.1. Effects of prolonged bed rest, immobilization, and inactivity on the development of joint contractures.

clinical principle in managing chronically ill and disabled patients is prevention of adverse effects of immobility and further decline in physical and psychosocial functions (Table 6.1).

This chapter will stress the significance of early recognition and prevention of these complications and will also stress the need for conditioning of the chronically ill and disabled.

Musculoskeletal Complications of Disuse

The musculoskeletal system, under control of the CNS, provides two basic physical functions, which are mobility and the ability to perform activities of daily living (ADLs). To maintain these functions, all components of the musculoskeletal system need to be intact. Muscle weakness or joint stiffness due to disuse will reduce the musculoskeletal function of mobility and ADLs, whereas maintaining normal muscle strength and joint flexibility will preserve it. Energy consumption in the upright position is 16–19 percent greater than in the supine position. Walking and running may greatly increase energy consumption up to 50–100 times, with muscle blood supply increased 15–20 fold. Standing, walking, and jogging are activities that are necessary to maintain or improve musculoskeletal and cardiovascular function and fitness. The normal cardiovascular and musculoskeletal response to physical activity and work may fall to dangerous levels if the stimulus of physical activity is not of sufficient intensity, frequency, and duration. Optimal or increased use of the musculoskeletal system will increase the functional capacity of the musculoskeletal as well as cardiovascular systems (8).

TABLE 6.1

Effects of Prolonged Bed Rest on Body Systems

Muscle weakness and loss of endurance, atrophy, joint and muscle contractures, immobilization osteoporosis, and hypercalcemia in children.

Orthostatic hypotension, cardiovascular deconditioning, redistribution of body fluids, thromboembolism.

Pressure ulcers.

Negative nitrogen, calcium, carbohydrate, and protein balance, insulin, parathyroid, androgen, corticosteroid and growth hormone alterations.

Ventilatory dysfuntion, upper respiratory infections, hypostatic pneumonia, pulmonary embolism.

Urinary stasis, stones, urinary tract infection, urinary voiding difficulties.

Constipation, loss of appetite, weight loss, hypoproteinemia.

Sensory deprivation, anxiety, depression, confusion, congnitive dysfunction, incoordination, motor/perceptual control.

TABLE 6.2

Histochemical Change in Disuse Muscle Atrophy

* Antigravity (type I) muscle atrophy (reduction in size of single muscle fiber up to 42 percent)
* Oxydative enzyme activity reduction (succinyl dehydrogenase, creatine phosphokinase)
* Reduced storage of glycogen and creatine

ATROPHY AND WEAKNESS

The effects of bed rest and inactivity on muscle strength and endurance have been clearly demonstrated in many studies. After 3 weeks of continuous bed rest, muscle strength is significantly diminished, predominantly in the antigravity muscles of the lower extremities. In a study by Gogia, the gastrocnemius muscle showed a 26 percent reduction in strength, knee extensors 19 percent, and elbow flexors 7 percent following 5 weeks of strict bed rest (6). Similar results have been shown in earlier studied by Deitrick (3), in which immobilization of the elbow for 5 weeks by a cast in healthy individuals caused a 35–41 percent reduction of elbow extension strength.

Slow-twitch muscle fibers show a greater atrophy than fast-twitch fibers during strict bed rest, which can explain why the antigravity muscles of the lower extremities become predominantly weaker (11). Also, the content of the oxidative enzyme of slow-twitch muscle fiber is significantly diminished by immobility. In some cases, type two muscle fiber might be more atrophic than type one when lack of use is related to the specific muscle groups in the upper extremities. The oxygen utilization and mitochondrial function in the disuse atrophy is markedly decreased (Table 6.2).

The physiological changes in neural control of an immobilized subject also contribute to deterioration of muscle strength and endurance. The ability to activate all motor units during muscle contractions is diminished in inactive patients. Maintaining normal function and coordination of striated muscles requires daily use of the upper and lower extremities and trunk for ADLs, locomotion, and work.

With complete bed rest, a muscle may lose about 10–15 percent of strength per week, and an individual who is bedridden for 3 to 5 weeks may lose half of his or her strength. Muscle strength (not endurance) can, however, be maintained if daily muscle contractions are performed at 30 percent of maximal tension several seconds per day in addition to ordinary daily self-care activities.

Inactivity may affect muscle endurance even more than muscle strength. Reduced activity produces profound changes in muscle blood supply, utilization of oxygen, and metabolic muscle activity. The oxidative enzyme activity and content, and consequently extraction of oxygen in the muscle, is decreased. Motor unit recruitment is diminished, although fatigability of a single motor unit was not demonstrated after prolonged bed rest. Disuse atrophy and weakness are manifested by reduced tolerance to exercise, physical activity, and work. Maximal or submaximal oxygen uptake for maximal or submaximal activities, as a measure of endurance and physical fitness, is significantly reduced. During continuous bed rest, a progressive reduction of cardiac reserve occurs. Maximal oxygen consumption (VO_2 max) 10 days and 20 days after bed rest is decreased by 6.1 percent and 27 percent, respectively.

The reduction of maximal strength and endurance is proportional to the length of bed rest. It is more prominent in the large muscles of the trunk and lower extremities than in the small muscles of the hands and forearms. The debilitating effects of inactivity on endurance can be diminished, but not prevented, with supine exercises if bed rest must be prescribed. For example, isometric leg exercises performed on a daily basis may reduce the loss of strength in all major muscle groups of the lower extremities, but have no effect on endurance. Only isotonic exercises of adequate intensity, frequency, and duration are sufficient to restore impaired endurance. The reduction of functional capacity is invariably associated with the loss of muscle proteins, due to either slower protein synthesis or protein breakdown, whereas activity will increase the strength through the increase in the number of muscle fibers and their cross-sectional size. The recovery from immobilization atrophy takes approximately 4 weeks, which is slower than recovery from direct muscle trauma. The normal muscle cells around the injured muscle fibers provide the condition for the fast recovery in contrast to that of disuse atrophy.

Prolonged disuse of muscle may cause pain in muscle and in the other musculoskeletal structures. Clinical observations have shown that prolonged bed rest is a cause of low back pain as well. This pain is presumably related to tightness of back muscles and hamstrings, combined with weakness of the back and abdominal muscles. Any shortening of these muscles alters spinal alignment and posture. Abdominal and spinal muscle weakness contribute to the increase in spinal curvature and weight bearing on the small apophyseal lumbar joints. Immobilization osteoporosis of the spine is another possible contributor to the development of back pain. Abdominal muscle strengthening, as well as strengthening and sensible stretching of paraspinal and hamstring muscles with pro-

TABLE 6.3

Exercise for Disuse Weakness and Deconditioning

* Isotonic assistive or manual resistive exercises to the very weak muscles for 30 minutes.
* Progressive resistive exercises (PRE) to weak muscles for 30 minutes daily by increasing weights (loads) and the number of repetitions. Increase the load for 10–12 lbs when 10–12 repetitions are performed with ease and comfort.
* Functional training in mobility and self-care activities, e.g., ambulation with or without assistive devices, on level surfaces and stairs.
* Brisk walking, stationary bike, jogging 20–40 minutes, three times a week, 2–3 months preceded by warm-up and followed by cool-down exercises. Maintain the pulse rate 20 beats above the resting during the exercises.

gressive general aerobic conditioning, may prevent repeated lower back pain conditions in unfit subjects.

Acute low back pain has often been treated with bed rest of varying duration. However, the therapeutic value of this inactivity has recently been disputed. Patients with acute and chronic low back pain placed on 2 days of bed rest subsequently had less time lost from work than patients who received 1 week of bed rest, although there was no difference between the two groups in respect to mobility and ADLs. Thus, prolonged bed rest should not be considered as a therapeutic tool in the treatment of low back pain syndrome.

Muscle weakness secondary to disuse is an indication that the administration of therapeutic exercises is necessary. In general, therapeutic exercises are indicated in a partial neurogenic paralysis and in the weakness caused by disuse. Progressive resistive exercises using weights or contemporary exercise machines are preferred for the muscles with antigravity strength. For the muscle with a trace or poor strength, active assistive and manually resistive exercises are done by a therapist. (Table 6.3)

FLEXIBILITY AND CONTRACTURE

Joint flexibility and full active or passive ROM of a joint are necessary to maintain optimal physical functions of mobility and ADLs. The reduced motion of joint due to immobility or immobilization may precipitate or be the only cause of joint stiffness and joint contracture. Even in some contractures with a specific cause, e.g., congenital contractures, or burn-induced, ischemia or bleeding into the muscle, the prolonged immobility is a precipitating and contributing factor in their development. Any pathological conditions affecting the joint cartilage, capsule, soft tissue around the joint and ligaments, muscle, skin or subcutaneous tissue which crosses the joint and when coupled with immobility and lack of stretch may initiate or accelerate the development of contracture.

In a person with normal mobility, the loose connective tissue in the capsule and intramuscular spaces is sufficiently stretched during daily activities to maintain full ROM. During inactivity or immobilization in a flexed position, the loose connective tissue may change in order to adapt to the new limb position. These changes start with rearrangement of collagen fibers, development of new interfiber cross-links and formation of thick bands of collagen fibers. The dense connective tissue loses normal elongational characteristics and becomes shorter in length, setting the stage for a progressive limitation of joint range of motion (ROM). The collagen tissue of a single muscle fiber that is located in the sarcolemma and myofibriles contributes initially very little to this disuse shortening. The deprivation of stretch during immobilization, immobility, or lack of exercises, associated or not with paralysis, is the most frequent single cause of contractures.

The chronic patients with functional limitation are especially prone to developing contractures. In the case of extensor muscle paralysis, the flexors are unopposed, deprived from stretch and will develop a shorter resting length. In LMN paralysis, the muscle fibers degenerate and become replaced by connective tissue. If such muscle is deprived from stretch and ROM, the contracture will develop. It should be emphasized that muscle that is undergoing atrophy is very prone to develop contracture. The relative increase in connective tissue coupled with lack of stretch leads to the same consequences as in paralytic muscles. The spastic muscle may also keep the joint in a prolonged flexed position, and if stretch is limited, fixed contracture may result. The clinician in the field of chronic care should appreciate the significance of the physiological stretch for maintenance of full joint flexibility.

Collagen tissue is usually stretched during standing and locomotion. In relaxed standing, the center of gravity falls behind hip (0.5–1.0 cm), in front of knee (3–5 cm), and at the center of the tarsal arch; consequently, passive stretching is provided to hip and knee flexor, hamstrings, and gastrocnemius muscles. Balance in relaxed standing is made possible by triceps surae with intermittent activity of anterior tibialis muscle. During normal or fast locomotion, all these muscles are well stretched. With prolonged immobility, the contractures of hips, knees, or ankles may cause significant problems in standing and ambulation. The hip flexion contracture will decrease the stride of the step, slow down ambulation, and increase lumbar lordosis. The knee flexion contracture will shorten the leg stride, forcing the patient to walk on the forefoot, and increase quadriceps energy consumption. Plantar flexion contracture will create problems during standing and ambulation as well. The gait is characterized by circumduction, external rotation during the swing phase, and knee hyperextension at stance phase.

In summary, if a joint is immobilized, two important factors must be considered in terms of prevention: limb position and length of immobilization. Immobilizing a joint in a flexed or extended position for a prolonged period of time may result in temporary or permanent limitation of ROM regardless of whether or not the joint is normal or involved with additional pathology. Mild contracture at any joint may reduce mobility and ability to perform activities of daily living, especially in persons with neuromuscular conditions. The types of contracture and treatment for each are summarized in Table 6.4 and below.

Joint Contractures Due to Immobility

The site of primary pathological change in arthrogenic contracture is in the cartilage, and later in the capsule and adjacent soft tissue. Damaged cartilage due to trauma and degenerative joint disease may cause joint incongruency and pain

TABLE 6.4

Prevention and Treatment of Contractures

ARTHROGENIC CONTRACTURE	SOFT TISSUE CONTRACTURE
1. Management of pain, inflammation	1. Active and passive ROM with terminal stretch
2. Ultrasound heating to capsular	2. Prolonged stretch structures for 30 with heating (superficial, deep)
3. Proper positioning at rest	3. Dynamic splinting, proper positioning at rest
4. Strengthening exercises for joint stability	
5. Manipulation for some capsular contractures	

INTRINSIC MYOGENIC CONTRACTURE	EXTRINSIC MYOGENIC CONTRACTURE
1. Passive and active ROM, flexibility exercises	1. Treatment of spasticity; medication (e.g., baclofen), motor point or nerve blocks
2. Specific stretching of two-jointed muscles	2. Functional Electrical Stimulation (FES)
3. Prolonged stretch for 30 minutes using low tension and muscle heating	3. Passive ROM, local ice application
4. Progressive dynamic splinting or serial casts	4. Strengthening of opposing muscles
5. Surgical release, tendon lengthening, transposition of a muscle	5. Dynamic splinting

with subsequent splinting and ROM limitation. Synovial proliferation due to inflammation and pain may also result in reduced ROM. Effusion into a joint causes overdistention of the capsule, resulting in pain during minimal motion. In all these situations, pain causes prolonged joint splinting and change in collagen tissue arrangement, forcing the joint to assume a fixed, immobile position. The increased fibrosis that develops after trauma or inflammation determines the final degree of joint contracture.

Normal cartilage provides smoothness to joint surface and absorbs external stresses during motion. Resistance to wear and tear is provided by collagen tissue in the cartilage. In the deepest zones of cartilage, collagen fibers (type II) form bundles that run in a perpendicular direction to the joint surface. Close to the surface, the collagen fibers form smaller bundles of type IX collagen that curve and run parallel to the joint surface in all directions, providing strength and smoothness.

Cartilage is maintained by diffusion from synovial fluid and subchondral blood vessels and is dependent on frequent joint motion. Immobility may lessen diffusion of nutrients to the cartilage. Animal studies have shown that immobilization leads to the destruction of cartilage and degenerative joint disease due to compression of the cartilage on the side of contact. These degenerative changes in joint cartilage have an effect on progressive fibrosis of the joint capsule. Arthrogenic contractures associated with immobilization are characterized by fibrosis of intracapsular and periarticular connective tissue, along with cartilage thinning, fragmentation, vascular engorgement, and adjacent trabecular bone resorption.

In inactive but otherwise healthy subjects or in chronically ill patients with mobility impairment, the joint capsule, soft tissue, or ligament tightness is characterized by a gradual reduction of the optimal resting length, and collagen fiber shortening and fibrosis. Amiel found that 9 weeks of immobilization of the knee caused a reduction of water and glycosaminoglycan content in the ligaments and alteration in collagen crosslinking (1). In this study, collagen mass was the same before and after immobilization, indicating that the collagen turnover rate did not change. Newly formed fibers were laid down in densely arranged bands, reducing the ability to achieve full ROM. Other investigators, however, found that overall collagen mass in the ligaments was reduced, suggesting that synthesis was either reduced or breakdown was increased during prolonged immobilization.

Immobilization joint contractures are frequently encountered in the shoulders, hips, spine, and knees. The initial changes in the shoulder are usually in the tendon and sheaths of the rotator cuff or long head of biceps or adjacent capsule following trauma and inflammation. Associated pain, with splinting, and position of the humerus in adduction and internal posture lead to a progressive reduction of ROM. The initial inflammation may spread to the entire capsule, causing shoulder capsulitis with a complete loss of ROM (frozen shoulder). Contracture of the hips is found following prolonged bed rest, sitting in a wheelchair, or after hip surgery and associated immobility. The knee flexion contracture is usually caused by posterior capsule fibrosis and associated hamstring muscle shortening. If a flexion contracture of the knee is 30 degrees or greater, the quadriceps, hamstrings, and gastrocnemius muscle must work harder during the stance phase of gait. The work of the quadriceps muscle with 30 degrees knee contracture is increased by 50 percent.

Soft Tissue Contracture Due to Immobility

The advanced soft tissue contracture might be difficult to differentiate from arthrogenic contracture because the initial changes may not be known. The contracture of soft tissue located in periarticular, subcutaneous, and cutaneous tissue, which restrict ROM are also due to increased collagen fiber density and fibrosis. New collagen tissue production with proliferation and subsequent formation of a large fibrous band is characteristic of burn contractures. If the affected joint in a burn patient is not frequently stretched, soft tissue contracture may rapidly progress to severe forms. Heterotopic ossification should also be considered a soft tissue contracture; when the soft tissue is replaced by the new bone tissue. The new bone is laid down between layers of muscles or around the joint and has no physical connection to adjacent bone and periosteum.

Muscle Contractures Due to Immobility

It is important to determine if ROM limitation is caused by muscle and tendon shortening. In those cases ROM exercises and stretching should be directed to the muscle belly or its tendon. It has been known that muscle fiber contributes very little to the initial shortening in myogenic contracture and that collagen fibers in the epimysium, perimysium, and endomysium are the main culprits.

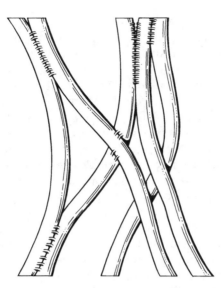

FIGURE 6.2. Development of cross-links in newly arranged collagen fiber meshwork.

Myogenic contractures may begin with intrinsic muscle changes, such as inflammation or degenerative process, and later with increased fibrosis. Contractures are precipitated by extrinsic factors, such as peripheral or central nervous system conditions, or by positional biomechanical forces. When a limb is held in a flexed position for 2–3 days, first adaptive shortening of the muscle belly begins. This adaptive shortening can be easily stretched during several sessions of ROM exercises. However, if a muscle is kept immobilized at shorter than optimal resting length for 5–7 days or longer, temporary and later permanent myogenic contracture may occur. For instance, collagen fibers of the muscle belly, whether in the endomysium, epimysium, or perimysium, will shrink, and their optimal resting length will diminish if immobilized in a flexed position. The loosely arranged collagen fiber (type III) of the connective tissue, which allows full ROM, may gradually become dense connective tissue (type I), with increase in the interfiber cross-linkage (Figure 6.2).

In paralytic contractures, a denervated muscle provides no opposition to its antagonistic muscle, whereas in spastic contracture the muscle imbalance is produced by increased muscle tone resulting from upper motor neuron lesions. Both conditions may produce a prolonged malpositioning of the joint. A study on preventive measures for spastic contractures in cerebral palsy patients indicates that gastrocnemius contracture will be prevented if the muscle is stretched by walking above its own minimal passive resistance for at least 6 hours per day. When the muscle was stretched by walking for only 2 hours or less per day, the gastrocnemius muscle contracture did occur. Stretching is a physiological necessity for the connective tissue and its collagen to maintain its function as a mechanical support to the musculoskeletal system. When the muscle is not stretched, such as in cases of immobility, structural changes in the collagen and muscle fibers may follow. The number of sarcomeres of a single muscle fiber is reduced (40 percent) when the joint is kept in a flexed position over several weeks.

Other studies have proven that repeated stretching and passive elongation of the muscle over a period of time produces an increase in protein synthesis and an increase in the number of sarcomeres in series of a single muscle fiber.

It is important to emphasize that improper joint position may alone cause muscle contracture. For example, the position of the body in a soft bed may produce hip flexion contracture. Two-jointed muscles, such as hamstrings, rectus femoris, and back muscles, are the first to become shortened in inactive individuals. Gastrocsoleus contracture is frequently found in the spastic hemiplegic leg as well as in the unaffected leg due to limited exposure to sufficient stretching during ambulation. In muscular dystrophy, for example, plantar flexion contracture is a product of dystrophic muscular changes and inadequate gastrocnemius muscle stretching. The hip extensors become very weak, forcing these patients to walk with excessive lumbar lordosis and on their toes in order to position the center of gravity in front of the knees. Walking on the toes prevents natural stretching of the triceps surae and promotes plantar flexion contracture.

In plantar flexion contracture, adjacent knee and metatarsal joints are subjected to greater stress during the stance phase of gait. A tight gastrocnemius muscle forces the knee and the metatarsal joints into hyperextension during the push-off phase to compensate for the plantar flexed position of the ankle. Furthermore, plantar flexor contracture causes an absence of heel strike and reduces the push-off strength of the muscle, contributing further to the abnormal abducted and externally rotated type of gait.

Principles of Contracture Treatment and Prevention

The basic therapeutic principles of contracture prevention involve adequate stretching (ROM exercises), proper positioning of the joint to prevent shortening of fibrotic or spastic muscles, and to provide strengthening exercises to the opposing muscles. The daily treatment of mild and moderately severe contractures with the use of ROM exercises and heating (e.g., ultrasound) and mobility training (e.g., progressive ambulation) is very effective. Inflamed joints and edematous soft tissue do not tolerate stretching, so stretching and heating are contraindicated. The superimposed spasticity should be treated with Baclofen, alone or in combination with Valium, Dantrolene sodium, Clonidine, or with neurolytic subarachnoid, paravertebral, peripheral nerve, and motor point blocks. Dynamic splinting or serial casting is used to maintain the gains after ROM exercises, keeping the joint in a position that would provide continuous stretch for 2 or more hours. The fixed contracture may require a surgical release procedure such as tenotomy, tendon lengthening, or tendon transfer.

IMMOBILIZATION OSTEOPOROSIS AND HYPERCALCEMIA

A lack of muscle pull and gravity on the trunk and lower extremity bones invariably causes disuse osteoporosis. This is another consequence of prolonged bed rest and immobility. The balance between bone production and resorption is disrupted within just a few days of bed rest, first cancellous, then later in cortical bone. Urinary calcium loss increases in the first week of bed rest and may reach 100 µg/day by the sixth week, plateau for several weeks, then gradually decrease, but never return to a normal level. Calcium loss is, however, greater than can be actually determined from urinary excretion, because calcium is also lost through the gastrointestinal system. The loss of calcium continues for months, even after resumption of physical activityy (10).

Radiographic signs of osteoporosis can be seen when at least 40 percent of the calcium is lost from the bones. The bone scan is positive, particularly at the site of long bone metaphysis of axial skeleton, due to an increase in blood flow and metabolic activity. Blood levels of calcium are normal in bedridden patients, although children and young adults may develop hypercalcemia that causes serious complications. Approximately 50 percent of healthy children with single fractures of an extremity develop hypercalcemia following a month or more of immobility. Immobilization osteoporosis is not possible to prevent by calcium and phosphorus intake, single skeletal compression, or with increase in orthostatic blood vessel tension. However, exercise can slow down and prevent its development. The literature on immobilization osteoporosis clearly demonstrates the sparing effect of exercise. Calcaneus bone demineralization that is connected with bed rest is diminished if the gastrocnemius muscle is exercised daily, whereas non-exercised legs showed signs of osteoporosis. Individuals with limb paralysis and lost mobility showed advanced disuse osteoporosis. Pathologic fractures due to innocent falls are common in such patients.

Patients with lower back pain who are prescribed prolonged bed rest (27 or more days) show a diminution of L2, L3, and L4 lumbar spine bone content at an average of 0.9 percent per week. This indicates that the use of "therapeutic" bed rest may cause a substantial vertebral bone demineralization. It takes weeks, even months, before calcium can be restored by resumption of normal activity. Reambulation of patients with lower back pain after 1 week of bed rest results in restoration of mineral bone content in about 4 weeks.

Cardiovascular Complications of Disuse

The neuromuscular and cardiovascular systems are closely interrelated. Decrease in functional capacity in one system produces a decrease in the other. For the same level of physical activity, well-conditioned persons (compared to deconditioned individuals) will have much smaller responses in heart rate, blood pressure, and stroke volumes. Furthermore, the conditioned person has a greater cardiac reserve and can do exercises and work at a higher intensity and duration. The inactive person with a sedentary lifestyle may end up with a cardiac reserve that is reduced to the level at which it may become difficult to perform daily activities or physical work.

During prolonged inactivity, a gradual reduction in cardiovascular functional capacity occurs, regardless of whether or not cardiac pathology is present. Recent literature in cardiac rehabilitation indicates that inactivity and a sedentary lifestyle is an independent risk factor for development of coronary heart disease.

Cardiovascular complications due to bed rest and inactivity include: inability to assume upright position (postural hypotension), impairment of cardiovascular functional capacity (cardiovascular deconditioning), reduction of plasma and blood volume (dehydration), and development of thromboembolic complications (Figure 6.3).

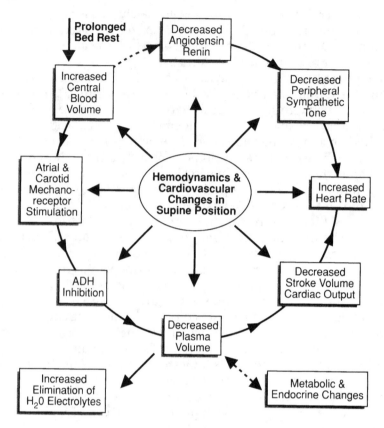

FIGURE 6.3. Cardiovascular changes induced by prolonged bed rest.

POSTURAL HYPOTENSION

Postural hypotension is a typical cardiovascular complication that may occur during prolonged bed rest when assuming a sitting or full upright position. The drop in blood pressure depends on the duration of recumbency. The increase in heart rate and drop of blood pressure are due to several factors. Initially, an excessive shift of the blood (700 cc) from the thorax into the legs occurs with reduction of the central hydrostatic pressure in the large veins of the thorax and right atrium. A transient or prolonged reduction of the end-diastolic ventricular volume and fall of stroke volume and cardiac output occurs. Secondly, the drop of blood pressure upon standing is aggravated by the inability of the peripheral vasculature to respond promptly with vasoconstriction. Thirdly, reduction of plasma and blood volume also contribute to orthostatic hypotension. This inability of the circulatory system to maintain normal blood pressure in an upright position may pose a great problem to chronically ill or disabled persons who are beginning to be remobilized in the process of rehabilitation.

In normal subjects, the ability to adapt to the upright position may be completely lost following 3 weeks of recumbency. In such cases, significant increase in heart rate (more than 20 bpm) and drop of systolic pressure (more than 20

TABLE 6.5

Therapy for Postural Hypotension

* Tilt table (gradual increase in standing position up to 20 minutes at 70°).
* Early ambulation using elastic stockings, abdominal binders.
* Bed rest should not be accepted as a part of the patient's treatment strategy unless specifically indicated.
* Increase fluid and salt intake, Ephedrine, Fludrocortisone (Florinef).

mmHg) may occur. In patients with chronic illness and functional impairment who are placed on strict bed rest for any reason (e.g., pressure sore), orthostatic hypotension should be suspected even after a week of recumbency. Near-syncope or syncope may occur due to beta adrenergic hyperactivity, which can be prevented by the use of propranolol.

The reconditioning process often lasts longer than that of deconditioning. The return of pre-bed resting heart rate and blood pressure levels upon assuming an upright position may take from 26 to 72 days. Dehydration is tolerated poorly in older persons who may show signs of blood pressure and heart rate changes sooner and for longer periods of time than middle-aged subjects.

Vigorous exercises performed daily in the supine position do not prevent orthostatic intolerance to the upright position. To prevent this complication, hydrostatic pressure created by the blood columns in the blood vessels of the abdomen and lower extremities appears to be the principal physiological stimulus within the circulatory system to help regain and maintain the normal blood pressure when assuming the erect position. The use of a tilt table is necessary to provide this stimulus in the patients with orthostatic hypotension. In medically stable patients, early mobilization and progressive ambulation will prevent these signs of deconditioning. During the process of mobilization for orthostatic intolerance, exercise of the lower extremity muscles, including the thighs and abdominals, may help as an adjunct therapy. Use of elastic stockings and an abdominal binder is recommended in quadriplegic and paraplegic patients (Table 6.5).

IMPAIRED CARDIOVASCULAR PERFORMANCE (DECONDITIONING)

The term *deconditioning* refers to the state of physical fitness in which the reduced cardiovascular functional capacity is produced by inactivity in a presence or absence of acute cardiac disease. Cardiovascular deconditioning presents itself as an altered response to exercise or physical work. A well-trained individual will respond to submaximal work with a moderate increase of heart rate and stroke volume. The deconditioned individual responds to the equivalent submaximal workload with greater increase in heart rate, blood pressure, and cardiac output. There is also a slower return of these parameters to resting level after cessation of the activity. Work capacity and tolerance to activities of a deconditioned person are compromised. The reduction of capacity is proportional to the period of inactivity. During strict bed rest, cardiac reserve gradually declines, and the pulse rate increases 1/2 to 1 beat per minute per day. Cardiovascular rehabilitation programs provided during the hospital or community-based outpatient phases of recovery are designed to increase cardiovascular functional capacity and fitness.

REDISTRIBUTION OF BODY FLUIDS

When supine, 700 ml of blood shifts to the thorax; there is an increase in end-diastolic volume and in cardiac output of 24 percent. This increase in central blood pressure and pulmonary blood flow of 20–30 percent suppresses antidiuretic hormone release, causing diuresis and reduction in total body fluid. During bed rest, there is a progressive decrease in total blood volume with maximal reduction at 2 and 6 days and lasting until the end of the first month of recumbency. Reduction of plasma volume is, however, much greater than the loss of red cell mass, leading to hemoconcentration and increased blood viscosity. This reduction occurs within a few days of recumbency and may reach 12–13 percent by the fourth day of bed rest. This effect can be reduced by active isometric exercises (5,12), which help to redistribute blood volume peripherally.

THROMBOEMBOLISM OF IMMOBILITY

Studies of factors related to the occurrence of thromboembolic events reveal a direct relationship between the frequency of deep vein thrombosis and the duration of bed rest. Virchow's triad consists of stasis, increased blood coagulability, and damage to the blood vessel wall. Two of these three factors are influenced by prolonged immobility. Stasis of blood flow in the lower extremities is directly related to the reduced pumping effect of the calf muscles and hypercoagulable state is induced by plasma volume reduction and an increase in circulatory fibrinogen. The incidence of DVTs in spinal cord injury patients is 12.5 percent. In Warlow's study of stroke patients, the incidence of DVTs in hemiplegic legs was 53 out of 65 cases, compared to 5 out of 76 cases in non-hemiplegic legs.

═══ Skin Complications

PRESSURE SORES (DECUBITUS ULCERS)

Pressure sores are a costly secondary complication of prolonged immobility. Pressure sores are a result of direct external pressure over bony prominences; persons who are bedridden are prone to develop them at high frequency. Spinal cord injury, head injury, and multiple sclerosis patients with an inability to perform independent bed mobility or pushups in a sitting position are among the groups at greatest risk for pressure sores. When the skin and subcutaneous tissue over bony prominences is exposed to prolonged external pressure, a localized tissue necrosis of varying size and depth will develop (Figure 6.4). Subjects with

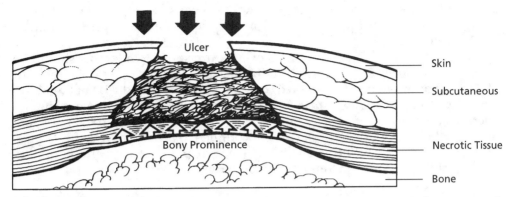

FIGURE 6.4. The necrotic tissue is formed in a space between the external pressure and the bony prominence.

normal, independent mobility rarely develop this complication. The patients with severe mobility and ADL impairment due to either neurological, musculoskeletal, or cognitive conditions may be at high risk for the development of pressure sores. Studies have shown that approximately 20 percent (2.6–35 percent) of persons admitted to nursing homes develop pressure sores. Reviews of the functional status of all these individuals suggest that the common denominator was impairment of mobility and self-care.

The incidence of pressure ulcers in acute hospital settings is about 3 percent, but in long-term facilities it may be as high as 45 percent. The length of stay of paraplegic patients without pressure sores in a hospital is approximately 1 month, in contrast to those with pressure sores who may stay an average of 8 months. Medical costs for the management of pressure sores in the United States exceeds $12 billion per year (4).

Because of the multiple risk factors and economic significance, pressure sores are usually discussed as a separate issue from immobility and prolonged bed rest. Only the basic principles of pressure sore development and prevention are discussed here.

Risk Factors

The factors that may cause pressure sores, such as direct external pressure, shear, and friction, are all related to immobility. On the other hand, the ability of the skin to withstand long periods of external pressure without developing ischemia depends on blood supply, skin temperature, humidity, and the metabolic condition of the patient. These all must be kept in mind for prevention of pressure ulcers. Albumin and pre-albumin should be checked and, if low, should be treated as part of the overall nutritional plan.

Patients with a diminished blood supply due to prolonged lying or sitting and increased external heat over bony prominences (often caused by specific wheelchair cushions) may have increased skin metabolic demand and have an increased risk of skin breakdowns. The incidence of pressure sores in patients with urinary incontinence and mobility impairment is as high as 15 percent;

the incidence is 3.7 percent for those who are continent. The percentage of patients with bowel incontinence who develop pressure sores is as high as 39.7 percent.

To understand the pathogenesis of pressure sores, two factors should be appreciated—one is the magnitude of the pressure, and the other is duration. In the sitting position, pressure exerted on the skin that is over the ischial tuberosities ranges from 150–500 mmHg, and supine pressure on the skin covering the sacral bony ranges from 10–50 mmHg. Sacral, trochanteric, and heel pressure sores are the most frequent in the patient confined to bed. Ischial tuberosity pressure sores are mainly found in the wheelchair patients with inappropriate pushup ability for pressure releases and cushions.

Natural History

Immediately after the removal of external pressure, the skin becomes edematous and red for more than 24 hours. Ulceration may appear in a few days. The process of demarcation of the necrotic tissue may last weeks unless surgically or chemically removed. Necrotic tissue debridement enhances the healing process, which begins with growth of the granulation tissue on the base of the ulcer. The growth could be optimized by keeping the ulcer free of infection and pressure. Epithelialization begins at the skin edges of the ulcer, which eventually covers the newly formed granulation tissue. The ultimate result of pressure sore healing is scar tissue formation covered by a thin epidermis.

Classifying pressure sores according to the depth of ulcer is more clinically useful in deciding whether to treat it surgically or conservatively. Five grade classifications of tissue involvement are the most frequently used to describe the nature, size, and depth of pressure ulcers (Table 6.6).

Prevention

Education of patients or caregivers should include an understanding of the risks of immobilization. They should be aware of the importance of frequent and consistent change in body position, proper nutrition, appropriate use of sitting devices or bed mattresses. Inspection of the skin for redness, induration, and skin abrasions must be stressed as well (Table 6.7).

The most important principle in the prevention of pressure sores is to limit prolonged confinement to bed without a turning program, or sitting in a wheelchair without effective pushups. Strategies must be developed to help patients avoid excessive direct or sheer pressure over bony prominences.

Treatment

The treatment of pressure sores should begin with frequent changes (at least every 2 hours) of the patient's position in bed with provision of a special bed or mattress if necessary. Without exception, external pressure should not be allowed. Necrotic tissue must be debrided because it promotes bacterial growth. The debridement procedure includes three basic approaches:

TABLE 6.6

Pressure Ulcer Treatment

	APPROACH	MONITORING
Grade I Erythema > 24 hr	No sitting, lying on the site (for all grades)	Monitor redness daily
Grade II Break in epidermis (superficial ulcer)	Opsite, dry dressing for blisters. Pulsed low- intensity direct current	Monitor/measure epidermal defect
Grade III Transdermal ulcer	Debridement (chemical surgical). Opsite, duoderm for protection. Pulsed low- intensity direct current	Monitor for size, excessive wetness, necrotic tissue
Grade IV Transdermal, fascial and muscle involvement	Debridement (surgical, chemical, mechanical). Wet and dry dressing. Expose to air several times/day. Special bed	Monitor for size, new necrotic tissue. Plastic surgery: debridement, rotation flaps
Grade V Involvement of underlying bone (with osteo- myelitis)	Debridement. Deep ulcer packing. Wet and dry dressing. Antibiotic if systemic signs are present. Special bed	Monitor size. Plastic surgery interventions. Rotation flap with removal of bone.

TABLE 6.7

Skin Inspection and Prevention for Bed and Wheelchair Bound Patients

A. Assessment

Assess the tolerance to lying position, sitting, and to pressure from prosthetic/orthotic devices.

*Check redness on 15 min, 30 min, 2 hr, and 24 hr

1) Sitting for 15 min, 30 min, 45 min, 1 hr, 2 hr, 4 hr, and 6 hr

2) Lying for 2 hr, then for 4, 6 hr check redness

B. Prevention

Progressive sitting, lying. Slow progress with daily increments from 15, 30, 45 min to 1,2,4,6 hr for sitting and from 2 hr to 4, 6 hr for lying in bed time. If redness after sitting or lying does not fade within 1 hr, reduce skin time by half.

C. Goals

Patient's goals: 4-8 hr of sitting for community function; 4, 6 hr for lying.

1. the use of chemical agents such as elase, collagenase (Biozyme-c), proteolytic enzyme (Traveze), and trypsin granules;
2. repeated surgical debridement; and
3. mechanical debridement by wet and dry dressing or water (whirlpool).

Surgical flaps provide skin and subcutaneous tissue, which has its own blood supply and sensation. Musculocutaneous flaps bring subcutaneous tissue and muscle layer for extra protection. Surgical flaps are preferred management techniques for grade 3 and 4 pressure sores.

Disuse Metabolic and Endocrine Changes

Basal metabolic rate after 6 weeks of bed rest is decreased approximately 6.9 percent. Deitrick's study on immobilized healthy subjects with leg casts showed a reduced basal metabolic rate, starting on the second day of recumbency and lasting for 3 weeks after 6 weeks of immobilization (3).

Energy expenditure at rest comes from carbohydrates and fat, yet daily loss of nitrogen increases during strict bed rest. The major storage of nitrogen is muscular tissue and reduced physical activity may increase the breakdown of protein or reduce protein synthesis. Body weight during bed rest often does not change, but there may be a significant reduction in lean body mass and an increase in total body fat.

The loss of nitrogen during immobility in a healthy person may reach 2 grams a day, and if associated with starvation or systemic disease, may increase tenfold. Increased nitrogen loss is usually noted on the fifth or sixth day of recumbency, with a peak in the second week. It takes one week to repair a negative nitrogen balance if the patient has been remobilized after being bedridden for 3 weeks. Inactivity may lead to hyperproteinemia and changes in autoimmune system (8).

Trauma, infection, and inflammatory conditions accelerate the development of a negative balance of nitrogen. Appropriate diet, full activity, and exercise will slow and arrest these adverse effects.

Urinary calcium excretion begins to increase on the second or third days of recumbency, with a peak loss during the fourth and fifth weeks, and lasts during the entire period of immobility. It takes longer to restore calcium after resumption of physical activity than to restore nitrogen balance. Total calcium loss following 7 weeks of bed rest may reach 14.0 grams and it may take several months to restore it to the pre-bed rest level (Table 6.8). Serum parathyroid hormone is increased during immobilization and influences the development of hypercalcemia during immobility in children.

After 7 days of bed rest, insulin plasma levels increase, and there is a paradoxical increase in plasma glucose levels. The hyperglycemia due to inactivity is not due to the reduced effect of insulin on suppression of hepatic glucose production, but rather due to a substantial reduction of insulin action on glucose uptake by the tissue and changes in insulin receptor and post-receptor activity. The insulin levels in bedridden patients are usually twice as high as those in ambulatory patients. Pro-insulin, C-peptide concentrations are also increased, indicating that the release of insulin from the pancreas is normal, but the insulin effectiveness is diminished (9).

TABLE 6.8

Effects of Bed Rest on Metabolic Systems

	ADVERSE EFFECTS	ONSET PEAK AND DURATION
Nitrogen	Increased excretion; Hypoproteinemia	Fifth or sixth week; entire recumbency
Sodium	Increased excretion	First and second day, normal level later
Potassium	Increased excretion	End of first week; normal level later
Sulfur, phosphorous	Increased excretion	Entire recumbent period
Calcium	Increased urinary excretion	Second and third day; peaks at fourth and fifth weeks; lasts months, to years after remobilization

Reports on corticosteroid levels in the serum during bed rest have been contradictory. However, urinary cortisol excretion is consistently increased. In studies of patients where bed rest lasted more than one month, ACTH levels were three times higher than baselines levels and required about 20 days of activity to return to normal levels. The adrenal glands become less responsive to the release of ACTH following prolonged recumbency.

During immobility, cholesterol levels are increased and the high density lipoprotein levels are decreased. Lipoproteins return to normal approximately 14 days after remobilization. Decreased androgen levels and decreased spermatogenesis have also been reported (Table 6.9).

Disuse Urinary and Gastrointestinal Tract Dysfunctions

Increased excretion of urinary calcium and stasis of urine in the renal pelvis, as well as difficulty in emptying the bladder during prolonged inactivity, promote the development of renal and bladder stones and infection. The increased excretion of phosphorous also promotes stone formation. In a recumbent position, it is more difficult to initiate voiding and to completely empty the bladder. Increased residual urine can lead to bladder distention, infection, and urinary incontinence (2).

Gastrointestinal complications of prolonged bed rest and inactivity are usually mild and infrequent and often attributed to causes other than immobilization.

Poor appetite for protein-rich food and reduced gastrointestinal peristalsis, which possibly is related to the increased adrenergic activity, may result in an inadequate absorption of protein and hypoproteinemia. Constipation is a common complication and is also related to plasma volume reduction and dehydration. A

TABLE 6.9

Effects of Bed Rest on Metabolic and Endocrine Systems

HORMONES	ADVERSE EFFECTS	ONSET/PEAK & DURATION
ADH	Inhibition with secondary diuresis, dehydration	Second or third day; entire recumbency
Insulin	Increased serum levels	Entire bed rest
Parathyroid	Increased blood levels	
Thyroid	Increased diurnal variation	
ACTH	Increased adrenal unresponsiveness	
Androgens	Decreased	Entire bed rest
Spermatogenesis	Decreased	Entire bed rest
Cholesterol	Increased	
HDL	Decreased	Not known
Cortisol	Increased urinary excretion	

bowel training program can be used to prevent and treat constipation due to immobility. Such a program includes a fiber-rich diet, scheduled post-meal toileting, stool softeners, suppositories, and bedside commodes for toilet usage.

Swallowing difficulties may increase in the recumbent position, especially in the elderly. Patients with swallowing difficulties should be seated in an upright position with their head kept in a slightly flexed position during eating. Aspiration of mucous secretions or gastric content is more likely to occur when lying down, particularly in patients with associated paralytic swallowing disorders.

Respiratory Restrictions and Complications

Mechanical restrictions of rib cage in the recumbent position may cause a temporary reduction of tidal volume, vital capacity, and minute volume. Clearance of secretions is also more difficult. Breathing tends to be shallow, aeration of the parts of the lungs adjacent to the bed mattress is diminished, and alveolar tension with normal blood perfusion is decreased, causing hypoxia. Cases with severe bed mobility impairment may develop atelectasis and hypostatic pneumonia. During protracted bed rest, development of a fixed contracture of the costovertebral joints may contribute to development of permanent restrictive pulmonary disease. In the supine position, only 32 percent of tidal volume is due to rib cage motion. In standing, rib motion contributes 78 percent. This can explain why the effective cough is also reduced.

Stroke patients confined to bed are at risk for pneumonia, which is also related to duration of recumbency. For instance, 13 days or more of bed rest increases the risk of respiratory infection by two- to threefold in stroke patients. The frequency of pulmonary emboli is increased and is also related to duration of immobility and bed rest (2,9). Prevention of this devastating complication should include Heparin subcutaneously, 10,000 i.u. twice a day, and early remobilization whenever possible.

Nervous System Complications

At first glance, it might be surprising to find problems of bed rest and immobility in the central nervous system. However, the adverse effect of inactivity does not spare the central nervous system. A whole spectrum of CNS dysfunctions have been found in bedridden individuals. The studies of healthy subjects during reinforced bed rest, space flight, or in patients with severe immobilization demonstrate a wide range of problems. First, a confinement to bed produces sensory and social deprivation, then gradually alterations in sensory perception, confusion, disorientation, and reduction of discrete intellectual functions. If prolonged bed rest continues, anxiety, increased dependency, emotional lability, and depression follow. These complications are attributed to the reduced exposure to the environmental and social cues with regard to time, place, people, and purpose. Similar changes occur in those who are socially isolated. However, if social isolation is associated with a lack of physical activity, these dysfunctions are more pronounced. Studies clearly show that intellectual functioning begins to deteriorate, especially when physical inactivity is present in conjunction with social isolation. Such persons manifest difficulties in problem-solving abilities, judgment, concentration, attention span, and focusing; they have reduced alertness, demonstrate the loss of interpersonal communication skills, and decreased pain threshold, and have emotional lability. If social and physical inactivity persists, other cognitive dysfunction may appear, including memory deficits, learning difficulties, auditory and tactile hallucinations, psychomotor retardation, incoordination, and reduction of fine motor skills. Thus, prolonged confinement to bed and social isolation lead to "cognitive deconditioning," dependence, and psychological disability, which reduce motivation and the ability to participate in rehabilitation (9).

Conclusion

The prescription for bed rest should include how many hours per day a patient should stay in bed, how frequently a patient's position should be changed, as well as which specific activities should be encouraged during bed rest. Only affected parts of the body need to be immobilized and other parts should remain mobile.

Problematic side effects should be anticipated and recognized so that preventive measures can be immediately applied. Any subject with impaired mobility should be periodically monitored for adverse effects to ensure the optimum restoration of function.

═══ References

1. Amiel D, Woo Sly, Harwood FL, Akeson WH. The effect of immobilization on collagen turnover in connective tissue: A biochemical-biomechanical correlation. *Acta Orthop Scand* 53:325–32, 1982.
2. Browse NL. *The physiology and pathology of bed rest.* Springfield, IL, Charles C. Thomas Publishers, 1965.
3. Deitrick JE, Whedon GD, Shorr E. Effects of immobilization upon various metabolic and physiological functions of normal man. *Am J Med* 4:3–36, 1948.
4. Donovan WH, Garber SL, Hamilton SM, Krouskop TA, Rodriguez GP, Stal S. Pressure Ulcers. In: DeLisa JA (Ed.). *Rehabilitation medicine: Principles and practice.* Philadelphia, J.B. Lippincott, 1988, pp. 476–491.
5. Downey JA, Darling RC. *Physiological basis of rehabilitation medicine.* Philadelphia, W.B. Saunders, 1971, pp. 8–11.
6. Gogia, PP, Schneider VS, LeBlanc AD, Krebs J, Kasson C, Pientok C. Bed rest effect on extremity muscle torque in healthy men. *Arch Phys Med Rehab* 69(12):1030–32, 1988.
7. Halar EM, Bell KR. Contracture and other deleterious effects of immobility. In: DeLisa, JA (Ed.). *Rehabilitation medicine: Principles and practice.* Philadelphia, J.B. Lippincott, 1988, pp. 448–62.
8. Kottke FJ. The effects of limitation of activity upon the human body. *JAMA* 196: 117–22, 1966.
9. Sandler H, Vernikos J. *Inactivity: Physiological effects.* San Diego, Academic Press, 1986.
10. Schneider VS, McDonald J. Skeletal calcium homeostasis and counter measures to prevent disuse osteoporosis. *Calcif Tissue Ont* 36:5151–54, 1984.
11. Spector SA. Effects of elimination of activity on contractile and histochemical properties of rat soleus muscle. *J Neurosci* 5(8):2177–88, 1985.
12. Taylor HL, Erickson L, Henshel A, Keys A. The effects of bed rest on the blood volume of normal young men. *Am J Physiol* 144:232, 1945.

7 Mobility

Walter C. Stolov, M.D., and Ross M. Hays, M.D.

Dictionaries define ambulation in part with a description of walking. To address the disabled patient's needs for independent and functional mobility, this concept must be broadened to encompass all methods by which an individual moves from one place or position to another. It is important to discard the concept of ambulation as the sole criteria for mobility. Even nondisabled people do not depend solely on ambulation for movement from place to place. A wheelchair is a device that conserves time and energy in much the same way that an automobile or an elevator or escalator does for nondisabled people.

The progressive mobility of a patient ranges from the simplest to the most complex movement activity he or she can perform. The position of least mobility—lying in bed—is the same for all. The end point of the mobility spectrum, however, is not as precise, depending on the intrinsic ability of the individual. To some, it is being able to ascend Mount Everest. To an elderly person recovering from a fractured hip or to a class IV cardiac patient, it may be the ability to negotiate the stairs leading from street to front porch, a determining factor in whether his/her future will extend beyond home confinement.

This chapter discusses general characteristics of mobility, the mobility spectrum, and methods for remobilizing a patient through that spectrum.

Characteristics of Mobility

1. *Each activity on the mobility spectrum depends on a preceding one.* In the normal infant and toddler, ambulation develops as the culmination of a sequence of developmental skills. The young baby begins with independent head control, moves on to control of the upper extremities and trunk, eventually demonstrates sophisticated reciprocal movement of the arms and legs in crawling, and then—with increasing developmental progress and strength—stands upright and walks independently. Similarly, the stages of rehabilitation and restoration of mobility are cumulative with each activity of the mobility spectrum depending on the attainment of a preceding, less complex skill. Independent sitting is unlikely to occur without the attainment of bed mobility. Independent transfer from bed to

wheelchair will not be possible without the attainment of trunk control necessary for sitting. Patients who do not have the skill or strength required to transfer from one sitting position to another will rarely demonstrate the strength and coordination necessary for ambulation.

2. *The ability to function depends ultimately on the physical layout of the environment in which the activity is to be performed.* The problems that astronauts have with extravehicular activity illustrates this point. It is not that they do not know how to use a wrench or to turn a nut, but rather that they cannot as effectively turn the nut in zero gravity. Similarly, walking down a hospital corridor is not the same as walking on a highly polished floor, one cluttered with scatter rugs, or on grass or gravel.

3. *Independence in performing an activity in a given physical environment can be categorized into four levels.*

First-Degree Independence —The person can perform the task independently without requiring human assistance for safety or efficiency.

Second-Degree Independence—The patient is physically able to perform the activity independently, but requires standby assistance either for safety or to provide verbal cues to help in sequencing and planning. In time, the assistant's tasks may be replaced with adaptive strategies.

Third-Degree Independence—The person is physically able to perform most, but not all, of a particular task. Partial physical assistance is required either because the physical environment cannot be optimally altered or because the task at hand necessitates more strength, coordination, or endurance than the patient has presently. This patient differs from the patient with second-degree independence because actual physical help is required.

Fourth-Degree Independence—The person requires total physical assistance for the activity to occur. This may include assistance in transfers from bed to wheelchair, bathing, and toileting, although the person may still have independent mobility with the use of adaptive equipment, such as a motorized wheelchair.

4. *Because patients in all but the first-degree level of independence require some assistance, their performance depends on another factor—the social environment.* In planning, one must therefore know who will be available to assist the person should help be needed. If there is a mismatch between the patient's needs and the assistance available, the person may suffer a greater loss of mobility than necessary.

To some extent the social environment is affected by the age of the patient. A young disabled child who is totally dependent will obtain assistance readily from a parent with minimal disruption to home and family life. An elderly patient requiring the same amount of assistance may be forced to leave his or her present living situation and consider placement in a nursing home.

5. *The degree of independence in performing an activity is not necessarily fixed.* Training, exercise, instruction in proper technique, appropriate use of adaptive equipment, and manipulation of the environment can broaden the ability to function and thereby increase the level of independence.

6. *The geriatric patient's ability to adapt to minor changes in physical condition or environment is diminished.* A change in either of these factors may throw the person into a state of increased dependence and even trigger secondary

medical complications. Learning to do familiar activities in new ways is not easy for these patients, and it becomes even more difficult if range of motion (ROM) in the joints and muscle strength have been lost through bed rest or disuse. Physical restoration decreases with age. Moreover, altering the physical environment of elderly persons is difficult because of emotional ties to familiar surroundings and reduced financial means. Finally, people who can provide the physical assistance that the geriatric patient requires may not be available. The following case study illustrates the reduced ability of the geriatric patient for physical and social adaptation.

A 72-year-old widow, who lives alone, lost her footing on a wet street when her cane slipped. The fall caused a nondisplaced fracture of the left humeral head. She was taken to the emergency room of a local hospital and her arm was put into a sling. She was told to return in 10 days, at which time early mobilization of the arm would be considered. The physicians in attendance recognized that she used her cane in the left hand to compensate for the residual hip weakness from a right hip fracture incurred 5 years earlier. They therefore arranged to have the taxi driver assist her into her home and ensured that a rented wheelchair would be simultaneously delivered.

The patient managed successfully at home for the first 3 days. On day 4 she ran out of groceries. Because the local store was next door to her apartment building, she thought she could get there using her cane, even though she had to carry it in her right hand. She had to negotiate five steps to get out of the apartment building. Although her stair-climbing technique had been excellent before her shoulder injury, she now had to use an entirely new pattern. At the last step, she lost her footing, fell, and refractured her right hip. Because of the two fractures, ambulation was never again achieved.

In this case the patient's intrinsic ability was affected by the shoulder fracture, but her ultimate loss of independent ambulation was a result of the physical and social environment. Had she resided in an accessible environment without stairs, the accident might have been avoided. From a social perspective, if another person could have gotten the groceries for her, she may not have been placed in a position of risk for subsequent injury.

The Mobility Spectrum

The mobility spectrum can be divided into three phases:

1. bed mobility;
2. breadth of transfer skills; and
3. travel, of which walking is but one example.

BED MOBILITY

Raising the head and limbs and turning in bed are the most primitive mobility functions. These functions help to protect the patient from decubitus ulcers, phlebitis, and atelectasis. The ability to rise to a sitting position at the edge of a bed and to maintain free-standing balance with the back unsupported is next in importance and is necessary to perform transfer skills independently.

To assist the patient in turning from side to side, the bed should have a firm mattress or bed board. Although an overhead trapeze may help the patient perform this maneuver, it is better to develop the ability to push and to press the arms into the bed for bed-turning skills. Usually, any patient who can learn to turn with the trapeze can also learn to maneuver without it, thereby avoiding the need for one at home.

A patient with a unilateral arm or leg problem can learn to rise to a sitting position at the edge of the bed sooner on the uninvolved side than on the involved side. A patient with left hemiparesis does not have enough strength in his or her paralyzed arm to help complete the task of moving from a supine to a sitting position at the left edge of a bed. The same patient can complete the task using only his or her right arm when rising to a sitting position on the right (uninvolved) side. The arm, pushed against the bed, provides for trunk elevation to complete the task. Attempting this function with an overhead trapeze may be unsuccessful. The patient may grab hold of the trapeze and become hung up in mid-air; or, if the trapeze is released while halfway up in order to shift his or her hand to the bed for support, the patient will usually fall backward.

Before sitting is attempted, it is essential to drop the legs over the edge of the bed. Most elderly patients are unable to maintain the long-sitting position with the knees extended because of tight hamstrings and a relatively immobile back.

TRANSFER SKILLS

The transfer spectrum includes movements from bed to wheelchair; wheelchair to toilet, bathtub, shower, or to car; and from wheelchair, regular chair, or toilet to a standing position.

The wheelchair-to-bed transfer can be done in two ways:

1. by a standing-pivot transfer; or
2. by a sliding transfer.

In the standing-pivot transfer, the patient slides to the edge of the chair, places the feet under him or her, leans forward, and pushes on the arms of the chair to rise to a standing position. The patient then pivots on his or her legs—usually about 90°—before sitting again.

In the sliding transfer, the patient removes one armrest from the wheelchair, pushes downward with one hand on the other armrest and one on the bed, and then slides sideways off the chair onto the bed. A patient will be unnecessarily dependent if he or she can do only a sliding transfer and if the wheelchair does not have removable arms. Transfer is facilitated when the bed and the chair heights are equal (about 20 inches from the floor), while the likelihood of a successful sliding transfer is reduced if these heights are unequal. The patient must set the wheel brakes before either type of transfer is attempted.

Skill in transfers is assured when the patient has free-sitting balance and good strength in the shoulder depressors and elbow extensors in at least one upper extremity. Either transfer technique may be used when sitting is both the initial and final position. The sliding technique may be used when strength of hip and

knee extensors is insufficient, or when severe hip and knee joint flexion contractures are present.

Wheelchairs with large wheels in front restrict the performance of transfers.
If the patient does a sliding transfer, he or she must vault over the wheels; with
a standing-pivot transfer, the patient must move around the wheels. Appropriate
prescription of a wheelchair specifically designed to meet the patient's needs is
necessary when it is to be his/her only mode of travel and transfer.

A person who otherwise could be independent in transfers is made totally
dependent by an inadequate physical environment. A high bed that makes nursing care simpler when a patient with a stroke is confined to bed complicates the
ability to transfer onto the bed when s/he is ready to be more mobile. Often the
wheels must be removed from the legs of a hospital bed in order to reduce the
height sufficiently to allow successful bed transfer.

Environmental modifications useful for toilet transfers are a properly placed
grab bar and the adjustment of the wheelchair and toilet seat to the same height.
(Toilet seat extensions are inexpensive and simple to install.) Environmental
changes useful for tub transfers include placing a chair in the tub and a grab bar
on the wall. The use of a hand-held shower head allows for safer bathing.

A patient with disturbances in memory function or visual perception may
require standby assistance. For example, if a patient in a wheelchair does not consistently lock both brakes before a transfer, he or she may need someone standing by to provide the necessary verbal cues and hence ensure a safe transfer.

TRAVEL SKILLS

Patients may require standby, partial physical, or total physical assistance in
bed mobility and transfer skills but be totally independent in travel skills. The
degree of independence in travel varies with the environment. The environments
of importance are the home, its immediate vicinity, and the community at large.
A person may be totally independent in walking within his or her home and in
the immediate vicinity, but require standby or partial physical assistance when
traveling in the community. Each environment must be considered separately
when evaluating a patient.

It is important to emphasize the concept of functional mobility and to discard the term "wheelchair bound." The goal is time- and energy-efficient mobility. For many patients, independent ambulation is possible for short distances
within a classroom, office, or the home. For longer distances a manual
wheelchair will be more efficient. In some cases, a power wheelchair will be the
most appropriate choice to provide speed and efficient mobility.

Precise seating and positioning are essential for efficient use of a wheelchair
and must be carefully considered in the prescription of this equipment. Inappropriate, ill-fitting wheelchairs, originally intended for other patients, hinder
mobility by creating risks for secondary disability such as skin breakdown or musculoskeletal complications.

An inadequate physical environment can produce dependence in a patient
who otherwise would be independent. Environments are increasingly being
modified to accommodate wheelchair use, but a precheck of new locations is
often helpful to avoid problems of accessibility.

The most successful users of manual wheelchairs are those who have relatively normal upper extremity strength, motor control, and alignment. However, wheelchair travel can be achieved even if a patient has only one functioning arm and leg. Coordinated use of the arm on the wheel and the leg on the floor pulling backward and toward the side of the affected arm permits a hemiplegic patient to develop directional control. This technique is usually simpler to learn than is the use of a one-arm driven chair. One-arm drive or electric wheelchairs become necessary only when a patient has lost the use of one arm and both legs.

Level, smooth, hard surfaces are easiest to negotiate in wheelchair travel. Traveling over ramps and soft or uneven surfaces requires more skill and wheelchair modifications. A wheelchair with a thin tire moves easily on level, smooth surfaces; those with balloon tires are easier to maneuver over deep-pile carpeting, grass, or gravel.

The majority of patients will be able to use the newer ultralight–frame wheelchairs originally designed for wheelchair athletes. Most of these frame designs will now accommodate adaptive seating to meet the needs of nearly all individuals. Disabled people who are interested in sports may choose from a wide variety of adaptive wheelchairs that enable them to compete in road racing, basketball, and a variety of athletic activities.

For patients with significant motor impairment but the cognitive skill necessary to control mobility, a power wheelchair is often the appropriate recommendation. Microswitch technology has enabled patients to obtain independent mobility with a minimum of motor control. Miniature switch interfaces allow patients to achieve independent mobility using only the muscles of the mouth. Patients with inconsistent motor control may be able to take advantage of microchip coding interfaces that allow them to steer using Morse code or other electronic signals. It is even possible to control a power wheelchair with an eyelid switch.

WALKING

Free-standing balance is necessary before walking can be considered a realistic goal. Predicting a patient's ability to master free-standing balance is based on the combined effect of several deficits of sensory or motor function. These include functional deficits of the following:

1. all afferent stimuli (i.e., visual, kinesthetic);
2. vertical perception;
3. sensorimotor coordination;
4. motor strength; and
5. learning potential.

Whether or not a patient can attain standing balance cannot usually be predicted until after at least a 2-week trial of daily training, and progress has been evaluated after sitting balance is achieved.

Loss of full passive ROM in the hip and knee extension or ankle dorsiflexion may contribute to the inability to attain standing balance. With loss of hip

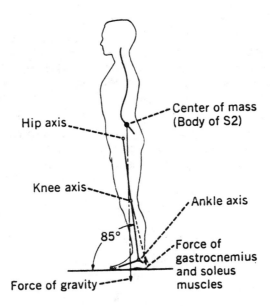

FIGURE 7.1. Relaxed standing position. Force of gravity through center of mass falls posterior to hip axis and anterior to axis of knee and ankle. Angle between tibia and floor is about 85°; hence, foot is in 5° of dorsiflexion. Stability of stance at ankle is provided by contraction of gastrocnemius and soleus muscles.

extension ROM (such as seen in hip flexion contracture), the force of gravity falls anterior to the hip joint and requires active contraction of the hip extensor muscles. With loss of knee extension ROM, the force of gravity is posterior to the knee joint, requiring forceful quadriceps contraction to maintain standing balance. Quiet standing is possible using little or no muscle strength if the center of gravity can be carefully balanced with the hips and knees in extension (Figure 7.1).

Weakness of the leg can fortunately be compensated for by braces that stabilize a joint or substitute for a specific muscle weakness. For example, weakness in the gastrocnemius and soleus muscles makes it difficult to resist falling forward. A short leg brace fitted with an ankle joint that prevents ankle dorsiflexion ROM will compensate for this weakness and stabilize standing balance.

Patients who are unable to extend hips and knees due to soft tissue contractures will either suffer loss of ambulation skills or will ambulate with excessive energy expenditure, reducing speed and endurance. Muscle strength may be lost as a consequence of atrophy associated with bed rest and illness. Joint contractures may also occur during long periods of immobility, and will thus have to be addressed prior to successful retraining for ambulation. In order to assure early ambulation, specific exercises should be performed during bed rest to maintain hip extensor (hamstrings, gluteus maximus) and abductor (gluteus medius and gluteus minimus) strength. Similarly, exercises should be implemented to increase knee extension strength, including quadriceps femoris and gastrocnemius–soleus to maintain better upright support with knees in extension.

Several general rules may be followed in the use of assistive devices for walking. In the case of pain or weakness of the lower extremity, a cane or crutch support is used in the hand contralateral to the affected lower extremity. Thus a patient with injury to the right ankle will be assisted by the use of a cane in the left hand. A cane should be used for balancing rather than weight bearing. When a force—greater than 30 to 40 pounds—is carried on the cane, an alternative aid, such as a forearm crutch, may be more appropriate. If stability at the shoulder is also a problem, the axillary crutch is a better choice. Axillary crutches should not be used in a manner that requires the axilla to support the person's body weight. If wrist pain or triceps weakness results in weight bearing at the axilla, the platform crutch should be used to prevent brachial plexus and radial nerve injury. If ambulation is slow and the hand must bear significant weight, a broad-based cane may be preferred. Patients should be cautioned that this type of walking aid is difficult to maneuver on stairs and grades. Patients requiring greater assistance and those who have difficulty with motor control (including ataxia and instability) may use a walker. Young patients (including ambulatory children with cerebral palsy) will frequently benefit from a posture-control walker, positioned behind the patient. Older patients will benefit from the use of a nonwheeled walker maneuvered in front.

═══ Summary

Progressive mobility is, in the broadest sense, the sequential development of bed mobility, sitting balance, transfer skills, wheelchair mobility, standing balance, and walking. An understanding of the patient's previous and current function is essential. The potential for independent mobility depends not only on the patient's intrinsic abilities but also on his/her physical and social environments. A program of exercises to prevent the loss of joint ROM and muscle strength during illness is a necessary prerequisite to the restoration of mobility.

After the patient has recovered from the acute phase of disability, the degree of independence should be reexamined so that plans may be made for an effective program of remobilization therapy. Such a program of training, exercise, instruction, and adaptive techniques will be most useful when combined with the use of assistive equipment and modifications to the social and physical environment. The goal of an effective mobility rehabilitation program should be the creation of a new equilibrium between the patient's performance and his or her environmental needs.

═══ Annotated Suggested Reading List

Brubaker CE. Wheelchair prescription: An analysis of factors that affect mobility and performance. *J Rehab R & D* 23:19–26, 1986.
Ergonomic, physiological, and anatomical factors that affect wheelchair mobility and performance.
Butler C. Augmentative mobility–controversial issues. *Phys Med Rehab Clinics of North America.* In press, 1991.
This article introduces the concept of augmentative mobility. Functional mobility is described as an integral part of both habilitation and rehabilitation.
Butler C, Okamoto GA, McKay TM. Motorized wheelchair driving by disabled children.

Arch Phys Med Rehab 65:95–97, 1984.

Documentation of effective wheelchair use by even young disabled children.

DeLisa JA, Greenberg S. Wheelchair prescription guidelines. *Am Fam Phys* 25:145–150, 1982.

A brief introduction to wheelchairs, useful for primary care.

Fisher SV, Gullickson G Jr. Energy cost of ambulation in health and disability: A literature review. *Arch Phys Med Rehab* 59:124–133, 1978.

Excellent, comprehensive review of energy expenditure in ambulation.

Stolov WC. Normal and pathologic ambulation. In: Rosse C, Clawson DK (Eds.), *The musculoskeletal system*. New York, Harper & Row, 1980, pp. 315–334.

A description of normal walking and abnormal gaits.

Williams M, Lissner HR. *Biomechanics of human motion*. Philadelphia, W.B. Saunders, 1962.

Detailed analysis of the biomechanics of gait.

Wilson AB. *Wheelchairs: A prescription guide (2d ed.)* New York, Demos, 1992.

A thorough review of factors to consider in selecting wheelchairs.

8 Neurogenic Bladder and Bowel

Diana D. Cardenas, M.D.

The normal function of the bladder and bowel should be viewed from the total aspect of the person's ability to function in the society in which he or she resides. It is anticipated that a person need not void more than once in 3–4 hours, will be able to sleep 8 hours, will need to evacuate the bowel daily to every other day, and will remain continent of both urine and feces. Any neurologic lesion that results in incontinence will decrease a patient's social and vocational potential. Interventions to alter the malfunctioning of these systems must have as their primary goal the return of the patient to her or his previous total functional state.

Neurogenic Bladder

The bladder may be considered as an inverted muscular sac, which resides in the bony pelvis in the adult, and is suspended in place by the urogenital diaphragm. The detrusor is a three-layered smooth muscle that forms the fundus and the internal sphincter of the bladder and through which, in a diagonal fashion, run the ureters to emerge in the trigone of the bladder. Parasympathetic end organs are scattered throughout the bladder with a greater concentration in the fundus than elsewhere and are terminations of the pelvic nerve (n. erigentes). These end organs are under acetylcholine control. Their preganglionic neurons are located in the S2–S4 segments of the spinal cord (see Figure 8.1). Both alpha and beta sympathetic end organs are scattered about the fundus and the vesical neck. The beta receptors are more prominent in the fundus and are antagonists to the parasympathetic end organs. The alpha adrenergic receptors are more prominent in the trigonal and proximal urethral area. They are terminals of the hypogastric postganglionic outflow from T11–L2 (see Figure 8.2).

The detrusor continues caudally and forms the bladder neck or internal sphincter and in contraction pulls upward, thus opening the "internal sphincter" or bladder neck. The trigone is a clinically distinguishable area at the base of the bladder. The urethral orifices pierce the extreme of its base and the orifice of the "internal sphincter" constitutes its apex. There are parasympathetic end organs in the bladder neck but they are of minimal clinical significance. A major concentration of postganglionic alpha receptors, the neural transmitter being norepinephrine, is situated in this area. The action of these receptors is to contract the vesical neck and the proximal urethra. The external urethral sphincter is supplied by the pudendal nerve arising from the S2–S4 levels (see Figure 8.1).

The central pathways consist of four arcs or loops (see Figure 8.2). The first pathway is the cortical-pontine-mesencephalic loop, the primary function of which is inhibition. The cerebrocortical areas in Loop I include the supermedial portion of the frontal lobe, the anterior portion of the cingulate gyrus, and the genu of the corpus callosum. This circuit includes contributions to and from the anterior vermis and fastigial nucleus of the cerebellum, thalamic nuclei (dorsalis medialis), and subthalamic portions of the basal ganglia. Neurons in the pontine-mesencephalic reticular formation are the final common pathway for the neural pathways from the frontal cortex and subcortical nuclei and form the detrusor reflex center. The pontine-mesencephalic area thus synchronizes input from the cerebellum, cortex, thalamus, and basal ganglia, and allows for the inhibition of the detrusor muscle. Lesions of this center in the brain stem result in loss of the detrusor reflex. Lesions in the cerebrocortical areas result in a loss of inhibition with a low threshold detrusor reflex and small bladder capacity.

The pontine-mesencephalic-sacral nuclei constitute Loop II. Its primary function is detrusor contraction and duration. These afferent and efferent columns in the area of the reticulospinal tract allow for the efficient contraction of the detrusor. Lesions along this tract result in an uninhibited inefficient voiding pattern. The pelvic and pudendal nuclei constitute Loop III. The primary function of this complex arrangement of afferent and efferent somatic and autonomic neurons, axons, and dendrites is to sort out, pass on, and initiate sensation, inhibition, and excitation of their end organs and integrate stimuli from cephalic centers. The pathway between the motor cortex and the pudendal nucleus constitutes Loop IV. Its prime function is voluntary control of the external sphincter.

Normal adult bladder capacity varies between 350–550 cc and micturition can be initiated or halted voluntarily. After voiding, residual urine is absent. During gradual filling with water or CO_2 (Figure 8.3a), the intravesical pressure remains quite low until capacity is reached. Uninhibited contractions do not occur unless a neurologic lesion alters the cerebrospinal inhibitory pathways.

Examples of lesions that can produce an uninhibited neurogenic bladder are cerebral thrombosis, brain tumors, brain damage secondary to trauma—which are typically Loop I lesions—and multiple sclerosis, typically a Loop II lesion. In such cases the bladder capacity is usually decreased. Voluntary initiation is usually present but may be impaired and inhibition of micturition is usually defective. Residual urine after voiding is usually absent or low. Cystometry (CMG) demonstrates uninhibited detrusor contractions (Figure 8.3b). The uninhibited neurogenic bladder may be further subdivided into the following: 1) Efficient: without residual urine and of almost normal capacity (brain-damaged patients, either traumatic or vascular may suffer from this type of bladder); and 2) Inefficient: with varying amounts of residual urine. The major neurological disease entity in this group is represented by multiple sclerosis.

If a lesion transects the spinal cord above the conus medullaris (sacral segments), a reflex neurogenic bladder results. Causes include trauma, infection,

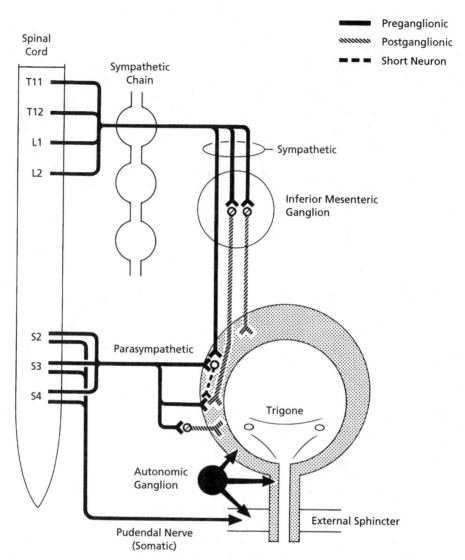

FIGURE 8.1. Peripheral nerve pathways of the bladder and external urethral sphincter.

tumor, and ischemia (Loop II, III, IV lesions). Voluntary initiation of micturition is absent. Residual urine is possible due to some decrease in the efficiency of the detrusor, but more probably secondary to increased resistance to voiding by virtue of spasticity and increased tone of the external urethral sphincter. Unlike the normal situation in which the external urethral sphincter relaxes reflexly as the detrusor contracts, in the reflex neurogenic bladder a condition known as detrusor-sphincter dyssynergia may occur in which the external urethral sphincter actually contracts when the detrusor contracts, thus preventing micturition. There is a shift of the CMG curve to the left with uninhibited contractions (Figure 8.3c). Rarely is vesical sensation present. Of course, an incomplete lesion that spares some voluntary control can produce variable findings.

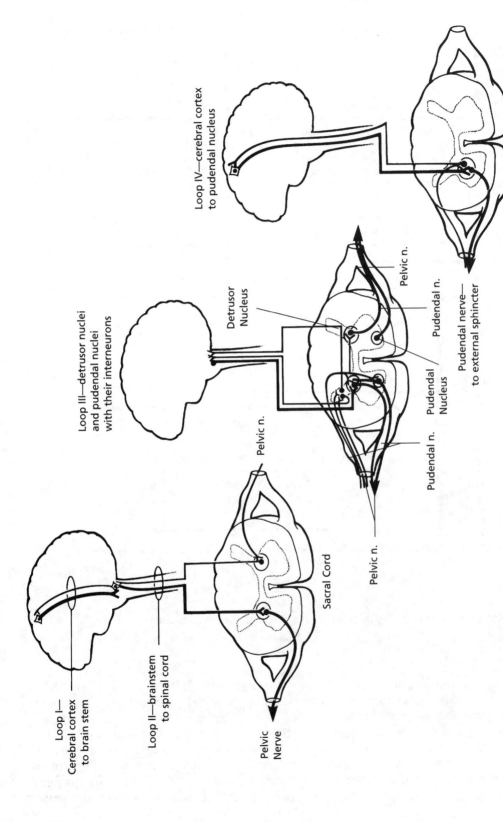

Loop IV—cerebral cortex
to pudendal nucleus

Loop III—detrusor nuclei
and pudendal nuclei
with their interneurons

Detrusor
Nucleus

Pelvic n.

Pudendal n.

Pudendal
Nucleus

Pudendal n.

Pelvic n.

Pudendal nerve—
to external sphincter

Loop I—
Cerebral cortex
to brain stem

Loop II—brainstem
to spinal cord

Pelvic
Nerve

Sacral Cord

Pelvic n.

FIGURE 8.2.   Central pathways involved in micturition.

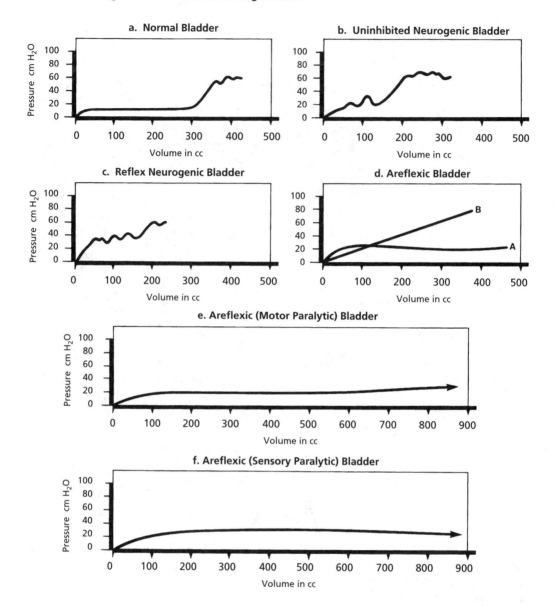

FIGURE 8.3. Cystometry patterns of normal and abnormal bladders.

Interruption of the spinal reflex through both afferent (sensory) and efferent (motor) fibers by damage at the level of the sacral segments or cauda equina may produce an areflexic neurogenic bladder. Causes include trauma, tumor, and myelomeningocele. Voluntary initiation of micturition is lost and residual urine is usually increased, with voiding occurring by external compression of the bladder (Credé expression) or Valsalva. Clinically one may confuse overflow incontinence due to the areflexic bladder with incontinence secondary to uninhibited detrusor contractions. CMG shows a shift to the right with increased cystometric capacity and low intravesical pressure (Figure 8.3d, A). Sometimes, with thickening of the detrusor wall, one finds a linear relationship on CMG rather than a persistently low intravesical pressure with filling. This is called a low-compliance bladder (Figure 8.3d, B). Two subtypes of areflexic bladders occur: 1. the motor-paralytic bladder, which results when there is a failure in the efferent limb of the reflex arc but the afferent limb is intact as is seen in poliomyelitis, herpes zoster, and extensive pelvic surgery or trauma (Figure 8.3e); and 2. the sensory neurogenic bladder, which results from any disease that selectively interrupts the sensory fibers between the spinal cord or the afferent tracts to the brain such as in diabetes mellitus, tabes dorsalis, and pernicious anemia (Figure 8.3f).

Determination of the amount of urine retained in the bladder after voiding can be obtained by catheterization immediately after voiding. Portable ultrasound equipment is also available for noninvasive estimation of bladder volume. Urodynamic evaluation is extremely helpful in determining the presence or absence of voiding dysfunction and the type of neurogenic bladder. A urodynamic evaluation should consist at a minimum of a simultaneous recording of intravesical pressure, intraabdominal pressure, and electromyographic monitoring of either the external urethral or anal sphincter. The simultaneous recording of intravesical and intraabdominal pressures allows the examiner to differentiate pressure increases generated from detrusor contractions from that transmitted from increased intraabdominal pressure. Electromyographic (EMG) monitoring of the sphincter either anal or urethral permits the recording of sphincter response to detrusor contraction.

The management of the neurogenic bladder depends in part on its classification and urodynamic characteristics. Anticholinergic drugs and smooth muscle relaxants that increase the threshold of the detrusor contraction are often used for the uninhibited neurogenic bladder. Care must be taken to titrate the dampening of the detrusor response to stretch with the emptying potential. The goal is to provide the patient with a balanced bladder without creating an unacceptably high residual urine volume. Drugs include oxybutynin 5 mg po and propantheline 15–30 mg po with increasing doses as needed. Another useful drug is imipramine, 50–75 mg po qhs. These drugs are also useful for the reflex neurogenic bladder.

Manual technique, such as suprapubic tapping, may trigger the detrusor to reflexly contract. In some patients this technique is sufficient to produce adequate emptying. In males reflex voiding may necessitate the use of an external collecting device. Alpha-adrenergic drugs, which block the sympathetics and help open the vesical neck, may also assist voiding. If obstruction is found at the vesical neck, transurethral vesical neck resection may be indicated. More frequently obstruction is found at the external urethral sphincter and external sphincterotomy may be the preferred option. However, urinary incontinence will result and necessitate chronic use of a condom catheter with either or both surgical procedures. Hence the optimal choice for the patient with a reflexive bladder with sufficient upper extremity function to perform self-intermittent catheterization (SIC) may be to perform SIC and use anticholinergics to remain dry between catheterizations.

Insertion of one or two fingers in the anus and gentle dilation or stretch of the anal external sphincter will result in the inhibition of this sphincter and the simultaneous inhibition of the external urethral sphincter. This combined with a Valsalva or Credé maneuver will, in many cases, allow micturition. Anal sphincter stretch may be used without intermittent catheterization after attaining a "balanced bladder" (i.e., a bladder that has a residual volume of urine no greater than 20 percent of average capacity). The limitation is the ability of the patient to perform this maneuver independently. This limits its usefulness in practice to a high paraplegic person or a low level quadriplegic. A "Hoke" corset will make the Valsalva more efficient in a high paraplegic or quadriplegic person. Anal sphincter stretch is a nonsurgical option for patients with detrusor-external urethral sphincter dyssynergia.

Unlike the uninhibited or reflex neurogenic bladder, the areflexic bladder may benefit from the use of cholinergic agonists. When the detrusor has been shown to respond at evaluation to bethanechol, it should be administered at large initial doses up to 50–60 mg by mouth and then reduced to the lowest effective dose. Bethanechol is frequently ineffective. The truly denervated bladder will respond to simple extra-vesical pressure, produced either by crede or the Valsalva maneuver. The patient will have to learn to void "by the clock," using either or both of the above maneuvers. This will prevent unexpected incontinence associated with sudden increases in intraabdominal pressure, which overcomes the resistance at the sphincters. If the patient with an areflexic neurogenic bladder is unable to void to low post-void residuals, then intermittent catheterization is recommended. The value of intermittent catheterization is to reduce the residual volume of urine and thus the risk of bacteriuria and consequently pyelonephritis and calculi formation.

The indwelling catheter allows for satisfactory drainage for any form of neurogenic bladder but is associated with numerous serious long-term complications (reflux, hydronephrosis, calculi). The caliber of the catheter should be less than that of the urethra, but large enough to allow a free flow of urine. In the male it should be strapped over the abdomen to prevent erosion of the urethra at the penoscrotal junction. A silastic catheter is fairly inert and can be left in place for 3–4 weeks; however, all patients will soon develop a bacteriuria. The use of a silastic catheter will reduce accumulation of calcium incrustations.

Long-term follow-up evaluations are important to prevent the insidious loss of renal function. Annual evaluations of the neurogenic bladder allow one to determine if the current choice of management is still appropriate. The evaluation should include excretory pyelography (IVP) at least every 2 years, an annual 24-hour urine collection for creatinine clearance, or an effective plasma renal flow scan and urine cultures whenever symptoms of urinary tract infection occur. Renal ultrasound, plain X-rays, cystourethrograms, and urodynamics are also selectively used. Attention to catheterization schedules, compliance, catheters, and appropriate treatment of urinary tract infections are equally important. With proper management the patient with a neurogenic bladder can enjoy a much healthier life.

▬▬▬ Neurogenic Bowel

The term *neurogenic bowel* applies to the alteration of bowel habits caused by neural pathology associated with trauma, neoplasms, demyelinating diseases, and sequelae of any surgical procedure that involves the peripheral neural distribution. The peristaltic action and mass movements of the bowel depend on postganglionic parasympathetic innervation. The external anal sphincter is innervated by the S_2–S_{3-4} somatic outflow via the pudendal nerve. The internal anal sphincter is supplied by the sympathetic and parasympathetic nervous system. Parasympathetic stimulation inhibits the internal anal sphincter, as does distension of the rectum. The external anal sphincter contracts reflexly during rectal distension. In neurologic conditions affecting the lower motor neurons, the rectum becomes a passive receptacle and the external anal sphincter is patulous and atonic. Reflex activity is lost except that mediated by the vagus. With good abdominal muscles some patients with lower motor neuron lesions may be able to expel part of the rectal contents by straining.

In diseases or injuries that affect the spinal cord above the sacral segments, the rectum can be trained to evacuate reflexively using a bowel program. Bowel programs utilize the gastrocolic reflex; that is, eating or drinking a hot liquid to stimulate peristalsis in addition to local stimulants such as glycerine, Dulcolax suppositories, or digital stimulation. The latter helps initiate the defecation reflex and rectal emptying. Increased dietary bulk and stool softeners help prevent constipation. A corset may assist in straining and increasing intraabdominal pressure. A regular time of day and performing the bowel program in a sitting position are also important. Because sensation as well as voluntary sphincter control may be impaired, the patient with a neurogenic bowel may be unaware of fecal material passing into the rectum and be unable to stop the chain of events by voluntarily contracting the external anal sphincter. Bowel accidents, however, can be avoided by regularly emptying the bowel contents up to the sigmoid colon. The frequency of bowel programs is individualized but often every other day programs are sufficient.

Conclusion

A neuroanatomic and urodynamic understanding of micturition serves as a guide to the management of the neurogenic bladder, but ultimately the optimal choice for any one patient will depend in large part on his or her total functional state.

The neurogenic bowel is largely autonomous in its function. By following simple guidelines, the vast majority of patients can obtain good evacuation and avoid fecal incontinence.

Annotated Suggested Reading List

Bradley WE, Timm GW, Scott FB. Innervation of the detrusor muscle and urethra. *Urol Clin NA,* 1:3–27, 1974.
　A classical article yet to be supplanted that describes, with copious diagrams, central and peripheral neural control of bladder and sphincter, and the various Loops discussed in this chapter.
Clinical Urodynamics—*Urol Clin NA* 6 (Feb):1979.
　The entire volume is devoted to clinical urodynamics. The authors are primarily

from Great Britain. While there is a proliferating literature on the subject, for the casual reader this will provide all one needs or wants to know on the subject.

Guttmann L, Frankel H. The value of intermittent catheterization in the early management of traumatic paraplegia and tetraplegia. *Paraplegia* 4:63, 1966.

A classic article describing the use of intermittent catheterization.

Raz S. Pharmacological treatment of lower urinary tract dysfunction. *Urol Clin NA* 5:323–334, 1978.

In 10 concisely written pages, Dr. Raz, a recognized authority on the pharmacology of the bladder, provides theory, practice, and choice of drugs that are available in the treatment of the neurally defective bladder. He offers a bibliography of 32 articles for those interested in specifics.

Yalla SV, McGuire EJ, Elbadowi A, Blaivas JG. (Eds.), *Neurourology and urodynamics: Principles and practice.* New York, Macmillan, 1988.

Recent text that describes basic anatomy, physiology, and techniques of assessment of urologic dysfunction. Excellent discussion of urethral pressure profiles, outlet obstruction, psychogenic voiding dysfunction, and the artificial urinary sphincter.

9

Sexuality and Physical Disability

Jo Ann Brockway, Ph.D.

Sexuality is but one among many health concerns of individuals with physical disabilities and is not necessarily the most important one. At least two studies (2,4) have suggested that sexual function is less important to hospitalized individuals with new disabilities than are ambulation and bowel and bladder control. This is particularly likely to be true in the immediate post-traumatic period and during the early stages of rehabilitation. Nonetheless, at some point during their hospitalization, most individuals with disabilities and/or their partners will have questions and concerns about their sexuality and future sexual functioning. At least one member of the rehabilitation team should therefore have the knowledge and skills necessary to provide helpful sexual counseling.

This chapter will familiarize the reader with the issues of sexuality and sexual functioning in persons with physical disability, provide a framework within which to view sexuality and disability, and provide information regarding sexual functioning in individuals with physical disabilities. Clearly, physical factors contribute to the sexual functioning of the individual with physical disabilities. It is essential to know the physiological concomitants of different disabilities with respect to sexual functioning in order to provide sexual counseling to such persons. It is important to emphasize here that the presence of the physiological basis for sexual problems does not preclude there being a psychological component to the problem, just as the presence of the psychological basis for dissatisfaction does not indicate that physiological factors are not also operative. Sexual functioning is a result of the complex interaction between physiological and psychological processes. Either—or more often both—may contribute to the sexual dissatisfaction of the individual with a physical disability. It is therefore important to know some of the factors that may influence sexual functioning in the individual with physical disability.

The sexual response cycle will be briefly reviewed in order to provide a framework within which to discuss sexuality and physical disability. The effects of various physical and psychological or emotional factors on sexuality and sexual functioning will then be considered, followed by a brief summary of some of the effects of selected specific disabilities on sexual functioning. We will also discuss providing sexual counseling to individuals with physical disabilities. Finally, case studies will be presented to illustrate some of the sexual concerns of individuals with disabilities.

Definition of Sexuality

While it is always important to consider sexuality from a broad perspective when providing intervention for sexual dissatisfaction, this is particularly essential when working with individuals who have physical disabilities. "Sexuality" includes, but is not limited to, genital sexual functioning (e.g., penile-vaginal intercourse). It also encompasses reproduction, contraception, and sensory experience (genital and nongenital), as well as one's perception of oneself and others as sexual persons, and one's feelings about sex roles and masculinity/femininity, the ability to achieve an intimate relationship, one's gender identity, and one's sexual preferences. Sexuality is a part of all one is and does, and each person has a different mode of expressing his or her sexuality. It should be emphasized that the inability to experience some aspects of sexual functioning does not preclude the experience of others, nor does it make one any less a sexual being. For example, the individual who has lost sensation in his/her genitals, or is unable to have penile-vaginal intercourse, may still have a sexual relationship which is satisfying to both him/herself and his/her partner. Since most of what makes up sexuality and sexual behavior in humans is learned, it can be revised or relearned to achieve greater sexual satisfaction.

The Sexual Response Cycle

While sexual behavior varies among individuals, their physiological processes involved in sexual responses are comparatively similar. Masters and Johnson (3) were the first to conceptualize and describe the sexual response cycle, which is usually divided into four phases: excitement, plateau, orgasm, and resolution.

The excitement phase is characterized by feelings of sexual excitement and sensations of sexual pleasure. The onset of genital vasocongestion is manifested by erection in men, and by vaginal lubrication and expansion of the vagina in width and depth in women. Other characteristics of the excitement stage are increased heart rate, blood pressure, and respiration.

The plateau stage is essentially a state of increased arousal occurring immediately prior to orgasm. The vasocongestive response is at its peak. In the male, the erection is firm, the penis is at its maximum size, and the testicles have become engorged with blood. In the female, there is swelling and coloration of the labia minora, the uterus has ascended from the pelvic floor, and the outer third of the vagina is widely ballooned. Just prior to orgasm the clitoris turns up 180° and retracts into a flat position.

The orgasm stage, considered the most intensely pleasurable of sexual sensations, is characterized by rhythmic contractions of the penis in men and of the circumvaginal and perineal muscles in women. Masters and Johnson (3) described the dual components of the male orgasm. The first consists of contractions of the internal organs and signals the sensation of "ejaculatory inevitability." The rhythmic contractions that follow immediately thereafter constitute the second component, and are experienced as the orgasm. After orgasm the male is refractory to sexual stimulation for a certain period of time. The characteristics of the orgasm are identical in all females, and clinical evidence suggests that female orgasm may always be triggered by some form of stimulation of the clitoris. The female does not become physically refractory to orgasm, and can often be stimulated to another and yet another orgasm until she is physically exhausted.

During the resolution phase, physiological responses abate and the entire body returns to its basal state. Somatic response to sexual stimuli diminishes. Heart rate, blood pressure, respiration, and vasocongestion all return to a resting state minutes after orgasm.

Physiologic Factors in Sexual Dysfunction

Several physiologic factors may impact on sexual functioning, including hormonal difficulties, vascular problems, neurologic impairment, damage to the genitalia, and medications.

Hormonal abnormalities are perhaps the rarest physiologic causes of sexual dysfunction. Testosterone probably plays a role in sexual desire, although the interaction between testosterone levels and erectile functioning is unclear. Low testosterone levels can result in low libido in men, as well as in decreased production of sperm cells. Elevated prolactin levels can result in low sexual desire, difficulty in achieving erection, and difficulty reaching orgasm. There is less information about the effect of hormone abnormalities on female sexual functioning. Estrogen deficiency can result in impaired vaginal lubrication and expansion, and atrophy of the vagina. There is some evidence that increased prolactin levels in females cause problems similar to those found in men with increased prolactin levels, including a lack of desire, difficulty with arousal, difficulty achieving orgasm, and poor vaginal lubrication.

Vascular difficulties affect sexual functioning primarily in the excitement and plateau phases. Vascular insufficiency in men may result in difficulty achieving erections. Risk factors for a vascular contribution to erectile dysfunction include hypertension, diabetes, cardiac disease, and smoking. There is less known about vascular factors and female sexual dysfunction, although it seems reasonable that both central and peripheral neurological causes exist.

Little is known about the effect of neurologic problems, that is, damage to the brain or the role of neurotransmitters in sexual desire. Injury or damage to the frontal and temporal lobes, diffuse cortical atrophy, and Parkinson's disease are all thought to affect sexual desire. There is considerably more known about the effects of peripheral neurologic functioning on sexual functioning, particularly with regard to men with spinal cord injuries. Neurologic factors may impair sexual functioning in a variety of ways: a decrease in or lack of sensation, particularly in the genital area; decreased physical mobility; and disruption of the physiologic mechanisms of excitement, plateau, orgasm, and resolution. Damage to the spinal cord may impair a male's ability to achieve erections and/or experience orgasm, and erections may not be as firm or as prolonged as prior to injury.

Damage to the genitalia by surgery or trauma can affect sexual functioning. Removal of one testicle does not generally reduce the testosterone level, but the loss of both testicles does result in hypogonadism; patients may experience low desire, erectile dysfunction, and difficulty in reaching orgasm. Men with a partial penectomy are often able to have erections, vaginal penetration, and orgasm, and orgasm has been reported even following total penectomy. In women, radical vulvectomy often results in exposure of the urethral opening, leading to localized discomfort and urinary tract infections. Reduced desire and difficulty becoming aroused are common. Loss of the vagina through reconstruction does not appear to have a physiological effect on sexual function.

Many medications have an impact on sexual functioning. Sedatives may decrease libido and sexual responsiveness. Anticholinergic drugs may cause erectile dysfunction, although they do not affect libido. Antiadrenergic drugs often cause ejaculatory dysfunction; some may also result in decreased libido and erectile dysfunction. Phenothiazines may result in retrograde ejaculation in which semen is ejaculated into the bladder. Butyrophenones may decrease libido and produce erectile dysfunction. Antihypertensives may lead to decreased blood flow and thus to erectile dysfunction. Tricyclic antidepressants appear to cause decreased libido and erectile dysfunction, and may interfere with orgasm.

Emotional/Psychological Factors

Depression in individuals with a physical disability may be related to loss of pleasurable activities, grief over loss of function and aspects of identity, or a perceived social devaluation as an individual with a disability, and may lead to decreased interest in sexual activity.

Anxiety appears to impair sexual functioning by producing distracting thoughts about failure to perform, leading to an inability to focus on pleasurable sensations. Many individuals with physical disabilities develop anxiety over the effect of the physical aspects of the disability, thus further impairing sexual function.

Combined attendant/partner roles may impair satisfying sexual functioning. It is often difficult for partners to combine the role of sexual partner with that of attendant, which may include hygiene, dressing, bathing, and bowel and bladder care. This appears to be partly due to level of fatigue involved in providing caretaking. As important, however, appears to be a psychological difficulty in performing personal-care chores—particularly bowel and bladder care—and "switching gears" to an erotic interaction.

Many individuals with a congenital or childhood onset of disability, particularly those now in their mid years, experienced childhood and adolescence without having had the social experiences of their age peers who did not have a disability. Many attended special schools with other children with disabilities and thus did not always acquire the same set of social skills as their counterparts who did not have a disability. Many of those who did attend regular classes were excluded from many nonschool social activities, thus they may lack some of the basic building blocks of the adult social behavior expected by others. Additionally, because of the biases of parents and teachers that persons with disabilities were either uninterested in sex or were unable to engage in sexual activities, many of these individuals reached adulthood with limited information about sexuality, sexual behavior, and reproduction. A lack of social savvy and limited information about sexuality may combine to make it more difficult for these persons to find appropriate partners for intimate relationships.

Individuals with a post-pubertal onset of disability often have had most of the social experiences common to their age peers, and have achieved a level of social skills comparable to most others of their age. They may have also had some sexual experience prior to the onset of disability. Thus they often have a "reference point" of social and sexual activities upon which to build. Unfortunately, many of these individuals have acquired some of the negative biases of society toward people with disabilities. Often, prior to becoming disabled themselves, they had viewed individuals with disabilities as asexual and thus may feel that they have lost their own sexuality after the onset of disability.

People with a progressive disability have difficulties similar to those of people with either childhood or post-pubertal onset disabilities, but also have to contend with progressively declining physical functioning. The continued stress of uncertainty about the future, and the constant need to adapt to changing physical conditions, often results in a deterioration of marital relationships. Partners who retain interest in a sexual relationship may either feel that they have no right to request sexual activity from their ill partner or may worry that sexual activity would exacerbate their partner's disorder and cause further decline.

The more conspicuous the disability, the more the individual with a disability stands out as "different" from the rest of society. Many able-bodied individuals would, a priori, not view an individual with physical disability as a desirable partner. The individual with a physical disability may be seen in a stereotyped manner as unattractive, unintelligent, or dependent. Further, a prevalent misconception in our society is that the person with a disability does not have sexual needs or desires and is uninterested in sexual activity. Thus, the conspicuously disabled individual may not be seen as a potential sexual partner by a large proportion of the nondisabled population and therefore may have a restricted range of potential partners from which to choose. The ideal person in our society as portrayed in advertisements is not older or spinal cord injured or paunchy or wearing a leg brace. The individual with a disability, particularly the newly disabled person, may feel "less of a man/woman" because of changes in his or her physical appearance (e.g., loss of muscle tone, awkward gait, amputation), the inability to perform certain previously enjoyed and valued activities (e.g., skiing, repairing a car, playing a guitar), or changes in sexual functioning (e.g., an inability to achieve erection or a lack of pelvic mobility). The extent to which body image is a factor relates to the extent to which the individual was concerned about physical appearance prior to onset of disability, the extent to which physical appearance is impacted by the disability, and the extent to which he or she values other aspects of his or her functioning.

Some Effects of Selected Disabilities on Sexual Functioning

SPINAL CORD INJURY

In males, the higher the level of lesion, the more likely erection will occur. Those with complete upper motor neuron lesions are likely to have reflex erections from tactile stimulation (60–90 percent), but neither psychic (requiring input from brain and mediation through the spinal cord) nor spontaneous (from visceral input) erections; they are unlikely to have ejaculations (1–3 percent). Erections may be fleeting or may last. Males with complete lower motor neuron lesions are less likely to have erections, although some (10–30 percent) may have spontaneous or psychic, and often fleeting, erections; about half that number may ejaculate (5–15 percent). With incomplete lesions, the incidence of erection and ejaculation increases (10–20 percent). The incidence of fertility in men with spinal cord injury is low (0–5 percent). Men with incomplete lesions have a greater likelihood of fertility than men with complete lesions; men with lower motor neuron lesions have a greater likelihood of fertility than do men with upper motor lesions. Men who have lesions between T10–L1, and who are upper neuron for sacral segments but intact in the sympathetic segments, have the best chance for erections, emissions, ejaculations, and fertility. Both males and females with spinal cord injury may be inorgasmic. Both have, however, reported the experience of "psychological orgasm," described as a release of tension that is warm and satisfying. Both males and females may have limitation in coital positioning due to impaired lower extremity mobility. Spinal cord injury does not affect fertility in women. Most return to having normal menstrual periods within 6 months, and some experience no disruption of menses. Pregnancy should have no more complications than for an able-bodied woman except for obvious difficulties with mobility and transfers. Some women, depending on level and completeness of lesion, may not feel the onset of labor. Delivery can be normal but may be precipitous, may cause dysreflexia in quadriplegics, and in total leads to more C-sections. Psychological factors, such as problems with body image and loss of self-esteem, may be related to changes in physical appearance (e.g., loss of muscle tone), need for adaptive equipment (e.g., leg bags for urine collection), decreased genital sensation, and changes in physical abilities, and may contribute to diminished sexual satisfaction.

TRAUMATIC HEAD INJURY

Sexual dysfunction occurs with some frequency after head injury. Several classes of sexual difficulties are related to head injury. Self-sexual stimulation is often seen during acute recovery after a significant head injury. This may embarrass family and staff when it occurs in their presence, but it appears to be part of the normal recovery process rather than actual sexual dysfunction. Patients can be taught to discriminate between appropriate versus inappropriate contexts for this behavior. Later, the most frequently occurring type of sexual difficulty is inappropriate sexual behavior; that is, inappropriate verbal or gestural behaviors, or inappropriate touching of others. A third type of sexual difficulty is more truly a sexual dysfunction. Many patients report a loss of interest in sex after head injury. This seems to be related primarily to a general loss of initiation and motivation rather than to a primary loss of sex drive. Fertility is not likely to be affected by head injury. Choice of contraceptive method should take into account impairment in upper extremity function, as well as judgment and memory problems.

MULTIPLE SCLEROSIS

Decreased physical function and mobility may impair sexual positioning, and must also be taken into consideration in method of contraception. Decreased or unusual genital sensation may occur. There may be decreased vaginal lubrication in women with MS. Pregnancy may lead to an exacerbation of MS, which may later remit. Men with MS may experience erectile dysfunction.

DIABETES

Erectile dysfunction may occur, particularly in older diabetic patients; this may be progressive, whereas orgasm and ejaculation may remain normal. If retrograde ejaculation occurs, ejaculation is usually diminished. Women may experience orgasmic dysfunction. While organic factors can cause these dysfunctions, there appears to be considerable interaction between physiological and psychological factors in many diabetic patients with sexual difficulties.

HEART DISEASE

Heart disease may—but does not always—impede coitus in both men and women. When the patient has returned to mild to moderate physical activity, he or she can generally also return to the level of sexual activity experienced with the usual partner prior to onset of cardiac problems. Intercourse with the spouse or regular partner is apparently much less likely to lead to acute coronary insufficiency than is intercourse with a new or extramarital partner. Fear of a repeat coronary, on the part of both the patient and partner, may impair sexual function.

Providing Sexual Counseling

The extent of the health-care professional's involvement in providing intervention for the sexual concerns of patients with a disability depends on the nature of the patient's individual problems. Annon (1) has described the Permission, Limited Information, Specific Suggestions, Intensive Therapy (PLISSIT) approach to sexual counseling and therapy, a four-level hierarchy of treatment intensity that can be applied to the treatment of sexual concerns of physically disabled patients and their partners. The PLISSIT approach is based on the concept that not all sexual problems require the same intensity of intervention. Some require relatively short, superficial treatment, whereas others require more intense, in-depth therapy.

The first level of intervention in the PLISSIT model is the granting of permission to the patient and partner to have and to discuss sexual concerns or dissatisfaction, or to engage in sexual behavior. One way in which the health-care professional provides this permission is by initiating a discussion of sexual concerns rather than waiting for the patient or partner to do so. Permission to engage in sexual behavior may be indicated by saying something like "the best way to find out where you have sensation and what feels good to you is to experiment. Have your partner touch you (or touch yourself) in different ways all over your body, including the genital areas, and see what you feel."

At the second level of intervention, the health-care professional provides limited information to the patient or partner, usually of an educational and a general, nonpersonalized nature; for example, providing information about the sexual sequelae of a medical condition or the sexual side effects of a medical treatment. Statements such as the following may provide the information the patient and/or partner need to alleviate a specific concern:

- A spinal cord injury does not in itself interfere with a woman's fertility.
- People who have had a heart attack may resume sexual activity in much the same way as they resume any other exercise.
- Folding the catheter back and taping it to the penis before intercourse works for many men who use catheters; this does not cause injury to either partner.

The third level of intervention involves making specific suggestions that may help resolve a sexual problem/dysfunction specific to the individual patient and/or partner. The rehabilitation professional who provides this level of information should be knowledgeable not only in the areas of sexuality and the particular disability of the patient, but should have specific information about the patient's physiologic functioning and should also have taken a sexual history from the patient. Suggestions about coital positioning, sexual activities other than genital intercourse, the use of adaptive devices, and the use of sensory modalities other than touch to enhance sexual pleasure may be helpful. It is important to be sensitive to the patient's sexual values and to make any suggestions in a manner not in conflict with his or her ideas about sexual morality.

The fourth and most in-depth level of intervention is intensive therapy. Intensive therapy is appropriate when psychological or intrapersonal problems are at issue and generally includes individual and/or relationship counseling. Rehabilitation professionals who provide intensive therapy should have training in individual, relationship, and sexual counseling, as well as being knowledgeable about physical disability.

The following case studies illustrate some of the issues raised by individuals with physical disabilities, and the use of the PLISSIT approach to sexual counseling.

Gary is a 26-year-old married male, quadriplegic following a motor vehicle accident. He functions at essentially a C8 level, and has normal strength in upper extremity muscles except for some weakness in the small muscles in the hand. His is an upper motor neuron lesion, meaning that basic cord reflexes below the injury are intact; he has spasticity. Gary and his wife had a close relationship and were able to communicate well with one another prior to his injury. They reported having had an active and enjoyable sexual relationship. They now have questions about how Gary's injury may affect their sexual relationship.

With an upper motor neuron (UMN) lesion, Gary can expect to have erections of a reflex nature. However, he will not have psychogenic erections. His reflex erections are usually fleeting although rarely may persist. His chances of having successful coitus per se are considerably less than that of having erections, in light of the fleeting nature of the erection and its unpredictability. His chances of ejaculating are small, certainly less than 5 percent. Ejaculation, if it does occur, will probably be retrograde into the bladder. It is highly unlikely that he is fertile, due not only to difficulties with erection-coitus-ejaculation, but also to decreased sperm production possibly related to loss of normal temperature regulating systems.

The emphasis in counseling Gary and his wife was at the Limited Information and Specific Suggestion Levels of intervention. They were presented with the concept that sexuality entails more than traditional intercourse in the male dominant position. Counseling includes information regarding techniques to increase erectile ability (e.g., papaverine injections and penile prostheses) and artificial insemination. Sexuality ranges from the way we think about ourselves and our bodies to the way we interact with other people, both verbally and physically. Communication between the two is very important. The couple may need to spend time together learning what Gary can and cannot do, where he has sensation, and what feels good to both of them. They can continue to have a satisfying sexual relationship, although certain adaptations may need to take place and the goal for Gary may no longer be ejaculation.

Deborah is a 22-year-old woman who sustained a severe closed-head injury in a motor vehicle accident 2 years ago. While she has achieved considerable recovery of physical functioning and is independent in activities of daily living, she continues to have an awkward gait, very minor facial scars, impaired memory, and poor judgment. She is very aware of her awkwardness and is hypersensitive to her facial scars. She has become sexually active and came into the rehabilitation clinic asking for contraceptives. Both a gynecological and a psychology consult were requested. After consultation between the gynecologist, physiatrist, and psychologist, an IUD was recommended. Because of Deborah's poor memory and judgment, it was felt that she might not remember to take oral contraceptives regularly and could not be relied on to use foam or a diaphragm consistently. Additionally, Deborah's sexual activity appeared to consist largely of a series of short-term relationships in which she engaged in sexual activity as an attempt to gain affection. She became intensely emotionally involved in each relationship but the partner did not, with the result that Deborah felt worthless and unattractive. Counseling at the Intensive Therapy Level of intervention was begun, including AIDS education, to increase her feelings of self-worth and her knowledge of sexual function, pregnancy, and AIDS and other sexually transmitted diseases, with the goals of helping her to develop more rewarding relationships, which might include protected sexual activity but which also had mutual interests, affection, and friendship as a basis. The process of counseling involved much repetition of information and ideas to facilitate Deborah's learning.

══ References

1. Annon J. *The behavioral treatment of sexual problems. Volume I: Brief therapy.* Honolulu, Enabling Systems, Inc., 1975.
2. Hanson R, Franklin M. Sexual loss in relation to other functional losses for spinal cord injured males. *Arch Phys Med Rehab* 57: 291–303, 1976.

3. Masters W, Johnson V. *Human sexual response*. Boston, Little, Brown, 1966.
4. Phelps G, Brown M, Chen J, Dunn M, Lloyd E, Stefanik ML, Davidson JM, Perkash I. Sexual experience and plasma testosterone levels in male veterans after spinal cord injury. *Arch Phys Med Rehab* 64: 47–52, 1983.

▬▬▬▬ Recommended Reading

Becker EB. *Female sexuality following spinal cord injury*. Bloomington, IL, Cheever Publishing, Accent Special Publications, 1978.
Cole TM, Cole SS. Sexual adjustment to chronic disease and disability. In: WC Stolov, MR. Clowers (Eds.), *Handbook of severe disability*, U.S. Government Printing Office, 1981.
Green R (Ed.). *Human sexuality: A health practitioner's text*. Baltimore, Williams & Wilkins, 1979.
Masters WH, Johnson VE. *Human sexual inadequacy*. Boston, Little, Brown, 1970.
Rabin BJ. *The sensuous wheeler: Sexual adjustment for the spinal cord injured*. San Francisco, Multimedia Resource Center, 1980.
Schover LR, Jensen SB. *Sexuality and chronic illness: A comprehensive approach*. New York, The Guilford Press, 1988.

Common Disabilities Requiring Chronic Care

10

Stroke Syndromes

Andrew Gitter, M.D.

A cerebrovascular accident (CVA) or stroke is the sudden onset of a focal neuro-logic deficit resulting from infarction of brain tissue. In the elderly, stroke is the most common neurologic disorder that results in permanent disability. Because stroke is so prevalent, a basic understanding of the physical, cognitive, and func-tional limitations resulting from stroke and the rehabilitation interventions available for these patients is necessary to assist them in achieving their maximal level of independence.

Epidemiology

Approximately 500,000 new strokes occur annually in the United States, of which 40 percent result in death during the first 30 days. A declining incidence of stroke during the past 30 years has resulted from better treatment of risk fac-tors, with most of the decline attributed to better control of hypertension. Of the survivors of a new CVA, an estimated 70 percent will require rehabilitation in order to maximize their functional skills and level of independence.

Major risk factors for CVA include a prior transient ischemic attack (TIA), hypertension, diabetes mellitus, valvular heart disease (especially in association with atrial fibrillation), and smoking. The identification and treatment of modi-fiable risk factors is important to potentially decrease the incidence of subsequent stroke. The diagnosis of stroke in the elderly patient implies a high likelihood of coexisting cardiac and peripheral vascular disease as well as the need to concur-rently manage disability from these disorders.

Etiology

The major vascular etiologies of stroke are thrombotic, lacunar, embolic, and hemorrhagic. Each of these etiologies implies a different underlying pathogenesis, risk factors, diagnostic evaluations, and prognosis.

The most common cause of stroke is thrombotic occlusion of the carotid or intracranial arteries due to atherosclerosis. Because atherosclerotic lesions tend to occur at the bifurcations of large vessels, thrombotic events often result in extensive strokes that leave patients with significant disability. Preceding transient ischemic attacks occur in more then 50 percent of these patients. Following a TIA, the risk of a completed stroke is greatest in the next 3–6 months. A history of a TIA should prompt evaluation for surgically treatable carotid atherosclerotic disease. Unless contraindicated by other medical problems, these patients should be treated with aspirin to decrease the risk of further thromboembolic events.

Lacunar strokes, which account for 10 percent of all strokes, are small infarcts resulting from the occlusion of small penetrating arterioles in the basal ganglia, internal capsule, and brain stem. Microatheromas and hypertensive vasculopathy are the predominant underlying pathologic processes. Lacunes typically present with highly focal symptoms, with pure motor deficits being the most common. The majority of patients demonstrate good to excellent functional and neurologic recovery.

Embolic strokes account for 15–30 percent of all CVAs. Identifying the source of the emboli is frequently difficult, but a cardiac source is likely in the setting of valvular heart disease, atrial fibrillation, or acute myocardial infarction. Infarction results when an embolus traveling through the cerebral circulation lodges and occludes a vessel too small to allow it to pass. Most embolic strokes occur in the middle cerebral artery distribution. Emboli can fragment and migrate from the original site of occlusion, resulting in the reperfusion of infarcted brain tissue and subsequent intracerebral hemorrhage. The incidence of recurrence of emboli following the initial stroke is significant. For this reason, many experts recommend anticoagulation of these patients unless intracranial hemorrhage has occurred or the stroke is large.

Primary intracerebral hemorrhage (ICH) occurs as a result of the rupture of small penetrating arterioles. Due to the involvement of penetrating arterioles, most hemorrhagic strokes injure subcortical or basal ganglia structures. ICH accounts for approximately 10–15 percent of all strokes, and is usually seen in the setting of long-standing poorly controlled hypertension. The initial mortality is high, but if a patient survives the acute hemorrhage, the blood is resorbed, often leaving less residual disability than a comparably sized thromboembolic infarct.

Common Stroke Syndromes

The neurologic symptoms following stroke depend on the specific brain regions that are injured. Characteristic stroke syndromes result from infarcts that involve each of the three major cerebral vessels: anterior cerebral, middle cerebral, and posterior cerebral. An appreciation of these typical syndromes is important for localizing the lesion as well as for evaluating and implementing an appropriate rehabilitation program. The distinguishing features of these stroke syndromes are detailed in Table 10.1.

The clinical presentation of brain stem stroke is much more varied than that of cerebral infarction. Crossed long tract motor and sensory signs in conjunction with ipsilateral cranial nerve findings are pathognomonic for brain stem lesions. Cognitive and intellectual deficits are absent.

Management of the Acute Stroke Patient

Early management of stroke includes determining its etiology, evaluating the severity of the neurologic deficits, managing of medical problems, and prevent-

TABLE 10.1.

DEFICIT	ANTERIOR CEREBRAL	MIDDLE CEREBRAL	POSTERIOR CEREBRAL
Motor	Hemiplegia—leg affected more than arm	Hemiplegia—arm and face affected more than leg	Typically no motor involvement
Sensory	Absent or mild hemisensory loss	Hemisensory deficit common, varying degrees of visual field loss usually present	Hemianopsia. Bilateral occipital lobe injury results in cortical blindness
Memory	Poor short-term memory	With left brain CVA verbal memory impaired. With right brain stroke visual memory impaired	Poor short-term memory
Language	Impaired articulation may occur	Aphasia syndromes (Broca's, Wernicke's, global) occur with left hemisphere CVA	With left hemisphere stroke alexia without agraphia. Aphasia may occur
Spatial/ Perceptual	Typically not affected	Varying degrees of spatial and perceptual deficits with right hemisphere CVA. Constructional apraxia common	Visual-spatial deficits with right hemisphere stroke
Affective / Behavioral	Frontal lobe syndromes may be present, more common with bilateral strokes	With right hemisphere CVA, aprosodia may be present. Depression common especially with frontal lobe lesions	No characteristic disorder

ing complications. Despite considerable research, there are no medical interventions currently available that have been convincingly shown to alter the ultimate degree of neuronal injury or recovery that occurs following a cerebral vascular accident. Patient care therefore focuses on supportive measures.

Chronic hypertension is a common preexisting risk factor associated with stroke. Following an ischemic stroke, impaired cerebral autoregulation can decrease cortical blood flow if blood pressure is lowered too rapidly. Strict guidelines for the management of elevated blood pressure post-CVA do not exist, but most patients with mild to moderate hypertension can be monitored without intervention during the acute period.

Venous thromboembolic complications are common. Clinically significant deep venous thrombosis (DVT) or pulmonary emboli occur in approximately 30 percent of stroke patients. Preventive measures should be implemented in all patients placed at bed rest, including minidose subcutaneous heparin, range of motion (ROM) exercises for the lower extremities, and antiembolic stockings. The risk of DVT decreases substantially once the patient develops leg spasticity and begins to walk.

Delayed swallowing reflexes, impaired oral motor control, and a decreased level of alertness combine to cause dysphagia following stroke. Because of the associated high risk of aspiration pneumonia, oral intake should be restricted until adequate function of the swallowing mechanism can be documented by a speech pathologist or by radiographic swallowing studies.

Dysphagia can be improved by specific therapy. Meals should take place in a quiet, nondistracting environment with the patient positioned upright and the neck and head flexed to help protect the airway. A mechanical soft diet is better handled by the patient with poor oral control who has difficulty with bolus formation. Specific exercises for improving the strength and coordination of oral and facial muscles are of benefit in many patients. Most patients with cortical strokes recover sufficiently to allow oral intake to meet their caloric needs. Brain stem strokes are more likely to result in severe bulbar weakness and incoordination that necessitate the use of feeding gastrostomies or jejunostomies.

Rehabilitative Management of the Stroke Patient

Comprehensive stroke rehabilitation uses a multidisciplinary team approach to evaluate and treat the limitations of mobility, activities of daily living (ADL), language, cognition, and vocation following a CVA. The general principles and goals of treatment are:

- improvement of function by promoting natural recovery;
- training new compensatory skills;
- substitution of lost function with orthotics and adaptive aids;
- prevention of complications;
- modifying the patient's environment to maximize independence;
- family education and training; and
- modification of risk factors.

Not all survivors of a stroke will require comprehensive inpatient rehabilitation; 10 percent will have nearly complete spontaneous recovery of function while an additional 10–15 percent will have severe cognitive deficits that prevent intensive rehabilitation. The remaining patients are candidates for rehabilitation.

Early rehabilitation intervention should begin within the first several days following the acute stroke. Active and passive range of motion exercises are instituted to prevent contracture. Daily ROM also minimizes joint and muscle pain and assists in DVT prophylaxis. Positioning the paralyzed shoulder and arm in abduction and external rotation minimizes contracture formation and protects against traction injuries. Patients unable to roll and reposition themselves are turned every 2 hours to prevent the development of decubitus ulcers.

The length of time the patient should remain at bed rest is a controversial issue. Most clinicians favor early remobilization and active involvement in rehabilitation to prevent the complications associated with immobility. The remainder of this chapter will highlight the typical deficits seen following stroke and the rehabilitation approach to them.

Cognitive Defects

Mental status and intellectual changes are to be expected following strokes that involve the cerebral cortex. The ability to participate and benefit from a rehabilitation program is primarily determined by the level and extent of cognitive dysfunction. Alertness, cooperation, and learning are essential components of rehabilitation treatments. As such, patients with severe neglect and denial, the inability to follow commands (verbal or gestural), or who do not demonstrate carryover of learning from day to day will be unable to compensate for functional losses with rehabilitation.

Some degree of difficulty with directed attention, short-term memory, mental flexibility, and problem solving is seen following most cortical strokes. Specific differences between right- and left-brain strokes exist and require different rehabilitation management techniques.

APHASIA

The left cerebral hemisphere is responsible for language and communication skills. Injuries to this hemisphere can result in a variety of aphasia syndromes—disorders of speech production and comprehension. A generalized communication disorder usually exists, and impairments in verbal language skills will coexist with deficits in reading, writing, and processing symbolic information. Establishing a consistent means of communication is essential for patient participation in a comprehensive rehabilitation program.

Many classification schemes exist for aphasia. One clinically useful method is to characterize the aphasia by the type of patient-demonstrated verbal skills. Patients with fluent aphasia can produce well-articulated phrases and sentences with near normal rhythm and melody. The speech, however, is likely to contain nonsense words and phrases, jargon, neologisms, and paraphasic errors in which sounds and words are substituted for each other. Significant impairments in the comprehension of spoken language and reading are present. Fluent aphasias are more common after strokes in the temporal and parietal lobes.

Nonfluent aphasia is characterized by the effortful production of sparse or telegraphic speech that is poorly articulated. Broca's aphasia—the most common form of nonfluent aphasia—follows left frontal lobe strokes. Comprehension and reading skills are relatively well preserved in these patients. Global aphasia results in marked impairment in all language function.

Formal communication assessment by a speech pathologist is necessary to classify the aphasia and, more important, to identify preserved areas of language function. Specific aphasia treatment programs have been developed and are useful in selected patients. Communication with any aphasic patient can be improved by asking simple one-stage questions, augmenting spoken language with gestures, and anticipating the needs of the patient.

NEGLECT AND SPATIAL PERCEPTUAL DYSFUNCTION

Unilateral neglect and impaired spatial perceptual skills are most frequently seen with right (nondominant) parietal lobe strokes. Unilateral neglect is the inability to direct one's attention and awareness toward important sensory events in the surrounding world. Patients with neglect may fail to dress or groom on the affected body side, eat off only half of the plate, and bump into walls and objects on the left side during wheelchair use or ambulation. Denial of disability (anosognosia) and an inability to recognize the neglected, paralyzed extremity as belonging to oneself, are seen with more severe lesions. The lack of awareness, judgment, and impulsiveness that results from neglect and denial, can be major impediments to successful rehabilitation.

Right parietal lobe lesions also result in more severe and persistent perceptual problems than do corresponding lesions of the left brain. These patients perform poorly on two- and three-dimensional constructional and drawing tasks (Figure 10.1). Difficulties in judging distances and in assessing the shape, size, and relationship between objects in the environment are common problems. An impaired sense of midline and true vertical, difficulties in picking out visually important information from a complex background (figure ground deficits), and dressing apraxias are commonly seen during rehabilitation.

Verbal skills are well preserved, making it easy for families and even health-care providers to overestimate the abilities of these patients to function independently. The right hemisphere stroke patient learns poorly from mistakes. Those with persistent neglect, impulsiveness, and perceptual problems are more likely to have accidents and falls during transfers. Safety following discharge is a major concern. Driving and the use of dangerous equipment should not be allowed unless the appropriate skills are specifically evaluated.

Gross denial and neglect diminish by 3–4 months post-stroke, although milder problems with neglect and spatial perceptual disorganization frequently persist. Emphasizing the use of verbal and written cues during training in mobility and self-care activities will take advantage of the retained language skills seen in these patients. Additional treatment strategies include the use of visual scanning drills, mirrors, and biofeedback to improve vertical posture and to stress activities that cross the midline.

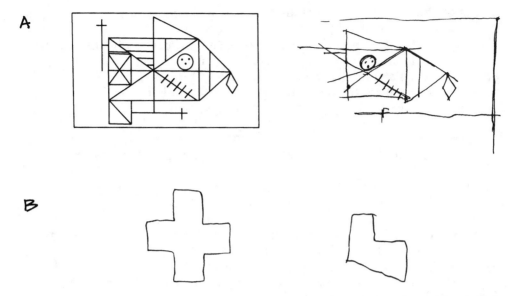

FIGURE 10.1. (A) Rey-Osterrieth Drawing. Note the left neglect and errors in spatial details in the drawing done by a former architect following a right parietal lobe CVA. (B) Severe visual spatial neglect and distortion in a patient with an extensive nondominant right fronto-parietal lobe infarct.

MEMORY

Some impairment of short-term memory is common after a stroke. The process of registering, storing, and recalling memories is complex and may potentially be influenced by a number of problems seen post-stroke. These include impaired orientation and attention, aphasia, visual searching and scanning, neglect, and depression. A systematic evaluation of these aspects of memory is important for adequate treatment. Memory impairment can be modality-specific with left brain lesions causing verbal memory dysfunction and right brain lesions resulting in spatial and perceptual memory problems. The treatment of memory dysfunction is the responsibility of all members of the rehabilitation team. Contributing problems should be addressed. The efficacy of specific interventions in improving memory deficits post-stroke is unclear but the empirical use of memory books and aids, minimizing distractions, and using repetition during training appear to help.

Emotional and Affective Disorders

DEPRESSION

Approximately half of all stroke survivors will experience at least one major or minor depressive episode. Because highest incidence occurs during the 6–24-month period following the acute stroke, it frequently is not clinically apparent during the initial inpatient rehabilitation. The incidence and severity of depression appears to be increased with left frontal lobe infarcts.

The assessment of mood disorders can be complicated by the limited awareness, denial, aphasia, and emotional lability, which can coexist with them. The only signs of depression may be unexpected poor recovery, unexplained regression in function, poor cooperation, anger, or anxiety. Both psychotherapy and antidepressant drug management are used in treatment.

DISORDERS OF EMOTIONAL PERCEPTION AND EXPRESSION

Patients with right cortical strokes may demonstrate varying degrees of aprosodia, the impaired understanding and expression of the nonlinguistic aspects of speech. These patients may have difficulty accurately displaying their internal emotional state and appear consistently confused, apathetic, or may demonstrate inappropriate jocularity. The patient can be incorrectly diagnosed as being depressed if apathy is the dominant emotional state displayed. Depending on severity, difficulties in understanding and following emotionally laden conversations may exist as well.

Although specific tests have been devised to assess aprosodia, they are not routinely used. Behavioral observations and family reports of changed personality traits should alert the rehabilitation staff to these problems. Family education is the most important component of treatment.

Mobility and Related Problems of Motor Control

Hemiplegia is the most obvious neurologic deficit following stroke. The motor deficits that occur are best considered as part of an "upper motor neuron motor syndrome" in which weakness is the result of abnormalities of cortical and extrapyramidal motor control and is associated with increased reflex activity, loss of rapid alternating movements, impaired fine motor coordination, and fatigability.

MOTOR RECOVERY

A typical sequence of motor changes is seen as patients recover from hemiplegia. The hemiplegic side is initially flaccid and lacks deep tendon reflexes. Over the next several weeks, reflexes become hyperactive and muscle tone increases. Movement recovers initially in synergy patterns in which multiple muscles in an extremity are activated together. These synergies give rise to the characteristic flexed arm and extended leg posture that is seen following a stroke. Finally, isolated, voluntary control over individual muscles occurs. Recovery can plateau at any stage along this continuum.

MOBILITY AND GAIT RETRAINING

Impaired mobility and ambulation resulting from hemiplegia has a major impact on the ability of the patient to return home. Mobility skills can be thought of in a hierarchy, beginning with bed mobility and progressing through sitting balance, transfers, standing balance, and ambulation.

Physical therapists use a series of progressive mobility activities and exercises to train stroke patients for independent function. The core components of early mobility training are strengthening exercises of the uninvolved extremities, teaching specific compensatory techniques, and the use of repetitive drills and mat activities to improve balance and transfers. Achieving independence in getting into and out of bed without supervision is an important goal, as it significantly lessens the physical demands placed on the long-term caregiver.

Wheelchair use should be taught to all hemiplegic patients and is critical in the nonambulatory patient. The hemiplegic wheelchair should have a lower seat to facilitate use of the unaffected leg for propulsion and steering. Removable arms and swing-away footrests ease transfers and in activities of daily living.

Unless the home is wheelchair accessible, the ability to ambulate indoors and climb stairs is a prerequisite for returning home. Acquisition of these ambulation skills marks a major psychological milestone for many patients and their families in the post-CVA period. Good standing balance and some voluntary hip and pelvis control are needed for successful ambulation. Gait training consists of a graduated series of balance and skill training exercises. The patient begins on the parallel bars, learning to shift weight and improve standing balance. Reciprocal movements of the extremities are trained. Because distal control and strength are more markedly affected, the use of an ankle-foot orthosis (AFO) to substitute for weak ankle muscles and to improve knee control is frequently required. The patient progresses from the parallel bars using a hemiwalker, quad cane, single-point cane, or no assistive device as skill permits. Sixty to eighty percent of hemiplegia patients will be independent short-distance ambulators.

APRAXIA

Approximately 25 percent of patients with left hemisphere strokes have apraxia, defined as the impaired ability to carry out a motor task on command despite having adequate strength, sensation, coordination, and comprehension. In apraxia, the basic motor elements of the requested movement appear to be inappropriately selected, or are produced in an incorrect sequence. To test for apraxia, the patient is asked to perform a variety of motor tasks either by verbal command or by gesture. The task complexity should progress from simple acts, such as licking the lips or waving goodbye, to multiple-stage commands, like having the patient imitate picking up a match, striking it, and then blowing it out.

Apraxia interferes with the acquisition of new motor skills and limits the ability to learn compensatory strategies needed for ADL and mobility independence. Specific treatment programs have not been systematically studied, although empirically repetition, the breaking down of tasks into small steps, as well as the use of imitation, are helpful.

SPASTICITY

Spasticity develops over a period of several weeks to months following a CVA. The increased muscle tone caused by spasticity frequently contributes to the development of contractures by holding joints in a fixed position. In the upper extremity, contractures of the shoulder in an adducted and internally rotated position can lead to shoulder pain and difficulties with dressing and hygiene. In the lower extremity, the most common adverse sequela is a plantarflexion contracture at the ankle. If severe enough, ambulation and transfers are affected. Treatment of spasticity is appropriate if an improvement in function can be expected or if it is the source of painful spasms.

Initially daily stretching is used to improve joint range. Resting wrist-hand splints and AFOs will maintain the respective joints in a functional position and help prevent serious contracture formation. Antispasticity drugs have a limited role in the treatment of spasticity post-stroke. Phenol motor point blocks or tendon releases of selected muscle may be necessary in selected patients who have severe spasticity.

Activities of Daily Living (ADL)

The loss of independence in the basic activities of daily living (ADL) is a demoralizing and frustrating experience for stroke patients. Occupational therapists evaluate and treat problems in self-care. Important areas to assess are personal hygiene, self-feeding, dressing, bathroom skills, and homemaking skills. Multiple factors contribute to impaired ADLs, including hemiplegia, sensory loss, neglect, spatial perceptual deficits, aphasia, and poor short-term memory. The loss of arm strength, sensation, and dexterity—especially of the dominant hand—limits the ability to learn compensatory skills. Initial treatment stresses upper extremity ROM exercises and the use of resting hand splints to prevent shoulder and hand contractures that could interfere with dressing and hygiene. Coordination and strengthening exercises are added as recovery occurs to promote and facilitate upper extremity motor return. Recovery of fine motor skill is unlikely unless voluntary isolated control of hand motion occurs within the first week post-stroke.

Specific training in compensatory techniques and the use of adaptive aids, such as specialized eating utensils, velcro closures on clothing, buttonhooks, and bath benches are usually needed to achieve optimal function. Sitting balance is required for independence in upper extremity dressing, grooming, and toileting. With good standing balance, independence in all bath transfers can be expected. Higher level ADLs include basic homemaking skills, shopping, management of finances, telephone use, and community transportation.

Vocational Loss

Vocational disability is less paramount in the stroke population because most survivors are of retirement age. For the younger patient interested in a return to work, further neuropsychological testing, mobility training, and workplace evaluation are necessary. An inability to drive or to use community transportation systems is a major block to successful employment. Like many persons with a disability, societal and employer misperceptions remain an additional barrier that must be overcome. Overall, 50 percent of young stroke survivors can return to some prior level of employment, homemaking, or schooling.

===== Management of Common Medical Problems

UPPER EXTREMITY COMPLICATIONS

Hemiplegic shoulder pain develops in as many as 85 percent of stroke patients and impairs functional use and recovery of the arm. Common causes of shoulder pain are brachial plexus lesions and shoulder-hand syndrome. Persistent muscle flaccidity, severe spasticity, contracture, or subluxation of the glenohumeral joint are frequently associated with shoulder pain and may be contributing etiologic factors.

SHOULDER-HAND SYNDROME

Shoulder-hand syndrome (SHS) is a form of reflex sympathetic dystrophy that occurs in 12–25 percent of the stroke population. The classic signs and symptoms of SHS are shoulder pain with movement, pain and tenderness in joints of the wrist and hand, edema, vasomotor changes, and a loss of range of motion. Since treatment is most effective when started early, early diagnosis is important; it is based on the clinical findings and the presence of increased uptake in the hand and wrist on radionuclide bone scan.

Initial treatment consists of pain control, beginning with non-narcotic drugs or transcutaneous electrical stimulation, control of hand edema with compressive gloves, and, most important, promoting both passive and active ROM and functional use of the affected arm. If a rapid response is not seen with these initial measures, the use of a short course of oral corticosteroids or, alternatively, a series of local anesthetic injections of the cervical sympathetic ganglia in conjunction with continued physical therapy, is appropriate.

SHOULDER SUBLUXATION

Subluxation at the glenohumeral joint of the shoulder is a common problem. It has been suggested that subluxation may lead to increased spasticity and pain, as well as contribute to traction lesions of the brachial plexus. The biomechanical changes resulting in subluxation are complex and not fully understood. Downward rotation of the scapula, weakness of the deltoid and supraspinatus, and the loss of passive restraint of the coracohumeral ligament all contribute. Subluxation may spontaneously reduce as hypertonicity develops.

The use of slings is controversial. These do not appreciably reduce subluxation, but do serve to protect the shoulder from traction during the period of flaccid weakness. The prolonged use of slings may contribute to flexion synergies and contractures. When patients are in wheelchairs, arm troughs and lap boards are adequate to position the arm.

BRACHIAL PLEXUS LESIONS

Improper positioning or traction on the hemiplegic arm during transfers may result in lesions of the upper trunk of the brachial plexus. An atypical pattern of motor return (distal greater than proximal) or excessive atrophy and flaccidity of the shoulder girdle muscles suggest a clinically important lesion. Electromyography can document the presence of denervation. Treatment consists of patient and caregiver education and protection of the shoulder from further traction. Spontaneous recovery frequently occurs over a 6 to 12 month period.

NEUROGENIC BLADDER DYSFUNCTION

Immediately post-stroke, bladder areflexia and flaccidity occur, resulting in urinary retention. Intermittent catheterization or an indwelling Foley catheter may be necessary to prevent bladder overdistension. Voiding trials followed by intermittent catheterization to document post-void residuals are usually started within the first 3–10 days post-CVA. During recovery, the majority of patients complain of frequency and urge incontinence. Urodynamic studies demonstrate detrusor hyperactivity and uninhibited bladder contractions resulting from decreased cortical control over voiding reflexes.

Incontinence is exacerbated by the impaired mobility associated with hemiplegia. The initial measures used to maintain continence are timed voids every 3–4 hrs, moderate fluid restriction, and the use of bedside commodes and urinals. Anticholinergic drugs decrease bladder hyperactivity and are beneficial in some patients. With use of these medications, post-void residuals should be checked to assure adequate bladder emptying. By one year post-stroke, only 15–20 percent of patients remain incontinent.

═══ Annotated Suggested Reading List

Rowland LP (Ed.), *Merritt's textbook of neurology.* Philadelphia, Lea and Febiger, 1984.
    The chapters on vascular diseases offer a concise review of the neurologic aspects of classification, diagnosis, and neuroanatomy of stroke syndromes.
Kaplan PE, Cerrullo LJ (Eds.), *Stroke rehabilitation.* Stoneham, MA, Butterworth Publishers, 1986.
    Comprehensive guide to the rehabilitative evaluation, treatment, and management of stroke in adults. The sections dealing with physiatric complications and the special role of nursing, occupational therapy, and physical therapy in the management of stroke patient are particularly useful in understanding the need for a multidisciplinary approach to care for these patients.
Garrison SJ et al. Rehabilitation of the stroke patient. In: *Rehabilitation medicine: Principles and practice.* Philadelphia, J.B. Lippincott, 1988.
    Excellent overview of basic rehabilitative principles used with stroke patients. The extensive reference list is a convenient place to begin searching for additional information on specific topics.
Albert ML, Helm-Estabrooks N. Diagnosis and treatment of aphasia, Part I. *JAMA* 7:1043–1048, 1988.
Albert ML, Helm-Estabrooks N. Diagnosis and treatment of aphasia, Part II. *JAMA* 8:1205–1210, 1988.
    Comprehensive yet succinct overview of current views on the diagnosis, classification, treatment stategies, and effectiveness of intervention in aphasia.
Cailliet R. *The shoulder in hemiplegia.* Philadelphia, F.A. Davis Company, 1980.

Short and highly readable text covering anatomy, pathophysiology, and treatment of common shoulder problems seen following stroke. The illustrations are especially useful in gaining a conceptual understanding of the altered biomechanics of the hemiplegic shoulder.

11

Head Injury

Sureyya S. Dikmen, Ph.D., and
Kenneth M. Jaffe, M.D.

Each year the disabling effects of traumatic brain injuries irreversibly change the lives of thousands of American citizens and their families. Although once referred to as "the silent epidemic," the past decade has seen great interest focused on the survivors of head injury. This chapter provides an introduction to this condition and its rehabilitation.

═══ Definition

The most comprehensive definition of head injury is the one adopted by the National Head Injury Foundation. It is defined as an insult to the brain caused by an external physical force, that may produce a diminished or altered state of consciousness of varying length, and which results in impairment of cognitive abilities or physical functioning. It can also result in a disturbance of behavior or emotional functioning. These impairments may be either temporary or permanent, and may cause partial or total functional disability or psychological maladjustment.

═══ Epidemiology

The annual incidence of brain injury in the United States is approximately 200 per 100,000, resulting in over 400,000 new cases each year. This figure includes hospitalized cases and those who die before reaching a hospital. It omits, however, unreported head injury cases, those treated in the emergency room and released, and those treated in private physicians' offices. The incidence is highest between age 15–24 years. Secondary peaks occur in early childhood and in the elderly. Males outnumber females by a ratio of two or more to one. Moving vehicle accidents (MVA) are the single largest cause of brain injury, followed by falls. Alcohol intoxication is a contributory factor in approximately 50 percent of the cases. Non-accidental trauma is the leading cause in children under the age of one year.

The Glasgow Coma Scale (GCS), a measure of depth of coma, is described in Table 11.1. Using this scale, approximately 70–80 percent of those admitted to a hospital have mild head injury (GCS 13–15) requiring a hospital stay of 1–3 days. Twenty to 30 percent have moderate to severe head injuries (GCS 3–12).

Types and Mechanisms of Head Injury

Head trauma can be divided into two major types based on the mechanism of impact. Missile injuries are those due to penetrating gunshot or exploding shell fragments that progress through the scalp, skull, and brain in a destructive trajectory. These penetrating injuries result in localized or focal lesions superimposed on diffuse brain dysfunction, a pattern more similar to that observed in cerebrovascular accidents or tumors than to nonpenetrating or blunt trauma, as described below.

Closed-head or nonmissile injury results from blunt trauma, in which either a moving object strikes and accelerates the stationary or slower moving head, or the moving head is decelerated by a stationary or slower moving object. Diffuse axonal injury results from the acceleration/deceleration and rotational forces that are transmitted to the brain (shear strain), usually stemming from high-velocity impact. This primary mechanism of brain damage in closed-head injury patients causes neuronal axons to be disrupted in predictable locations. Typically affected are the corpus callosum, the parasagittal white matter, the tips of the temporal lobes, and the dorsolateral quadrants of the midbrain. Diffuse axonal injury is responsible for the initial loss of consciousness and the subsequent loss of cerebral white matter exhibited on computerized axial tomography (CAT) or magnetic resonance imaging (MRI) as cortical atrophy and generalized ventricular dilitation.

Other than diffuse axonal injury, cortical contusions and lacerations are another form of primary injury associated with blunt cerebral trauma. These cortical bruises and tears, of varying depth, usually occur on the undersurface of the frontal and temporal lobes due to impact with the irregularly contoured base of the skull; they are also seen under depressed skull fractures. Unlike diffuse axonal injury, cerebral contusions can originate from relatively low-velocity impact, as seen with falls.

TABLE 11.1

Glasgow Coma Scale

Eye opening		Best motor response		Verbal response	
Spontaneous	4	Obeys	6	Oriented	5
To speech	3	Localizes	5	Confused conversation	4
To pain	2	Withdraws	4	Inappropriate words	3
Nil	1	Abnormal flexion	3	Incomprehensible sounds	2
		Extensor response	2	Nil	1
		Nil	1		

The primary cerebral damage due to diffuse axonal injury and cortical contusions/lacerations occur at the moment of impact. This damage is irreversible and is probably not mitigated by subsequent care or intervention. It is possible to prevent secondary cerebral damage that is due to resultant hypoxemia, hypotension, increased intracranial pressure, cerebral edema or ischemia, and intracranial hemorrhage. Skilled field management, rapid emergency transport, and neurosurgical intensive care are all interventions targeted to reduce these secondary complications and their consequences. Obviously, the overall severity of the brain insult is a product of both the primary and secondary cerebral damage.

Prognosis

Prediction of outcome is important clinical information needed by patients, their families, and treating health-care professionals, both for treatment planning and for planning the future. It is also important information for prudent allocation of health services for those who need and can benefit from it. Prognosis rests on the demonstrated association between severity of injury and outcome. Unfortunately, there is no simple, well-accepted system that classifies the overall severity of head injury and reliably predicts outcome. Rather, a number of risk factors and individual severity indices have been shown to be related to outcome, which provide only rough guidelines. Generally, outcome improves with younger age, shorter and lighter coma, and shorter duration of post-traumatic amnesia (PTA). Due to marked individual variability, there are no ranges or cut-off scores that will signify the likely outcome for an individual case. Therefore, prognostic estimates need to be made cautiously; because they improve with time, they must also be adjusted periodically. The following commonly used severity indices are associated with behavioral outcome.

SEVERITY OF THE FOCAL INJURY

Focal lesions involve contusions, lacerations, and hematomas. Although the relationships between focal lesions and behavioral outcome have not been firmly established, it is reasonable to expect that the size and location of the focal lesion has significant relevance for outcome.

SEVERITY OF DIFFUSE INJURY

Depth of Coma

The Glasgow Coma Scale (GCS) objectively quantifies the level of consciousness and correlates well with recovery. As shown in Table 11.1, this scale consists of three components: eye opening, motor response, and verbal response. The most sensitive of the three is the motor response. The scale is practical, reliable, and is therefore used extensively. An oriented awake patient would receive a score of 15. A patient who has no eye opening and no motor or verbal response to pain would be given a score of 3. It should be remembered that the GCS is a measure of depth of coma and should always be reported in relation to time from injury.

Length of Coma

A patient is in coma if he or she is unable to obey simple commands, does not open his or her eyes, and fails to utter recognizable words as defined in the GCS. A simple and reliable way to define length of coma is the time from injury to when the patient is able to consistently follow simple commands as defined by the GCS motor response.

Post-traumatic Amnesia

The duration of PTA is the time from injury to that when continuous memory returns. It is established retrospectively by asking the patient about his or her earliest memories after the accident and noting when they become continuous.

OTHER INDICES OF HEAD INJURY SEVERITY

Other clinical and nonclinical measures of focal and diffuse indices of head injury severity include intracranial pressure, eye movements, pupillary reactivity, cerebral blood flow, evoked potentials, and so on.

Consequences of Head Injury

PHYSICAL AND MEDICAL CONSEQUENCES

Head injuries do not always occur in isolation. Often, particularly with high-velocity impact, they are associated with extracranial medical and surgical complications. Almost any organ system can be affected, either during the early days after injury or sometimes even months later. The following section deals with some of the more common neurologic, physical, and medical problems that are due to extracranial injuries, as well as those due to the brain injury itself. Familiarity with these will hopefully lead to early recognition, prompt treatment, and reduced morbidity.

Nutrition and Feeding

Many patients with traumatic brain injuries are nutritionally compromised when admitted for rehabilitation. The presence of abnormal oropharyngeal muscle tone or sensation, as well as pathological reflexes, can also result in feeding and swallowing disorders. A multidisciplinary feeding team should perform a detailed nutritional and feeding-swallowing evaluation shortly after admission. With this information, appropriate decisions can be made about consistency, texture, and temperature of food, positioning requirements, methods of food delivery, and oral feeding techniques.

Fever and Infection

During the early recovery from traumatic brain injury, fever can signify a life-threatening central nervous system (CNS) infection, a trivial intercurrent viral infection, or hypothalamic damage (central fever). The last diagnosis can only be assigned after all other sources of infection have been diligently excluded.

Following a basilar or compound skull fracture, post-traumatic meningitis or brain abscess can occur. Prolonged nasotracheal intubation predisposes to an ipsilateral sinusitis. Urinary tract infections are common with indwelling Foley catheters or urinary stasis from incomplete bladder emptying. In the splenectomized patient, fever represents a true medical emergency requiring prompt broad-spectrum antibiotic coverage.

Endocrine Dysfunction

Posterior pituitary hyperfunction is common after head injury, and is indicated by the self-limited syndrome of inappropriate secretion of antidiuretic hormone. Diabetes insipidus is usually associated with more severe injuries, and can be transient or permanent. Because of the association of anterior pituitary insufficiency with diabetes insipidus, the anterior pituitary reserve should be carefully evaluated in its presence.

Heterotopic Ossification

Heterotopic ossification occurs commonly in patients with severe head injury, but its etiology remains obscure. Because it presents with warmth, redness, swelling, and pain, it can be easily confused with cellulitis, septic arthritis, fracture, or thrombophlebitis. The proximal joints of the upper and lower extremities are principally affected. Following diagnosis, passive range of motion (ROM) exercises, carried to the point of joint resistance, should be continued in order to prevent ankylosis. Surgery to remove ectopic bone can be undertaken to achieve specific functional goals.

Spinal Cord and Peripheral Nerve Injury

The diagnosis of spinal cord or peripheral nerve injury is frequently overlooked in the comatose patient. As alertness improves, all neurological and musculoskeletal complaints deserve careful investigation.

Spinal cord injury should be suspected if there is an absence of sacral or deep tendon reflexes, a differential response to pain in the upper versus the lower extremities, a dermatomal pattern of sensory loss, a flaccid symmetrical paraparesis or paraplegia, unexplained urinary retention or ileus, or priapism. Because failure to promptly diagnose spinal cord injury can further the disability—particularly with an unstable spine—a high index of suspicion must be maintained.

Pelvic fractures are associated with pelvic nerve and lumbosacral plexus damage. Brachial plexus injury must be ruled out in a patient with a flaccid arm, especially in the context of a clavicular fracture or high-velocity impact. As in stroke, proximal motor return precedes distal. Long bone fractures can damage the radial and peroneal nerves, whereas the ulnar nerve is particularly susceptible to direct pressure from prolonged bed rest—a preventable complication.

Basilar Skull Fractures

Fractures of the base of the skull are not always detected radiographically. However, the presence of periorbital hematoma (raccoon's eyes) and cerebral spinal fluid (CSF) rhinorrhea are pathognomonic for fractures of the anterior cranial fossa, and mastoid hematoma (Battle's sign) and CSF or bloody otorrhea for fractures of the middle cranial fossa.

Temporal bone fractures are noteworthy because of their proximity to important structures. The longitudinal type results in damage to the tympanic membrane and structures of the middle ear (hemorrhage, ossicular chain disruption). The post-traumatic perineural edema of the seventh cranial nerve following a longitudinal fracture results in a delayed, spontaneously resolving facial weakness or paralysis. Transverse fractures are less common, and are associated with vestibular dysfunction, profound sensorineural hearing loss, and the immediate onset of facial paralysis.

Post-traumatic Hydrocephalus

Post-traumatic hydrocephalus is uncommon even in the context of severe head injury. It must be distinguished from the ventriculomegaly due to diffuse atrophy or focal infarction (hydrocephalus ex vacuo). The classic signs of incontinence, gait disturbance, and dementia are usually not diagnostic in a severely disabled, low-functioning population. Failure to improve, deterioration, or more subtle changes in neurologic functioning should, however, prompt consideration of this entity.

Cranial Nerve Deficits

The olfactory nerve is susceptible to damage in head injury, but it is often not detected due to incomplete sensory screening. Partial or complete anosmia can result in alterations of dietary habits.

Optic nerve injury can result in monocular blindness, impaired acuity, or a field defect. An ophthalmologic evaluation should be conducted when it can be reliably performed. Traumatic ophthalmoplegia, due to damage of the oculomotor, trochlear, or abducens nerves or their brain stem nucleii, can result in dysconjugate gaze and diplopia. Surgical intervention is customarily delayed due to the high incidence of spontaneous resolution of this problem during the first year after injury.

Motor Deficits

The most common motor deficit following head injury is spasticity, with or without ataxia. Spastic hemiparesis or hemiplegia can interfere with fine motor function, particularly with an associated disturbance of discriminative sensory function or involvement of the dominant hand. Increased tone can also impair functional mobility and lead to contractures. Treatment is dictated by the specific clinical situation and includes physical modalities, positioning, range of motion, splinting, casting, and antispasticity medication.

Ataxia and postural and kinetic tremors occur less frequently. They can, however, be very disabling and challenging to treat.

Post-traumatic Seizures and Epilepsy

This is a frequent delayed complication following severe head injury. The incidence of post-traumatic epilepsy is 5 percent in civilian hospitalized head-injured patients. The probability of seizures increases with increasing severity of head injury, such as those involving depressed skull fractures and hematomas. The risk of developing post-traumatic seizures is highest during the first year after injury, but a higher than average risk persists for many years. Whether or not patients should be treated prophylactically with anticonvulsants to prevent the development of post-traumatic epilepsy has been controversial. Based on current knowledge, however, there is no firm evidence that anticonvulsant drugs prevent the development of post-traumatic seizures. Phenytoin, the most frequently used and the most extensively studied in this regard, does not appear to be effective in preventing the onset of seizures except during the first week post-injury (2). Additionally, it causes negative neurobehavioral side effects (1).

NEUROBEHAVIORAL CONSEQUENCES

Cognitive and emotional/behavioral difficulties occur frequently, even in the absence of physical problems, and are the major contributors to problems in resuming prior social roles and responsibilities. Such difficulties are not experienced by all head-injured patients. When they occur, however, they do so in varying degrees and combinations. In other words, the effects of head injury are not an all-or-none phenomenon, but rather quite diverse. This diversity is contributed to by multiple factors, including the nature of the head injury (e.g., severity, type, and location of brain lesion) and the premorbid characteristics of the patient (e.g., age, preexisting problems), and requires detailed and comprehensive assessments by experienced and competent neuropsychologists.

The neurobehavioral consequences of head injury may be grouped into three areas: cognitive, psychiatric, and psychosocial.

Cognitive Impairments

Cognition refers to functions, such as the ability to think, remember, and solve problems. Cognitive difficulties are quite prevalent following head injury and may involve a broad spectrum of functions depending on its severity. In mild head injury, the difficulties are likely to be subtle and selective. Correspondingly, they are likely to be severe and diffuse in those with severe head injury. Cognitive difficulties observed may involve the following skills.

ATTENTION AND CONCENTRATION: One of the most vulnerable to the effects of head injury is the ability to focus and sustain attention and resist distractors. Disturbed attention is thought to be one of the principal and selectively impaired abilities in minor head injury.

MEMORY AND LEARNING: A diminished ability to remember and learn new information is one of the most common complaints of head-injured patients. Depending on the severity and acuteness of the head injury, patients show problems in the acquisition of new information and in its storage, retrieval, and retention.

REASONING AND FLEXIBILITY IN THINKING: Patients with head injury may experience difficulties in analyzing new and complex situations, extracting the essence of a problem at hand, and systematically trying out various solutions. They may have difficulty in thinking out a problem from various perspectives and in abandoning unworkable solutions.

PERCEPTION, ORGANIZATION, AND INTERPRETATION OF SPATIAL AND TEMPORAL RELATIONSHIPS: Selective difficulties in these right cerebral hemisphere functions are not common unless that hemisphere is specifically damaged.

VERBAL LANGUAGE SKILLS: Basic language difficulties (i.e., aphasia) reflective of left cerebral hemisphere dysfunction are also uncommon unless the left cerebral hemisphere is specifically involved. Word finding difficulties, reduced verbal fluency, and decreased efficiency and conciseness of verbal expressions are more common. These are thought to be reflective of more general problems in attention, memory, and organized thinking.

REDUCED INFORMATION PROCESSING SPEED: This, and the breakdown of abilities in general as a function of the complexity of the task, are two important aspects of cognitive difficulties in head injury. However, head-injured patients are capable of all the cognitive functions described above if the complexity level and the speed requirements of the tasks are adjusted to the level of the individual.

Psychiatric Impairments

Psychiatric impairments include personality, emotional, and behavioral disturbances.

TRANSIENT SYNDROMES: Patients with severe head injury sometimes manifest transient syndromes as they emerge from coma. The most common include:

1. organic excitement consisting of increased energy, euphoria, rapid thinking, and speech and psychomotor agitation;
2. marked aggressiveness; and
3. a paranoid state represented by suspiciousness of the motives of others.

The occurrence of these transient, subacute reactions increases the risk of long-term psychiatric problems.

PSYCHIATRIC DISORDERS: Major psychiatric disorders involving psychoses or neuroses are rare but do occur. Affective disorders, such as depression, are more common than are thought disorders, such as schizophrenia. Neurotic disorders are usually diagnosed in patients with mild head injury who continue to experience excessive disabilities in the absence of objective difficulties attributable to the injury. Post-concussional syndrome, post-traumatic neurosis, accident neurosis, and post-traumatic stress disorders are some of the terms used to describe such conditions.

POST-TRAUMATIC SYMPTOMS: These, also called post-concussional symptoms, include complaints of headaches, fatigue, dizziness, irritability, difficulty with concentration and memory, and increased sensitivity to light and noise. These symptoms are reported by most head-injured patients soon after injury, including those with mild head injury. These symptoms typically subside with time in patients with mild head injury; however, a fraction of patients with mild head injury continue to have problems over a prolonged period of time. Some even develop the neurotic disorders mentioned above. There is considerable controversy regarding the etiology for the persistence of these symptoms, which often are not accompanied by objective findings. Multiple factors (both physical and nonphysical) probably contribute to the difficulties in individual cases.

BEHAVIORAL ALTERATIONS: Some forms of behavioral change in head injury create significant difficulties of adjustment. Depression is common, either as a reaction to loss, trauma, or biochemical alteration. It tends to occur early following mild head injury, but later as the severity increases. Also seen are inaccurate self-assessment, where the patient overestimates his or her abilities, and poor social awareness, manifested as socially inappropriate behavior. These difficulties occur with severe head injury and may be associated with frontal lobe involvement. Unrealistic self-appraisal, however, usually disappears with time, suggesting that this lack of awareness may be related to the patients' lack of opportunity to test out and realize their losses soon after injury. Increased irritability and low frustration tolerance occur commonly and are bothersome, especially for family members. Anger outbursts and losses of temper are particularly troublesome but occur less frequently. Impulsiveness (speaking or acting before considering the consequences) and emotional lability (changeability of mood) reflect a loss of control over one's reactions or emotions.

Psychosocial Disabilities

These refer to alterations in everyday life as they pertain to social roles and responsibilities. Higher level roles and responsibilities include work, leisure and recreation, interpersonal relationships, and independent living. The cognitive, physical, and psychiatric difficulties described earlier could impair psychosocial functions, depending on their severity and their combination. Employment difficulties are common, particularly among those with severe head injury. Due to cognitive difficulties, the patient may be unable to perform the same job or, still worse, become unemployable. Difficulty interacting with employer or coworkers also occurs. Loss of ability to live independently forces dependence on the family or public assistance programs. Disruptions in recreation and leisure pursuits are often due to loss of peer relationships and the physical agility necessary for participation in premorbid physical recreational activities. Finally, social and interpersonal relationships are frequently impaired or lost. Further, patients experience difficulties cultivating new friendships. Parents, usually mothers, assume the multiple responsibilities and the great burden.

═══ Management

The goal of rehabilitation is to achieve the highest level of functioning and independence possible in mobility, self-care, age-appropriate level of independent living, education, work, recreation, and interpersonal relationships. Ideally, the goal is to resume preinjury activities and responsibilities. The general approach to achieving this end is to facilitate recovery in the injured individual, and/or to alter the environment to accommodate those losses that are either permanent or only very slowly reversible. The highest level of functioning being the goal, and the target of treatment extending beyond the injured individual, the task of the treatment team is to carefully determine the following:

1. those premorbid activities and responsibilities that the individual is expected to perform;
2. injury-related impairments, and their implications for resuming prior activities;
3. prognosis as to whether and when the individual will be able to resume prior activities; and
4. available social and financial resources.

Injury-related losses need to be explored in the areas of physical and motor skills (e.g., ambulation, balance), self-care (e.g., dressing, feeding), communication (e.g., read, write), cognition (e.g., memory, reasoning), emotional status (e.g., depression, emotional lability), major role (e.g.,work, school, homemaking), leisure activities (e.g., sports, reading), and relationships with others (e.g., family, friends). After the evaluation process, the task of the rehabilitation team is to integrate the information gathered in order to formulate reachable goals and treatment plans to attain them. Periodically, briefer forms of evaluation are repeated to monitor progress and adjust goals.

The diversity of consequences that follow head injury may affect all aspects of life and requires the efforts of a multidisciplinary team. Depending on the severity and characteristics of the injury, as well as the preinjury activities and responsibilities of the injured individual, the treatment goals may include maximizing functions in motor skills (e.g., range of motion, balance, etc.), independent mobility, self-care, independent living, cognitive functions, interpersonal and social skills, vocational activities, and leisure activities.

The basic principles of treatment include the following:

1. affecting a close match between what is expected of the patient and his or her actual capabilities;
2. a gradual increase in demands imposed on the patient based on the successful performance of prior simpler steps;
3. retraining and/or facilitating the recovery of lost functions (e.g., strength, memory, balance);
4. if lost function is not recovered, capitalizing on strengths to cover for weaknesses (e.g., use of memory books, use of verbal mediation in pathfinding to compensate for disorientation in space);
5. use of environmental manipulations and restructuring to maximize function, (e.g., creating a simple, structured, and predictable environment to improve the orientation of severely impaired patients);
6. multiple practice trials on the to-be-learned tasks to improve speed, efficiency, and safety;
7. use of environmental aids to maximize independence when indicated (e.g., wheelchair mobility if walking is not possible); and

8. making treatment goals relevant to the needs of the patient in real life, and making sure that the gains made in the program are transferred to the outside.

During the inpatient rehabilitation stay, the focus is on getting medical aspects under control, improving mobility, and basic self-care skills. The focus of outpatient care tends more toward psychosocial issues and the reintegration of the patient into the community.

References

1. Dikmen S, Temkin N, Miller B, Machamer J, Winn HR. Neurobehavioral effects of phenytoin prophylaxis of post-traumatic seizures. *JAMA* 265:1271–1277, 1991.
2. Temkin N, Dikmen S, Keihm J, Wilensky AJ, Winn HR. A randomized double-blind study of phenytoin for prevention of post-traumatic seizures. *N Engl J Med* 323:497–502, 1990.

Annotated Suggested Reading List

Cooper PR (ed.). *Head injury* (3d ed.). Baltimore, Williams & Wilkins, 1993.
This book contains the latest theoretical and practical information relevant to the acute management of head-injured patients.
DePompei R, Blosser JL (Issue Eds.). School reentry following head injury. *J Head Trauma Rehab* 6(1). Frederick, MD, Aspen Publishers, 1991.
A compilation of articles covering school reintegration for the child with traumatic brain injury.
Dikmen S, Machamer J, Savoie T, Temkin N. Life quality outcome in head injury. In: Adams KM, Grant I (Eds.), *Neuropsychological assessment of neuropsychiatric disorders*. New York, Oxford University Press, (in press, 1994).
This chapter reviews information available on psychosocial (everyday life) outcome in adults and attempts to identify gaps in the literature.
Dikmen S, Levin HS. Methodological issues in the study of mild head injury. *J Head Trauma Rehab* 1993;8(3):30-37.
Dikmen SS, Machamer JE, Winn TR, Temkin NR. Neuropsychological outcome at 1 year post head injury. *Neuropsychology* (in press, 1994).
This paper provides 1-year neuropsychological outcome data for a large representative group of head-injured patients.
Jaffe KM (Issue Ed.). Pediatric head injury. *J Head Trauma Rehab* 1(4). Frederick, MD, Aspen Publishers, 1986.
Jaffe KM (Guest Ed.). Traumatic brain injury. *Pediatric Annals* 23 (1). Thorofare, NJ: SLACK, Inc., 1994.
Two compilations of articles covering many important aspects of pediatric head injury.
Levin HS, Grafman J, Eisenberg HM (Eds.), *Neurobehavioral recovery from head injury*. New York, Oxford University Press, 1987.
This book contains recent research on neurobehavioral outcome of head injury.
Levin HS, Eisenberg HM, Benton JL (Eds.), *Mild head injury*. New York, Oxford University Press, 1987.
This book contains a comprehensive discussion of current advances in the understanding, treatment, and management of mild head injury.

Rosenthal M, Griffith ER, Bond MR, Miller JD (Eds.), *Rehabilitation of the adult and child with traumatic brain injury* (2d ed.). Philadelphia, F.A. Davis, 1990.

A multi-authored authoritative text covering all aspects of head injury rehabilitation.

Ylvisaker M (Ed.). *Head injury rehabilitation: Children and adolescents.* San Diego, College Hill Press, 1985.

A practical guide for professionals seeking guidance on effective treatment strategies for children with head injuries.

12

Spinal Cord Injury

Catherine W. Britell, M.D., and
Margaret C. Hammond, M.D.

The rehabilitation of individuals with spinal cord injury (SCI) requires a well-coordinated, experienced interdisciplinary team, working in a setting that allows effective communication and interaction among team members. An SCI rehabilitation unit must be large enough to support the appropriate medical and rehabilitative programs as well as a social milieu that will achieve the goals of optimal health maintenance, maximal independent function, and effective psychosocial and vocational adaptation.

Incidence, Etiology, and Life Expectancy

Traumatic spinal cord injury occurs in approximately 55 people per million per year, 35 of whom survive to undergo rehabilitation. Nontraumatic injury, mostly due to cancer, is approximately twice as frequent and is seen primarily in patients over age 40. Almost half of all traumatic injuries occur in young people between age 15 and 24. Of these patients, 82 percent are male, with nonwhite men more heavily represented than in the general population. Forty-six percent of traumatic spinal cord injuries are the result of automobile accidents, with falls (16 percent), stab and gunshot wounds (12 percent), and diving accidents (10 percent) being less common etiologies.

Life expectancy after SCI has increased significantly over the past 10 years. Overall life expectancy is now 85 percent that of the general population. The major cause of death in SCI is pulmonary disease, with cardiovascular disease and genitourinary infection in fewer numbers.

Mechanisms of Neural Injury

The spinal cord is well protected by the bones, ligaments, and muscles surrounding the vertebral canal; SCI is therefore usually a result of significant trauma, with concomitant fracture and/or dislocation of vertebrae. This trauma usually results in instability of the spinal column; therefore, the spinal cord is particularly susceptible to further injury until either surgical or external stabilization has been accomplished.

When the spinal cord is injured, the release of multiple tissue factors causes edema and the acute inflammatory response. Edema usually peaks at 48–72 hrs, after which there is often some early recovery. One focus of current research is evaluation of various medications to decrease early edema and inflammation.

During the first few days to weeks after injury, there are no reflexes below the level of the lesion. This condition is called "spinal shock." When spinal shock resolves, reflexes return in muscles whose lower motor neurons are intact. This usually occurs when the bony injury is above T12, and is termed an *upper motor neuron lesion*. If the bony injury is at T12 or below, the conus medullaris or cauda equina is frequently injured, and reflexes in the lower extremities often do not return. This is termed a *lower motor neuron lesion*. Likewise, a lower motor neuron lesion can occur above this level if there is a multilevel crush injury of the cord. Spinal cord injuries may be complete, with total sensory and motor loss below the level of the lesion, or may be incomplete. Incomplete lesions may fall into any one of the following syndrome categories:

- Brown-Sequard Syndrome—Hemisection of the cord, with motor loss on the opposite side of the lesion, and sensory loss on the same side.

- Anterior Spinal Artery Syndrome—Lesion, usually by infarction, of the anterior half of the cord, resulting in loss of motor and some sensory function and preservation of position and vibratory sense.

- Dorsal Column Syndrome—Lesion of the posterior section of the cord, with loss of position and vibratory sense.

- Central Cord Syndrome—An injury, usually in the cervical area, of the central part of the cord, which usually results in greater weakness of the arms than of the legs, and often spares the sacral segments, which control bladder and bowel functions.

The motor level of the injury is defined as the lowest level at which useful motor function is spared. If the motor level is T1 or below, the condition is arbitrarily termed *paraplegia,* and if C8 or above, it is termed *quadriplegia* or *tetraplegia.*

After injury, the care of the individual with SCI falls into four overlapping phases: acute care, rehabilitation, treatment of medical complications, and sustaining health maintenance and ongoing maximization of function.

Acute Care

Because the patient with SCI has often sustained multiple trauma, initial management frequently includes establishment of an adequate airway and respira-

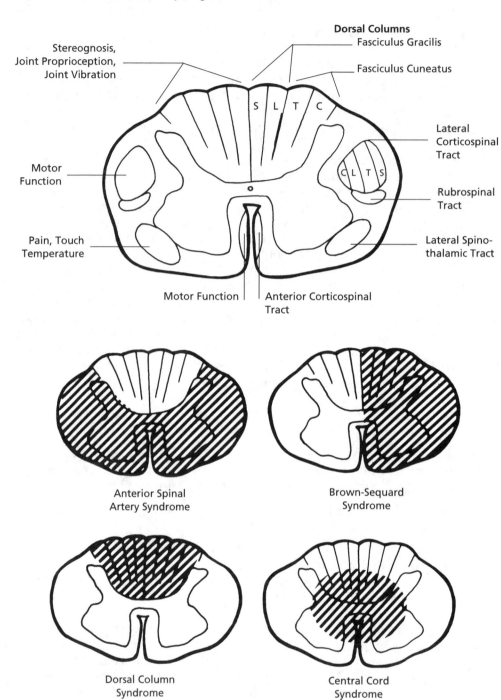

FIGURE 12.1.

tory support as necessary, hemodynamic resuscitation, management of other bony and visceral injuries, adequate bladder drainage, and careful maintenance of position of the unstable spine. For cervical fractures, application of traction via tongs inserted into the skull and management on a rotating bed or frame is performed while the patient's medical condition is stabilized. For thoracic and lumbar fractures, management on a frame or careful log-rolling on a bed is necessary to prevent further injury. Diagnosis of the bony and neural lesion is an early priority. Myelogram/computerized tomography and/or magnetic resonance imaging is routinely performed as soon as the patient is adequately resuscitated to tolerate these procedures. Careful daily neurologic examinations are essential for ongoing management decisions.

In the first hours to days following injury, attention to the following areas of concern will prevent further morbidity.

RESPIRATORY MANAGEMENT

Patients with cervical and high thoracic lesions will have some degree of respiratory compromise. Respiratory function in these patients is further threatened if there is an associated chest injury. A baseline chest X-ray and arterial blood gas determination, along with daily monitoring of breath sounds and bedside spirometry are indicated in order to ensure adequate ventilation.

Generally, a pCO_2 of greater than 40 mm Hg or vital capacity below 1000 suggests that ventilatory assistance may be needed. With all acute patients who are immobilized, aggressive pulmonary management by experienced nursing staff will be necessary to prevent atelectasis and resultant complications.

GASTROINTESTINAL CARE

Often there is an acute paralytic ileus, either from the spinal cord injury itself or from abdominal trauma. Because untreated trauma to the spleen or pancreas can prove fatal, one must first rule out these conditions in an acutely injured patient with abdominal distension.

If distension occurs, nasogastric intubation and gentle suction with careful fluid and electrolyte replacement are indicated. When there is no significant abdominal trauma, ileus usually resolves within a few days following injury. In cases of persistent uncomplicated ileus, a trial of metaclopromide may be indicated.

Another problem frequently seen, especially in those injured above the T5 level, is gastric ulceration and bleeding due to increased acid secretion, which is a result of unopposed vagal parasympathetic activity. The stool should be regularly tested for occult blood, and routine administration of cimetidine or ranitidine is generally carried out for the first 6 weeks following injury.

The stool must be evacuated routinely to maintain regular emptying and continence between planned bowel movements. This is best accomplished by daily bowel care, usually carried out shortly after breakfast or the evening meal, using digital stimulation and often aided by a bisacodyl suppository.

GENITOURINARY CARE

During the period of spinal shock, there is no reflex emptying of the bladder. The bladder must therefore be emptied mechanically in order to prevent over-stretching, urinary stasis, infection, and kidney damage. This is initially done by means of an indwelling catheter and closed drainage system.

When the patient is stable, generally not receiving IV fluid and medications, and able to maintain a steady oral intake, intermittent catheterization is initiated. At least 24 hours before beginning intermittent catheterization, the patient should be placed on a schedule of fluid intake of approximately 1600 ml per day: 300 ml with each meal and 240 ml each midmorning, midafternoon, and early evening (or alternatively may drink 100 ml per hour while awake). When a steady output pattern is achieved, intermittent catheterization using sterile technique is begun, starting at every 4 hours and adjusting intervals to achieve volumes of approximately 300–400 ml per catheterization (never exceeding 500 ml).

Urine cultures are followed on a regular basis. At this time there is no evidence that antibiotic prophylaxis or treatment of asymptomatic bacteriuria are effective in preventing serious infections or renal damage. If there is fever or leukocytosis, however, prompt, specific treatment is indicated.

SKIN CARE

A number of factors combine to make the acutely injured patient particularly susceptible to skin breakdown:

- lack of normal innervation of the skin and underlying blood vessels;
- hemodynamic instability and resultant periods of hypoperfusion; and
- the necessity of immobilization to attain spinal stability

In the acute phase, the sacrum, heels, and back of the head are areas at highest risk if the patient is lying supine; and the trochanters, knees, and malleoli take the greatest pressure when side lying. For patients with cervical fractures who are managed in tongs, skin integrity can be maintained by use of a constantly rotating bed or a stationary frame that can be turned to position the patient prone or supine.

If the patient has a thoracic or lumbar fracture or the neck has been stabilized adequately, careful positioning on a bed with a 4-inch foam pad over the mattress and turning every 2 hours by log-rolling will effectively prevent sores. Although a number of devices are available for pressure reduction and protection of skin, a program of careful positioning and bridging with pillows and frequent turning remains the most effective management approach.

VENOUS STASIS PREVENTION

Deep venous thrombosis and pulmonary embolism pose a significant threat in the first 3 months following injury. Regular calf and thigh measurement should be instituted immediately. A difference of greater than 1 centimeter is suggestive of a thrombus and requires further evaluation. A baseline duplex scan will often allow later noninvasive diagnosis if lower extremity swelling occurs. Contrast venography is relatively contraindicated because of its resultant irritation and inherent throm-bogenicity in this population, and is performed only when there is a contraindica-tion to anticoagulation and a definitive diagnosis cannot be made as required with the noninvasive tests. In general, prophylactic low-dose heparin is given subcuta-neously. Light support stockings are also routinely used, and many practitioners also favor the use of external pneumatic calf compression for prophylaxis. If a venous thrombus is diagnosed, full anticoagulation is undertaken with heparin, and sub-sequently with coumadin for 8–12 weeks post-injury. For venous thrombosis, anti-coagulation is usually continued for 3 months. If a pulmonary embolus is diag-nosed, anticoagulation is generally recommended for 6 months.

MAINTENANCE OF RANGE OF MOTION (ROM)

In order to prevent unwanted contractures, it is necessary that each extremity is brought through its complete range of motion twice daily by nursing and physi-cal therapy staff. This is usually done in the process of bathing or repositioning. During the first few weeks, spinal instability may impose limitations to complete ranging. Specifically, any twisting motions or asymmetrical movement of arms or legs are usually contraindicated while a spinal orthosis is in place. It is therefore necessary that spine stability precautions be determined and documented at the outset and periodically as the patient progresses. In some muscle groups, some degree of tightness is necessary for function, and so it is important that they not be overstretched. For example, in quadriplegics, it is important that some mild contracture of the finger flexors takes place in order to maintain an adequate grip; finger flexors must therefore never be taken through the full range of motion. Likewise, some tightness of hamstrings and lumbar paraspinals is necessary to maintain a good sitting posture and to keep the patient from falling forward while doing activities in the long-sitting position. Over-stretching of the ham-strings may severely inhibit independence in dressing activities and transfers.

SPINE STABILIZATION AND ORTHOSES

In order for mobilization and active rehabilitation to progress, the spine must be sta-bilized either surgically or by the use of an external fixation device. If initial evalu-ation shows bone or disk fragments in the spinal canal or of it is determined that proper alignment and healing is unlikely without surgery, an open reduction and fusion is usually performed. Following surgery, the patient is maintained in some sort of orthosis, usually for 2–3 months, depending on the degree of instability, the type of surgery performed, and the rate of healing. If surgery is not performed, the orthosis will be worn 3+ months following injury, depending on the injury and rate of healing. The types of orthoses most often used are the following:

Mid Thoracic to Lumbar Fractures—

A custom-molded TLSO (thoraco-lumbar-sacral orthosis) is a specially mold-ed plastic body jacket worn 24 hrs per day for 3 to 4 months until fusion is assured. It must be closely fitted over the sternum, pubic rami, and iliac crests to prevent thoracolumbar and pelvic motion.

High Thoracic Fractures (T5 and Above)—

A custom-molded TLSO with cervical extension is used because the high thoracic area cannot be controlled with neck movement. Fractures in this area require control of cervical flexion, extension, and rotation by use of the SOMI extension.

Cervical Fractures—

A halo vest, consisting of a ring with four bolts fixed into the skull attached firmly to a molded polypropylene thoracic jacket, provides the best stabilization for closed reduction or postoperative use when spine position is critical. It is usually worn 2–3 months, after which progression to a Philadelphia or soft cervical collar and then gradual weaning from cervical support is done.

There are a number of types of SOMI (sternal occipital mandibular immobilizer) available, the most frequently seen being the Minerva brace. The degree of immobilization provided depends on how closely fitted it is and varies inversely with how much mandibular motion is allowed. It is usually worn for 2-3 months until the fracture is healed. Temporomandibular joint pain is a frequent complication of its use.

The Philadelphia collar gives support but not immobilization. It is often used for those who will remain inactive until the fracture is healed or for whom immobilization is less important than support and protection from extreme movements.

The soft cervical collar may be used for neck protection and to prevent fatigue when another orthosis is being discontinued.

All spinal orthoses must be checked regularly for skin tolerance, and appropriate adjustments made whenever persistent erythema is discovered.

When the patient is in a spinal orthosis, precautions as regards spine stability usually include the following:

- All active motions should be performed bilaterally and symmetrically.
- An overhead trapeze should not be used on the bed.
- Independent rolling should not be done.
- Supervised falling and recovery from the floor should not be started until orthosis is no longer required.

===== Rehabilitation

The purpose of rehabilitation is to allow the patient to independently manage excretory function, skin care, and activities of daily living; to understand health promotion and prevention of complications as they apply to the specific needs of the person with SCI; and to maximize independent personal and community mobility, psychosocial and sexual function, and independent living and vocational potential.

Rehabilitation should start immediately after injury, with staff carefully explaining all treatments, bringing the patient in on decision making, and encouraging the patient to assist as much as possible with feeding, self-care, and hygiene activities. The degree of functional independence attainable by a patient with optimal rehabilitation depends primarily upon his or her neurologic level, as summarized in Table 12.1.

Other important factors in determining outcome are age, general health, family and social support systems, educational level, and preinjury personality and coping styles. A person who has been employed and has a secure place in the family and community generally has a better prognosis for independent living, health maintenance, and vocational rehabilitation than one who has had a dysfunctional lifestyle prior to his or her injury.

MOBILITY

The patient should be gotten out of bed as soon as spine stability and skin integrity allow. Initial mobilization should be in a manual reclining wheelchair with elevating leg rests. Postural hypotension should be anticipated, particularly in lesions above T6, and can be minimized by the use of support hose and Ace wraps, and by slowly progressing the patient to the upright position with feet initially elevated.

It is imperative that a cushion with maximal pressure relief be used during initial mobilization and that sitting times start very short (15 minutes) and progress slowly, with regular skin checks. Dependent pressure relief (by tipping the wheelchair carefully backward or reclining the back fully) should be done every 10 minutes until the patient is able to manage this consistently in an independent fashion. When the patient is able to sit in a wheelchair for 30–45 minutes at a time, active therapy programming can begin, working toward functional goals.

Mobility training may be limited at first by spine stability considerations as outlined above, so any necessary precautions must be carefully determined and documented before beginning. Mobility training usually progresses from bed mobility and transfers to wheelchair mobility and ambulation as the neurologic level allows. Integral to this process is teaching the patient to take responsibility for maintenance of range of motion by regular stretching and protection of his or her joints and extremities. At the same time, careful reeducation and strengthening of remaining muscles, as well as exercise conditioning, will allow the patient to maximally take advantage of his or her remaining neurologic function.

Community mobility is an important part of mobility training. The patient must learn how to plan travel within the community, using accessible routes and public transportation. Driver evaluation and training should also be undertaken if possible during the initial hospitalization, because this is important aspect of social functioning and employability.

ACTIVITIES OF DAILY LIVING

Simple tasks, such as self-feeding and basic hygiene, should be started while the patient is still in bed. A call system that the patient can operate independently is an essential first step in giving the patient control of his or her environment. Other bedside devices to control radio, television, and telephone are also useful in establishing a constructively independent attitude early on.

TABLE 12.1

Functional Spinal Cord Levels

NEURAL SEGMENT(S) AND FUNCTIONAL SIGNIFICANCE	IMPORTANT MUSCLES	RESULTANT MOVEMENTS
C1, C2 Uses mouthstick, head pointer, chin drive	Upper cervical muscles	Head control
C3, C4 Breathes without ventilator	Diaphragm	Inspiration
C5 Uses joystick to control wheelchair; feeds self, manipulates switches and keyboard with cuff or splint	Deltoid Biceps	Shoulder flexion and abduction Elbow flexion
C6 Positions hand precisely; forms tenodesis grip; writes, performs most ADLs; may use manual wheelchair; often drives van with lift	Pronator teres Extensor carpi radialis	Wrist pronation Wrist extension
C7 Transfers independently; independent in all ADLs; drives automobile	Triceps Extensor digitorum communis	Elbow extension Finger extension
C8 More precise manipulation of objects; slow keyboarding; strong grip	Flexor digitorum superficialis Opponens pollicis	Finger flexion Thumb opposition
T1 Precise keyboarding; playing musical instruments	Interossei	Finger abduction and adduction
T2–T6 Better pulmonary function	Intercostals	Forced inspiration; Expiration
T7–T12 Normal respiratory function; effective cough; good trunk stability; functional swing-through gait with KAFOs	Intercostals Abdominals	Forced inspiration; Expiration Trunk flexion
L1–L3 Reciprocal gait with KAFOs	Iliopsoas Adductors	Hip flexion Hip adduction
L3, L4 Gait with AFOs, crutches; wheelchair may not be needed	Quadriceps	Knee extension

(cont'd.)

Neural Segment(s) and Functional Significance	Important Muscles	Resultant Movements
L5–S1 Gait without orthoses or crutches; wheelchair usually unnecessary	Gluteus medius Tibialis anterior	Hip abduction Foot dorsiflexion
S1, S2 Running, jumping, climbing	Gluteus maximus Gastrocnemius	Hip extension Foot plantar flexion
S2, S3, S4 Normal excretory and sexual function	Anal and urethral sphincters	Bowel and bladder control

The patient should learn to be as independent in all aspects of self-care as possible, even if it would be more efficient to have an attendant perform many care activities, because the greater level of independence will allow greater self-esteem and make the patient more able to direct personal care and take charge of his or her lifestyle. In the course of rehabilitation, the occupational therapist and other rehabilitation members may also prescribe various assistive devices to enhance independence in self-care, care of the environment, and vocational ability. These may be as simple as a cuff to grasp pencils or spoons or as complex as a voice-actuated, personal computer-based robotic arm, with environmental control, communication, and other PC functions. Evaluation and modification of the home environment is an important part of the rehabilitative process and should be accomplished as soon as the eventual level of function is clear, so that essential modifications can be completed by the time of discharge.

BLADDER MANAGEMENT

The goal of bladder management is to attain continence or containment of the urinary flow with regular, complete, low-pressure emptying and to prevent infections.

Generally, indwelling catheters should be avoided if possible, because they are associated with chronic bacterial colonization, a higher rate of upper tract infection and renal damage, and a significantly increased risk of bladder cancer. Initially, the patient is managed in the hospital with regular sterile intermittent catheterization. The patient should take over this function as early as possible if hand function allows or, if not, should keep track of drinking and voiding schedules and be able to direct the process.

In patients with lesions above the sacral levels, as spinal shock resolves and reflexes return, there will be a return of reflex voiding. A major problem that often occurs at that time is detrusor-sphincter dyssynergy, which is characterized by simultaneous contraction of the detrusor and sphincter. This results in sustained high intravesicular pressures, hydronephrosis, and renal failure. A careful evaluation, including neurological examination, cystometrogram with sphincter EMG, and voiding cystourethrogram using X-ray contrast or ultrasound imaging,

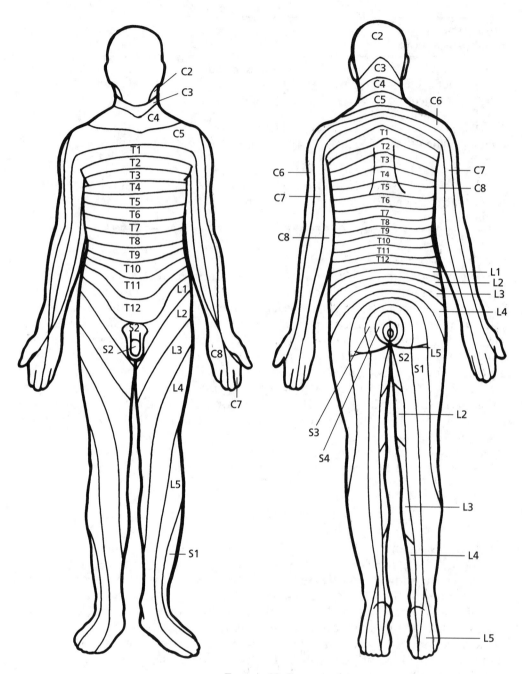

FIGURE 12.2

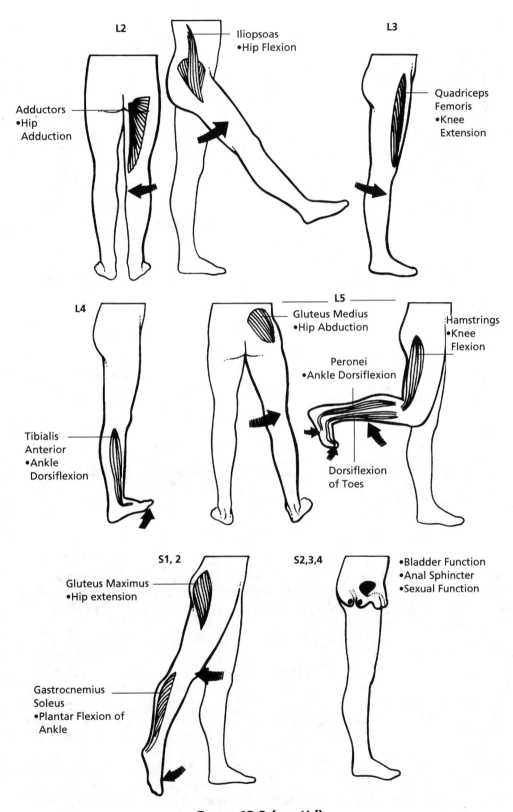

FIGURE 12.2 (cont'd)

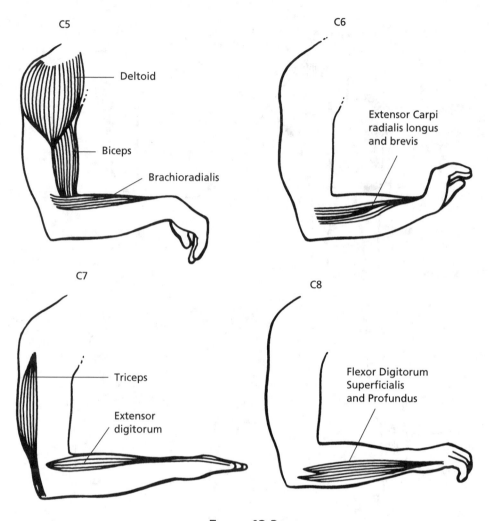

FIGURE 12.3

will assist in determining the best bladder emptying system for the patient. When this has been determined, the rehabilitation team will assist the patient and family in assuming independent management of bladder emptying and monitoring of function.

BOWEL CARE

In order to attain independent bowel control, the patient first must regulate diet and fluid intake, learning especially to avoid foods that produce diarrhea. Daily or every-other-day emptying is necessary to preserve rectal tone and prevent impaction or accidents. Bowel care is usually done after breakfast or dinner, on a toilet or commode-shower chair if possible. Evacuation is stimulated by stretching of the anal sphincter with a gloved finger, sometimes aided by a bisacodyl or carbon dioxide suppository if necessary. If adequate emptying is achieved, the patient will remain continent until the next bowel care is done. Sometimes a high-fiber diet, soluble fiber supplements, or stool softeners will aid in making the stools more manageable. Regular use of laxatives should be avoided.

SKIN CARE

Careful and effective attention to skin integrity is one of the most important skills learned in rehabilitation. First, the seating system must allow independent pressure relief, either through weight shift or a powered recline system. Measurement of pressures during sitting and weight shifting can be useful in determining the optimal weight shifting routine and teaching the patient the effect of sitting in various positions. It is important to teach the patient that no cushion or mattress can prevent pressure sores without regular weight shifts. Regular skin inspection using a mirror should be instituted early. The patient must be carefully instructed to get off the affected area if any persistent redness occurs, and stay off that area until the skin has returned to normal. Other concerns, such as proper hygiene, clothing, and care in transfers, must also become a part of the patient's behavior.

SEXUALITY AND REPRODUCTION

Sexual function, innervated at the same level as the bladder and bowels, is most often disturbed to some degree in individuals with spinal cord injury. Because sensation is abnormal or absent, orgasms are not experienced as they were before the injury, although many people report pleasant sensations and definite feelings of sexual release.

Three to 6 months following spinal injury, women begin to menstruate and are normally fertile. Normal vaginal deliveries are possible and usually done with ease except in high quadriplegics who may experience severe autonomic hyperreflexia.

For males, sexual and reproductive function is usually more significantly impaired. Approximately 54–87 percent of men are able to achieve erections after spinal cord injury, but they are often not sufficient for successful coitus. Only 10–20 percent ejaculate, and fewer than 5 percent are able to father children. This fertility impairment is due to a number of factors, including retrograde ejaculation into the bladder and poor sperm function due to chronic infection. Sperm collection using vibratory or electrical stimulation has been somewhat successful, particularly in those individuals with high incomplete cord lesions. A number of techniques and devices are available to enhance erections, including external prostheses, intracorporeally implanted devices, and injections to achieve erections. Any of these techniques should be part of a comprehensive interdisciplinary program of education and counseling, and the patient and significant other should have a careful psychological evaluation to explore their possible negative emotional and relational effects.

Following SCI, it is necessary for the patient to learn that many aspects of sexuality, including attractiveness, arousal, and the excitement of a positive relationship, are not altered by the injury. They will need to redefine the physical aspects of sexual functioning to complement a normal, healthy, positive attitude toward their sexuality. Rehabilitation programs should include effective education and counseling toward that goal.

PSYCHOLOGICAL FUNCTIONING

The process of adapting to the changes brought about by SCI is one that is ongoing. Most patients go through a "mourning" for lost function, including feelings of shock, denial, anger and hostility, depression and hopelessness, and finally reach a constructive acceptance of their condition. Some, however, do not evidence these feelings, but simply get on with rehabilitation and putting their lives back together. It is the job of the rehabilitation team to be sensitive to patients' reactions and to help them work through expected negative feelings to develop a positive attitude about themselves and their lives. Occasionally a patient will require ongoing, intensive psychotherapy to deal with these issues. The rehabilitation psychologist will be able to identify and treat these patients and also provide leadership to the rest of the rehabilitation team in providing a generally sensitive, appropriately supportive environment.

SOCIAL AND FAMILY FUNCTIONING

Family and community support are essential to the patient's successful reintegration into the independent setting. While the rehabilitation team is trying to promote independence and self-sufficiency, the family may at the same time have difficulty letting go of their loved one, who has been so severely hurt. Furthermore, the patient, who may have once held a place of authority and responsibility in the family, is now seen as an "invalid," incapable of contributing and being in control. Often the psychosocial team can be helpful in counseling the patient and family to support reestablishment of a positive role for the patient.

The practical matters faced by the patient and family may be overwhelming. The loss of income, accessibility needs, and physical care needs with which they are now presented will require a great deal of effort and adjustment. The social worker can be of great help to the patient and family in threading their way through agencies and bureaucracies in order to reestablish a functioning household.

VOCATIONAL REHABILITATION

Although vocational rehabilitation as such can rarely begin during the initial hospitalization, the idea of working again should be presented to the patient early and often. As functional goals are achieved through rehabilitation, it becomes more clear to the patient what he or she can do, and constructive planning for resuming work can be done. Before leaving the hospital, a plan for liaison with a vocational rehabilitation agency at a specific future time should be in place.

===== Medical Complications of Spinal Cord Injury

During and following the rehabilitative phase of treatment, a number of complications specific to SCI can occur. Prompt recognition and treatment of complications will allow the patient to continue maximal healthy functioning.

Autonomic Hyperreflexia

This condition occurs in quadriplegics and paraplegics with lesions above T6. It is characterized by a sudden onset of headache and hypertension, and may also have associated bradycardia, sweating, piloerection, nasal stuffiness, dilated pupils, or blurred vision. Because the hypertension can reach dangerous levels, this condition constitutes a medical emergency. The etiology of AH is the sympathetic reaction to noxious stimuli coming into the lower segments of the spinal cord. It is most often caused by bladder distension, and relieving the distension will usually alleviate the problem. Less frequently, AH occurs with bowel distension, injury to the lower extremities, or other causes. If the condition persists after emptying the bladder, control of the blood pressure by sublingual nifedipine followed by a methodical diagnostic and treatment process is indicated.

Spasticity

After spinal shock has subsided, the return of reflexes may be accompanied by increased muscle tone and severe hyperreflexia, caused by lack of upper motor neuron inhibition of the normal postural, protective, and stretch reflexes. Although spasticity can sometimes be useful in maintaining muscle tone, it often gets in the way of normal function and can make prevention of contractures very difficult. Generally, the first line of treatment for spasticity is regular adequate stretching. The muscle tone in spastic patients often subsides significantly after stretching. Useful medications include baclofen, diazepam, and clonidine. Because diazepam is a depressant and is addictive, it is usually added last to the regimen when the other two medications do not provide adequate control. With disabling spasticity that persists despite medications, early trials suggest that intrathecal baclofen via an implanted pump may be beneficial.

In cases of severe spasticity in nonfunctional limbs that significantly impairs positioning and overall function, many patients have benefited from a Bischoff's myelotomy, which consists of interrupting the connections between the sensory and motor portions of the reflex arc in the spinal cord. It is important to reassure the patient that the spasticity in itself is not a dangerous or negative thing unless it impairs function or positioning, and can simply be ignored if it is mild.

Heterotopic ossification (HO)

This is an extra-osseous collection of calcium usually in the tissues surrounding the hip, which has been reported to occur in 16–53 percent of patients following SCI. Rarely, it can occur in the knee, shoulder, or elbow as well. Its etiology is unknown. It is usually noted between 1 and 4 months following injury, and is characterized by swelling, increased temperature and possibly erythema of the affected joint, loss of range of motion, pain if sensation is spared, and frequently fever. HO can be mistaken for deep venous thrombosis or can coexist with DVT, so that condition must always be ruled out.

Hematoma, infection, and tumor are other possible diagnoses that can cause the same findings. X-rays will be positive only in the later stages after significant ossification has already taken place. The three-phase bone scan will be positive much earlier, and the serum alkaline phosphatase will be elevated during the active phase.

When HO is diagnosed, gentle but complete range of motion should be continued, and treatment with oral disodium etrodionate should be initiated.

PAIN

Almost all patients have abnormal sensations below the level of injury following SCI. Most patients learn to interpret these as a normal consequence of the neural injury and learn to ignore them. There are a number of patients, however, who interpret these sensations as frank pain, some of whom become severely disabled by chronic pain behavior and drug-seeking activities. The majority of these problems can be avoided by careful attention to pain management in the acute phase.

Directly following injury, many patients experience the expected post-traumatic pain and are treated with narcotic medications. At this time, it is crucial to carefully educate the patient to discern between true painful sensations and abnormal sensations or fear of pain. It is also important to be aware that short-acting narcotics can be a source of pain in themselves and that the patient may experience frequent relative withdrawal. Therefore, if the acute patient is requiring regular pain medications, it is often helpful to use a pain cocktail containing methadone, slowly decreasing the narcotic until it is discontinued.

For patients who present with chronic pain, tricyclic antidepressants are often the most useful medication. It is wise to avoid narcotics in these patients, because their effectiveness is limited. If pain behavior or drug addiction is established, a program of ongoing psychotherapy and physical treatment, including an exercise conditioning program, are indicated.

POST-TRAUMATIC SYRINGOMYELIA

This condition is a collection of fluid within the spinal cord at the site of injury that can dissect in either direction and cause further neural damage. It has been reported to occur between 6 months and many years following injury. The incidence of syringomyelia is suspected to be as high as 15–20 percent, but it is functionally significant in only 1–3 percent of individuals.

Pain and numbness are the most frequent presenting symptoms, with weakness appearing much later. Diagnosis is made by magnetic resonance imaging, and surgical treatment by drainage and shunting has resulted in resolution or at least stabilization of symptoms in some patients.

===== Sustaining Care of the Spinal Cord Injury Patient

The individual who has had a spinal cord injury has a number of unique medical problems that require ongoing care and monitoring. A careful program of preventive care will have a significant benefit to general health, physical function, and social and vocational effectiveness. Each individual with a spinal cord injury should have access to a primary care provider who understands the medical considerations particular to SCI and who is comfortable with patients with significant physical disability. Regular health maintenance screening should be done annually, or more often if there are specific problems. In addition to the usual adult health concerns, annual evaluation of the genitourinary system should include a sensitive measure of renal function, imaging of the urinary tract, and evaluation of voiding pressure and efficacy, as well as appropriate cancer screening. Because respiratory failure is the most common cause of death, pulmonary function should be monitored and screening for sleep apnea should be done. A neurologic exam, including careful sensory and motor testing and grip and pinch measurement, should be done yearly as well. A rehabilitative evaluation is indicated to determine whether functional independence is maximized, whether equipment is up-to-date and working well, and whether ongoing progress has continued as expected. At the same time, if psychosocial and vocational needs are identified, appropriate referrals can be made.

===== Conclusion

Spinal cord injury presents the health-care provider with an interesting and challenging set of problems and a unique opportunity to help people. Care of the SCI patient is an ongoing commitment, and the rewards to the practitioner increase as the health care relationship continues over the years. With optimal interdisciplinary care, the individual who has sustained a spinal cord injury can lead a full, healthy, productive, and rewarding life.

===== Annotated Suggested Reading List

Bromley I. *Tetraplegia and paraplegia: A guide for physical therapists* (2d Ed.). Edinburgh, Churchill Livingstone, 1981.
> A detailed "how-to" on maximization of muscular function and mobility, written for physical therapists, but also useful for physicians who must order or direct rehabilitative services.

Donovan WH, Bedbrook G. Comprehensive management of spinal cord injury. *CIBA Clinical Symposia* 34(2), 1982.
> A 36-page, well-illustrated introductory review of the medical considerations pertaining to spinal cord injury.

Hohmann GW. Psychological aspects of treatment and rehabilitation of the spinal cord injured person. *Clin Ortho* 112:81–88, 1975.
> Reviews in a sensitive and concise fashion the major psychological considerations in adapting to a spinal cord injury.

Merli, GT, Crabbe S, Paluzzi RG, Fritz D. Etiology, incidence, and prevention of deep vein thrombosis in acute spinal cord injury. *Arch Phys Med Rehabil* 74:1199–1205, 1993.

Staas WE, Formal CS, Gershkoff AM, et al. Rehabilitation of the spinal cord injured patient. In: DeLisa, JA (Ed.), *Rehabilitation medicine: Principles and practice.* Philadelphia, J.B. Lippincott, 1988.

This book chapter with 216 references covers most aspects of the medical and rehabilitative care of SCI.

Sugarman B, Brown D, Musher D. Fever and infection in spinal cord injury patients. *JAMA* 248:66–70, 1982.

This article concisely reviews the special considerations of evaluating the febrile spinal cord injured patient.

Trieschmann RB. *Aging with a disability.* New York, Demos, 1987.

A major portion of this book reviews the medical and psychological aspects of aging in the spinal cord injured patient.

Yashon D. *Spinal injury.* New York, Appleton-Century-Croft, 1978.

A comprehensive review of the surgical management of acute SCI, as well as related medical problems.

13

Low Back Pain

Stuart M. Weinstein, M.D.

Low back pain is pervasive. It is estimated that up to 80 percent of the world's adult population will experience at least one occurrence of low back pain in their lifetime. Various pain generators have been identified in the lumbar spine, including bone, soft tissue, and neurologic structures; yet the etiology of acute lumbar pain can be unclear. Further, as many as 70 percent of initial episodes of acute low back pain will resolve within three weeks, and 90 percent or more will resolve by three months. Temporally, persistent pain symptoms beyond twelve weeks defines a chronic process.

Chronic disease processes are usually associated with a variable degree of disability (i.e., impaired function) for work activities or activities of daily living. Disability due to low back pain predominates in Western, industrialized cultures. Under age 45, back pain is the most common disability in the industrial world, and it is the most expensive health care problem between the ages of 20 and 50. The estimated financial burden to society to manage low back pain has exceeded $50 billion per year in the 1990s. The relatively small percentage (i.e., less than 20 percent) of injured workers who remain off work more than 6 months accounts for nearly 80 percent of the total cost.

These sobering statistics have prompted extensive research in the past decade in such areas as risk factors for developing low back pain, psychosocial issues associated with persistent complaints of back pain and their contribution to delayed recovery, and treatment protocols for the management of low back pain. Medical factors identified to be positively associated with developing low back pain include poor cardiovascular fitness, a history of smoking, and prior back injury. The concept of low back "weakness" as a risk factor for injury is controversial; however, trunk strengthening definitely has a role in the rehabilitation process. The finding that psychosocial factors contribute to disability is commonly encountered when evaluating chronic low back pain, especially in the injured worker population. Understanding chronic low back disability as a syndrome—an aggregate of physical, psychological, and behavioral problems—rather than a single pathologic process may assist with treating this entity more appropriately and effectively.

Functional Anatomy

The lumbar spine is composed of a series of five articulated motion segments (Figure 13.1). Each consists of a three joint complex—one intervertebral disc situated anteriorly between the endplates of two adjacent vertebral bodies, and two facet joints posteriorly formed by the superior articular process of the vertebrae below and the inferior articular process of the vertebrae above. The disc is comprised of a central nucleus pulposus—a gel-like substance containing water, collagen fibers, and a mucopolysaccharide matrix—and the peripheral annulus fibrosis formed by concentric layers of obliquely oriented cartilaginous fibers. The facet joints are synovial in nature. Individual lumbar nerve roots exit bilaterally, just below the pedicle of each vertebral body and travel laterally a short distance in the

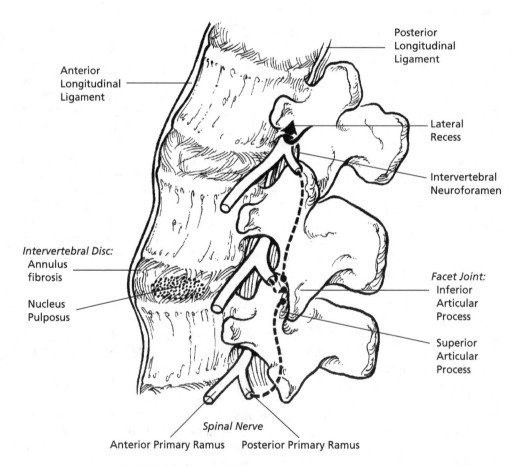

FIGURE 13.1. Lumbar motion segment—postero-lateral view.

intervertebral foramen before descending. The lateral recess should be differentiated from the intervertebral foramen, as the lateral-most portion within the spinal canal medial to the foramen. Lateral recess stenosis with nerve entrapment can occur.

Numerous structures intrinsic and extrinsic to the lumbar spine are innervated to varying degrees and thus can be pain-sensitive. Only the outer one third of the annulus fibrosis is innervated, whereas the remainder of the annulus and the entire nucleus pulposus are not. The lumbar facet joints are well innervated, with each joint receiving branches from up to three different segmental levels via the posterior primary rami. There also exists extensive ligamentous (i.e., posterior longitudinal ligament (PLL), anterior longitudinal ligament (ALL), ligamentum flavum (LF), supra- and interspinous ligaments (SSL, ISL) and muscular innervation (i.e., erector spinae and multifidi).

Normal lumbar spine motion includes flexion, extension, and axial rotation (i.e., torsion). Eighty to ninety percent of flexion and extension occurs at L5–S1 and L4–L5. Hip rotation contributes to full forward bending. The lumbar facet joints do not restrict motion in this sagittal plane, given their ninety degree orientation, but normally restrict rotation to two or three degrees, thereby protecting the disc. Control of the spinal mechanism is gained by the synergistic action of muscle and ligaments, with the primary goal of minimizing shear force at the intervertebral joint. This joint is subject to both compressive and shear loads. Compressive load is absorbed by the annulus fibrosis and vertebral body column. The nucleus pulposus is mostly ineffective in responding to acute loads, but assists in redistributing loads borne by the annulus. Intradiscal pressure varies with body position. Flexion oriented positions (i.e., sitting, bending, lifting) result in the greatest relative increase in pressure. In the setting of annular fiber disruption due to chronic or inadequate protection from shear stress, repetitive flexion loads may result in frank nucleus pulposus herniation through an incompetent annulus fibrosis. Thus, the system is most sensitive to shear, tolerates shear relatively poorly, and works to balance anterior and posterior shear forces at the intervertebral joint.

The hip extensors (i.e., gluteus maximus and hamstrings) produce the greatest extension force at the intervertebral joint. These muscles generate fifteen thousand inch-pounds of force, assisting in the maintenance of the upright posture, but they do not contribute much to counterbalance the anterior shear produced by lifting. The paraspinal muscles are weaker, due to their relatively shorter lever arms and small cross-sectional area, but their oblique orientation does provide a small component to posterior shear. The ligamentous system provides the greatest protection from shear loading. When passively stretched, the midline ligamentous structures (SSL, ISL, LF, PLL, and facet joint capsule) generate tension and posterior shear. However, activities that do not require lumbar flexion can inactivate the ligamentous contribution, as passive stretch does not occur and no tension is generated.

The trunk musculature, acting via the thoracolumbar fascia (TLF), can provide the counterbalancing extension force without developing shear stress (Figure 13.2). This mechanism is quite effective and can act regardless of the degree of spine flexion. Maintenance of intra-abdominal pressure and abdominal cavity dimensions is required to optimize the function of the internal oblique and transversus abdominis muscles. However, intra-abdominal pressure does not

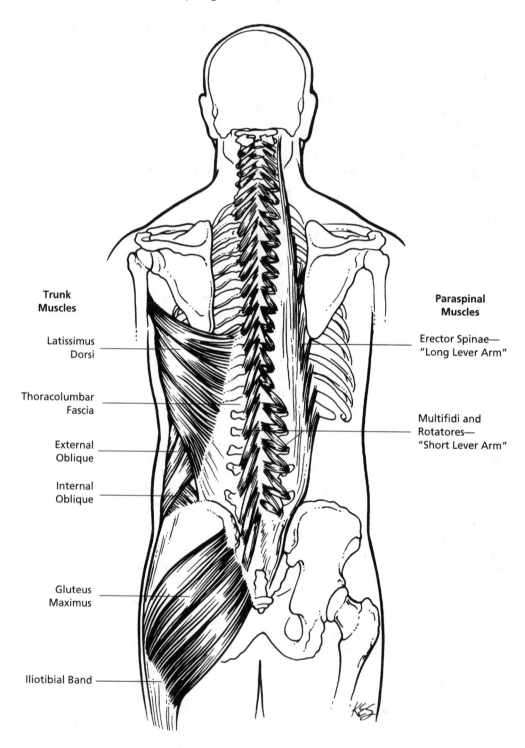

Trunk Muscles

Latissimus Dorsi

Thoracolumbar Fascia

External Oblique

Internal Oblique

Gluteus Maximus

Iliotibial Band

Paraspinal Muscles

Erector Spinae— "Long Lever Arm"

Multifidi and Rotatores— "Short Lever Arm"

FIGURE 13.2

itself decrease intradiscal pressure. It appears, therefore, that the combined stabilizing action of the trunk musculature and ligamentous structures is necessary for maximal lifting capacity and to minimize stress at the three joint complex.

Pathogenesis

The causes of low back pain are diverse and include many spinal and nonspinal etiologies. Pathologic and degenerative conditions involving the three joint complex are most common and will be addressed in detail. The differential diagnosis of low back pain, however, includes such entities as tumors, both benign and malignant (e.g., myeloma, metastases, neurofibroma), vascular disease (e.g., aortic aneurysm), inflammatory spondylopathy (e.g., sacroiliitis), gynecologic conditions (e.g., endometriosis), and other genitourinary or gastrointestinal illnesses. Understanding the natural history of degenerative lumbar spine disease assists with the proper diagnosis of various clinical presentations and the development of specific treatment plans. The lumbar spine motion segment will inevitably undergo degenerative change, frequently accelerated by traumatic events. Many early episodes of back pain will remit spontaneously, but the recurrence rate increases after each event. The treatment of acute disabling and chronic disabling back pain is often entirely different in scope.

One method of categorizing the degenerative process of the three joint complex is into three distinct stages—segmental dysfunction, segmental instability, and segmental stability. Each describes changes that affect both the intervertebral disc and facet joints, and the resultant interaction of these changes determines the specific clinical presentation. An overlap of stages frequently exists as these degenerative conditions occur as a continuum and are the result of the cumulative effect of excessive and abnormal physical stress. Usually the lowest two lumbar motion segments, L4–L5 and L5–S1, are affected first, as they are normally subject to the greatest loads. Acute presentation of low back and/or lower extremity pain can occur anywhere during this continuum. In this section, each stage will be presented in regard to pathomechanics of the disc and joint complex, presenting symptoms, diagnostic radiographic findings, and pertinent clinical correlates.

Phase I, segmental dysfunction, describes a state of abnormally reduced movement of the motion segment. Abnormally sustained muscular contraction, especially of the multifidi, which are relatively short segmental extensors and rotators, can lead to facet joint hypomobility and synovitis, and to tears of the superficial annular fibers (Figure 13.3A). This usually results in the classical "strain-sprain" syndrome, with initial symptoms primarily posterior element in nature (i.e., back pain worsened by static standing, walking, extension; better with flexion). Disc-mediated pain can occur throughout this stage. Disc protrusion or herniation may occur later, leading to discogenic pain, possibly with radiculopathy (pain and/or neurologic signs or symptoms limited to the anatomic distribution of a specific nerve root). Routine radiographs are frequently normal in this stage, particularly with first time occurrence of low back pain, although magnetic resonance imaging (MRI) may reveal early disc desiccation. Myelogram, computerized axial tomography (CAT scan), and MRI can all demonstrate disc herniation in later stages of phase I. The clinical significance of this

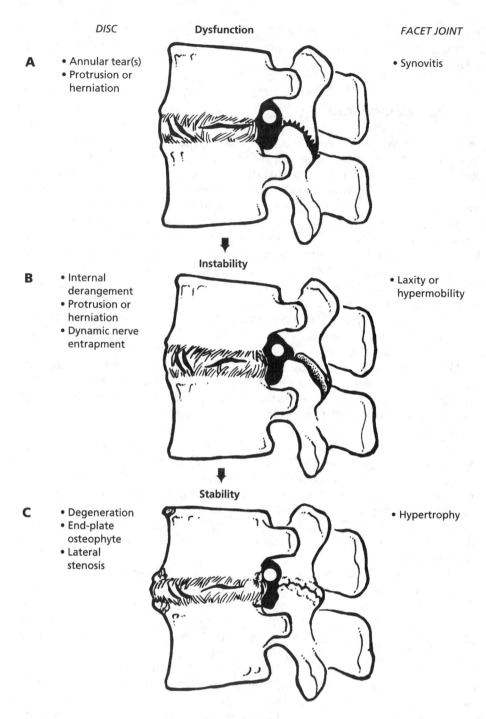

FIGURE 13.3

phase should not be underestimated, especially since lumbar muscle strain does not usually persist for greater than 6 weeks unless accompanied by disc and/or joint dysfunction.

Phase II, segmental instability, refers to a condition of hypermobility of segmental motion. The facet joint changes can induce capsular laxity and joint subluxation. Abnormalities of the disc lead to internal disc derangement and disc resorption (Figure 13.3B). The clinical symptoms are those of hypermobility, including both discogenic and posterior element symptoms, with poor tolerance for torsional loads. Radiculopathy can occur secondary to a variety of causes, including direct impingement on a root from a herniated disc, dynamic lateral entrapment due to narrowing of the lateral recess, and primary radiculitis due to neurochemical factors associated with an internally deranged disc. Imaging studies may reveal translatory motion with lateral-flexion-extension spinal radiographs, degenerative changes on MRI without disc herniation, lateral recess stenosis with myelogram/post myelogram CAT scan, and abnormal discograms. The early presentation of this phase is frequently misunderstood, usually when radiographic or imaging abnormalities are absent and frank instability is not demonstrable. A key physical examination sign is low back pain and/or dysrhythmia of lumbar motion, especially from forward bending to an upright posture.

Phase III, the final phase of segmental stability, again relates to segmental hyopmobility, but symptoms of back pain may actually decrease in this phase. Progressive degenerative changes result in facet joint hypertrophy and capsular fibrosis, severe disc resorption with collapse of the disc space and vertebral body osteophyte formation (Figure 13.3C). The main clinical presentation includes stiffness and inflexibility of the lumbar spine. Spinal stenosis leading to nerve entrapment is most common in this stage, resulting in neurogenic claudication (i.e., radicular symptoms such as burning and cramping in the thigh or leg associated with walking and standing; improved with flexion). Lumbar stenosis is the major radiographic abnormality resulting from marked degenerative changes. Occasionally degenerative spondylolisthesis (i.e., slippage of one vertebral body relative to another in the sagittal plane) occurs. Disc herniation is less common in the stability phase, as advanced degeneration decreases the susceptibility of the motion segment to torsional or shear stress.

The complexity of diagnosing a lumbar spine disorder cannot be understated. The stages of segmental dysfunction, instability, and stability cannot only overlap at any one lumbar motion segment, but different stages frequently occur simultaneously at adjacent motion segments. Thus, the resulting clinical representation is a conglomerate of various signs and symptoms. This complexity is further contributed to by the "nonmechanical" nature of lumbar spine pain mediation. As used here, the term "nonmechanical" does not refer to the extraspinal disease mentioned at the beginning of this section, but rather to the newer concept of chemically mediated inflammatory and pain generation. Within the past two decades, much clinical and experimental research has identified various enzymatic pathways and neurotransmitters (i.e., neuropeptides) that may account for "disc-like" clinical symptoms without evidence for disc herniation or nerve impingement on lumbar imaging. This new understanding of the biochemistry of lumbar spine disorders has resulted in the reevaluation of abnormalities such as annular tears and central disc protrusions, previously not widely considered to be painful conditions.

===== **Rehabilitation**

The rehabilitation approach to acute and chronic low back pain is significantly differenmt, although maintenance or restoration of function is a common goal. Acute and chronic lumbosacral pain and chronic low back pain syndrome can frequently be managed nonsurgically. While the treatment of acute back pain follows the common principles of musculoskeletal medicine (i.e., anti-inflammtory measures, relative rest, restoration of soft tissue and joint flexibility and strengthening), chronic low back syndrome with disability cannot be effectively managed by isolated therapy treatment. A multidisciplinary "pain management" model frequently is required.

One of the oldest treatment options available is rest, either absolute or relative. Most patients will respond to immobilization in 2–3 days at most. Prevention of secondary deconditioning effects and catabolic processes, including reduced cardiovascular performance expressed as decreased VO_2 max, negative nitrogen balance indicating decreased protein stores, and bony demineralization with excessive calcium mobilization, far outweigh the minimal benefit of prolonged bed rest. Anti-inflammatory control with medication is indicated and appropriate in the acute presentation. Judicious use of pain medication is often necessary, especially during the period of bed rest, when the central (i.e., sedative) effects do not significantly impact function. Long-term management of chronic pain syndrome with centrally acting medications is not appropriate and may actually impair the recovery process. Manual therapy techniques, including joint mobilization, help to decrease pain and improve motion, but should be used cautiously with segmental hypermobility.

Exercise has an important role in the rehabilitation of acute and chronic low back pain. Lower extremity flexibility exercises allow normal range of motion at the hip joints, decreasing excessive anterior or posterior pelvic tilt, and subsequently place less stress on the intervertebral joint. Flexion exercises serve to flatten the lumbar lordosis. These include posterior pelvic tilts, partial sit-ups, and knee to chest stretches. These may prove useful in the early stages of lumbar segmental dysfunction with primary facet joint pain, and also in later stages of segmental stability with lateral recess and foraminal stenosis. However, disc herniation with or without radiculopathy may be significantly worsened by flexion activities. Extension exercises promote maintenance of lordosis and lumbar extension range of motion, and decrease tension on the pain-sensitive PLL and nerve root. Once pain has "centralized" to the low back, indicating decreases nerve root irritation, progressive flexion range of motion is instituted in order to allow return to normal daily activities. Neither flexion nor extension protocols should be applied randomly and require careful diagnostic assessment.

Strengthening exercises have an important role in protecting the three joint complex from excessive stress, especially shear and torsion. As mentioned earlier, the abdominal and trunk muscles provide support for lifting maximum loads through their effect on the TLF. Day-to-day activities, however, do not always require maximum effort. Therefore, the paraspinal muscles must also be strengthened. The concept of "stabilization" exercises is often applied in regards to strengthening this "corset" of muscles.

Stabilization begins with adequate lower extremity flexibility and lumbar segmental range of motion, so that the spine and pelvis can attain a neutral relationship. This does not indicate absence of lumbar lordosis, but a position of minimized stress across the intervertebral joint. Extensive proprioceptive innervation of the muscles and facet joints provides feedback to maintain neutral spine positioning, through co-contraction of synergistic muscle groups (i.e., trunk flexors and extensors, hip flexors and extensors, and knee flexors and extensors). Basic stabilization routines focus on postural control in static positions such as supine and prone lying and kneeling and standing, progressing to advanced techniques emphasizing abdominal and trunk musculature in transitional and patterned movements typical of daily or recreational activities. Stabilization procedures emphasize exquisite trunk control. In a comprehensive exercise program, strengthening is followed by endurance training through aerobic exercise. Aerobic activities such as swimming and cross-country skiing can also selectively strengthen trunk musculature.

Selective spinal corticosteroid injection (i.e., epidural, nerve root sheath, and intraarticular facet joint injection) also have a role in the management of acute—and occasionally chronic—low back pain. These injections should always be coupled with a rehabilitation program. Use of selective injections in chronic pain syndrome should be addressed cautiously; injections alone cannot properly diagnose and manage the complex psychosocial issues that frequently accompany chronic back pain syndrome with disability. However, selective injections can occasionally reveal previously undiagnosed pathology, such as an atypical presentation of radiculopathy.

Management of chronic low back pain and chronic back pain syndrome is distinctly different from that of acute low back pain. Certainly, chronic low back pain presenting following an industrial injury or unsuccessful back surgery requires a thorough medical evaluation to rule out previously undiagnosed pathology, either spinal or extraspinal in origin. If discovered, this pathologic process may be amenable to physical therapy, selective injection, or even surgery. However, in many cases of chronic low back pain, no such process can be determined. A more appropriate diagnosis would then be chronic back pain syndrome. This is not a pathologic diagnosis, but a description of a process that implies significant impairment of normal function.

Conceptually, the key to understanding chronic back pain syndrome is to appreciate the poor correlation between nociception (i.e., the actual afferent impulses via pain nerve endings), the subjective feeling of pain, and pain behavior (i.e., any observable expression of pain and/or suffering). Chronic pain syndromes are also frequently associated with a variable degree of psychological dysfunction, usually depression. This is not to infer a psychosomatic state, but rather that psychological distress exists. The combination of a persistent physical complaint, pain behavior, and psychological distress, can yield a firmly disabled state, which often prevents gainful employment.

The clinical manifestations of chronic pain syndromes have common features, which include nonorganic physical exam signs and clinical symptoms. The findings are considered the clinical equivalent of psychological distress, indicating some degree of symptom magnification, possibly as an expression of suffering. Various psychological tests can assist with evaluating the psychological manifestations associated with chronic pain syndromes. An absence of objective clinical signs (i.e., muscle spasm, dural tension signs, and neurologic deficit) is common, but a chronic pain state can exist even in the presence of objective impairment.

The management of chronic pain syndrome usually focuses on behavioral modification. Often, a multidisciplinary pain management team is employed that includes a physician, nurse, physical and occupational therapists, psychologist, and vocational rehabilitation counselor. The goal of such programs is not specifically to reduce the subjective sensation of pain, but rather to restore function; a reduction in pain complaints frequently accompanies functional restoration. However, the behavioral approach positively reinforces "activity" and negatively reinforces pain behavior. The team's purpose is to provide comprehensive support to maximize physical restoration. Setting of short- and long-term goals upon entering such a program maximizes the outcome. These programs are not 100 percent successful, but, given the economic and social cost to society due to chronic low back pain, comprehensive treatment plans provide the maximum resources to manage ingrained disability problems.

===== Recommended Reading

Fast A. Low back disorders: Conservative management. *Arch Phys Med Rehabil* 69:880–891, 1988.
    A thorough review of nonsurgical lumbar spine treatment.
Fordyce WE, Roberts AH, Sternbach RA. The behavioral management of chronic pain: A response to critics. *Pain* 22:113–125, 1985.
    An excellent review of behavioral control theory in chronic pain management.
Gracovetsky S, Farfan H, Helleur C. The abdominal mechanism. *Spine* 10:317–324, 1985.
    An analytic explanation of the functional anatomic role of abdominal musculature regarding lumbar spine kinesiology.
Kirkaldy-Willis WH. *Managing low back pain* (2d Ed.). New York, Churchill Livingstone, 1988.
    A comprehensive and easily understood text of lumbar spine disease.
Mayer TG, et al. Objective assessment of spine function following industrial injury. *Spine* 10:482–493, 1985.
    A prospective study of multidisciplinary pain management to treat injured, disabled workers.
Nachemson AL. The lumbar spine: An orthopedic challenge. *Spine* 1:59–71, 1976.
    One of the first classical discussions of disc biomechanics.
Saal JA. Rehabilitation of sports-related lumbar spine injuries. *Physical Medicine & Rehabilitation: State of the Art Reviews* 1:613–638, 1987.
    Includes an excellent discussion of stabilization and strengthening techniques.
Waddell G. A new clinical model for the treatment of low-back pain. *Spine* 12:632–644, 1987.
    A well-formulated discussion of recognition and management of chronic back pain syndrome.

14

Chronic Pain: A Behavioral Perspective

Wilbert E. Fordyce, Ph.D.

This chapter describes the principles underlying the rationale for viewing chronic pain in behavioral terms, and sets forth in rudimentary form some tactical steps in case management.

Epidemiology

Chronic back pain is the most costly and prevalent disabling condition among adult workers. Back problems are estimated to interfere at some time with 80–85 percent of adults, irrespective of occupation, although a verifiable diagnosis explaining the report of pain is found in only approximately 12–15 percent of the cases. The numbers of injured workers is great but most resume normal function rapidly (1). It is the roughly 10–20 percent who linger into chronicity, continue to suffer, continue to be unable to work, and accrue enormous costs, who make up the core of the problem.

Neurophysiologic and Learning-Based Mechanisms of Pain

That which follows builds upon the neurophysiologic mechanisms that underlie the transmission and perception of pain. In addition to these mechanisms, understanding clinical pain also requires an appreciation and understanding of the plasticity of the human organism to the effects of experience, including basic sensory transmission and perception mechanisms. It is also essential to understand that experience, including that associated with injury and pain, is likely to influence the cortical component of pain perception and ensuing suffering. The cortical experience factor is likely to play a significant role in how much a person suffers from pain sensations that arise from injury or disease. Cortical experience is also quite capable of influencing the duration of the suffering and of generating pain related suffering in the absence of currently active nociceptive stimulation.

Physiologic mechanisms underlying the detection, transmission, and perception of pain are complex. The Gate Control Theory, first promulgated by Melzack and Wall (8), addresses the complexities of pain and its transmission and perception. Although some details presented in the initial discussions of the Gate Control Theory have been called into question by subsequent research, it is now evident that the nervous system has, in several complex ways, the capability of modulating the perception of pain and responses to it.

When adequately stimulated, peripheral somatic pain receptors activate A delta and C fibers; these in turn are received in Lamina 1 of the dorsal horn. Here these sensory inputs are modulated before transmission to the brain (5). But the system is more complex than that. Laminae 2 and 3 of the dorsal horn make up the substantia gelatinosa. These cells are also known to have a modulating effect on peripheral stimuli before transmission to the brain. Thus a system intervenes between peripheral stimulation and brain reception that is known to exert modulating effects. These modulating effects are influenced by the relative amount of activity in large- and small-diameter fibers. The former inhibit transmission of nociception; the latter facilitate it.

The spinal gating mechanism is also influenced by nerve impulses that descend from the brain and which implicate endogenous opioid peptides (8) as moderators of the pain experience. These neurochemical mechanisms are triggered by the brain.

It should be evident that vis-à-vis experience, prior learning, and expectations, the brain is ensured a role in the perception and experience of pain. In pain arising from uncomplicated injuries, particularly to the low back, chronicity frequently develops from problems of case management that derive from failure of the health care system to distinguish acute from chronic pain. This failure is also a failure to understand and utilize the implications of the learning process and the effects of experience on body processes, including pain-related matters. Pain problems are perceived, diagnosed, and treated as if all were acute. A study of the essential elements of "pain," however, indicates the basis for distinctions between acute and chronic. Those elements can be summarized as follows: (7)

- Nociception: Thermal, mechanical, or chemical energy stimulating specialized nerve endings, which then activate A delta or C fibers;
- Pain: Discrimination by the central nervous system that the impulse perceived is "pain"—not pressure, touch, proprioceptive, and so forth;
- Suffering: A negative affective response to the perception of a noxious stimulus, based on awareness or anticipation of adverse consequences, or ambiguity of those consequences;
- Pain Behavior: Actions of the person in response to perception of an aversive stimulus and anticipation of adverse consequences, and which are likely to convey to observers that the person is suffering or "is in pain."

The first two components—nociception and "pain"—relate to input from body parts implicated in a painful event. They are not the output; that is, elements of the response. The response consists of suffering and pain behavior. All four usually—but not inevitably—occur when there is an injury. We can sustain nociception without perceiving it or, if we do, without suffering or pain behavior. The logical reverse is also possible: to suffer and/or to emit pain behavior in the absence of nociception and, of course, its identification; i.e., perception of "pain." But the most important issue here is that the response elements, and perhaps also the stimulus identification of "pain," are influenced by learning or experience. The sensitivity of the central nervous system to learning or conditioning can, and all too often does, result in suffering and pain behavior persisting without currently adequate demonstrable nociceptive stimulation. The importance of the distinction between acute and chronic pain resides mainly in the fact that chronicity ensures that there will have been opportunity for learning or conditioning. The effects of learning and conditioning may—but do not always—result in suffering and pain behavior diverging or becoming somewhat autonomous from nociception. This is the conceptual basis for applying learning or behavioral concepts to clinical pain.

Pain problems originating with tissue injury can probably usefully be thought of as acute during healing time. If suffering and pain behaviors persist after healing time, and there is no (or insufficient) basis for inferring continuing peripheral nociception (i.e., failure of healing, residual structural defect), the problem is probably one of chronicity. It then becomes essential to understand whether, and, if so how, learning factors have entered the picture to carry out proper diagnosis and treatment.

Role of Learning

Learning is simply the residual effect of experience. Its role in clinical pain appears to focus on the following points.

First, as with all behaviors, pain behaviors are sensitive to consequences. Pain behaviors that are followed contingently by positive reinforcement are likely to persist, irrespective of the circumstances (e.g., nociception) that caused them initially. These conditioning effects, often termed *operant conditioning,* can be summarized by paraphrasing as:

- when pain behaviors are followed by "good" things that otherwise would not have likely occurred, direct positive reinforcement of pain behavior is likely; and
- when pain behaviors lead successfully to avoiding "bad" or aversive events that otherwise would likely have occurred, avoidance behavior is reinforced.

Second, automatic conditioning may occur when highly aversive stimuli are experienced. Just as ingestion of a toxic food may immediately result in persistent aversion to that food, so also a painful and/or frightening experience may immediately result in highly persistent behaviors designed to avoid repetition of the aversive event. Injection of highly aversive chemotherapeutic agents as part of treatment for a malignancy often leads to nausea, and even vomiting, when the patient is next presented with the prospect of another such injection. Whiplash injuries from being "rear-ended" in an auto may lead to a flareup of neck pain when next positioned to drive. In such instances, stimuli in the environment (e.g., sight of the clinic in which an injection is to be received, sitting behind the wheel of an auto) become sufficient to elicit suffering and pain behaviors. We can think of this form of learning as stimulus control.

Reasons for Pain Behaviors Past Healing Time

1. Nociception from an unhealed injury (possible but unlikely unless there is clear evidence of a residual structural defect);
2. Nociception from iatrogenic factors (e.g., scar tissue from surgeries);
3. Nociception from disuse, arising from prescribed - or practiced without prescription - prolonged overguarding of the involved body parts;
4. Contingently reinforced suffering/pain behaviors (direct or as avoidance learning); and
5. Pain behaviors confounded with suffering from other causes (e.g., depression, anxiety).

Options 3, 4, and 5 are corrected by activating the patient, not by conceptualizing the pain problem as reflecting a defect that must be repaired.

Communication with the Patient

In light of the foregoing, certain ideas need to be practiced by the physician and communicated to the patient. These can be summarized as follows:

- Hurt and harm are not the same.
- Healing is automatic, rapid, and promoted by properly paced motion.
- How much better the patient gets will depend mainly on what the patient does, not on what someone else does to him or her.
- To make "it" better, use it.

Evaluation of Behavior Factors in Chronic Pain

The evaluation of chronic pain is not a simple matter. An assessment of whether or not learning factors are playing a significant role can usually be determined by interviews of the patient and spouse (or significant other), or through such devices as activity diaries, Minnesota Multiphasic Personality Inventory (MMPI). An analysis of data bearing on items 3, 4, and 5 of the list noted above of reasons why pain behaviors may persist past healing time allows one to address the viability of explaining the persistence of pain behaviors in the relative absence of evidence of ongoing nociception from tissue defect by learning/conditioning effects. More detail can be found in reviews of this topic (2,3).

Perhaps the most practical implication in diagnostic or management issues of the foregoing is, until proven otherwise, that a pain patient whose symptoms persist despite the application of standard diagnostic and treatment methods should be assumed to have a problem that is being influenced by learning or conditioning, and those issues should be studied appropriately.

Treatment Based on the Behavior Change Model

Behaviorally based treatment methods have been in use for many years (6,9). In this brief chapter, description of treatment strategies implied by the foregoing can only be outlined. More detailed descriptions can be found in several reviews (2,4). That which follows assumes that the pain problem was trauma-induced, that medical evaluation indicates no significant residual structural defect, that sufficient time for healing has passed, that evidence indicates learning factors are playing a significant role, and that there are no medical contraindications to reactivation beyond those relating to complaints of pain per se.

One guiding principle is that treatment regimens should be designed to avoid contingently reinforcing pain behaviors with analgesics, rest, or other palliative treatment modalities. A second is that the patient and, as indicated, the family have been helped to understand that resolution of the pain problem has come now to depend on what the patient does, not what someone does to him or her. It follows from this as well that complaints of pain have by now become an insufficient basis for curtailing appropriately prescribed and paced activity.

The behavior change model, as distinguished from that of body defect, directs attention to: what behaviors need to be changed, what present reinforcing contingencies appear to be sustaining the behaviors to be changed, what rearrangements of behavior and consequences appear likely to be helpful, and what patient perceptions and expectancies about pain and illness need to be addressed. In the practical case, the problems more often are the use of analgesics long past healing time, protracted overguarding and adverse effects of disuse, failure of those persons around the patient to reinforce efforts at increasing activity and becoming reestablished in productive roles, and difficulties in finding opportunities to sustain the increased activity likely to develop with treatment. Each problem area will be addressed briefly.

MEDICATION MANAGEMENT

Patients presenting with heavy narcotic ingestion or with moderate amounts taken over long time intervals almost certainly will require a period of inpatient care to bring the medication problem under control. A shift to outpatient may then become an option. First, determine the actual medication intake via a 24–48 hour baseline or "drug profile," in which medications are taken prn, but with nurse monitoring to ensure that dangerous amounts are not taken. If the patient has been on injectables, shift to oral. Next, construct a pain cocktail composed of 10 cc volume per dose. Each dose consists of the Methadone equivalent of whatever narcotics were being taken, Phenobarbital equivalents for barbiturates, and cherry syrup sufficient to total 10 cc. Deliver this q4h if baseline ingestion has been frequent; otherwise, q6h.

If you are concerned about major toxicity until more modest ingestion levels are reached, taper narcotic and barbiturate levels from 10–20 percent per day. Thereafter, a 10–20 percent decrease per week is appropriate, always occurring concomitantly with reactivation. Full and open disclosure prior to beginning the pain cocktail regimen is quite appropriate.

REACTIVATION

Exercises selected to promote generalized conditioning as well as strengthening and use of the body parts specifically limited by the pain problem should be recommended. Patients should enter into each exercise a minimum of once, and preferably twice daily, or more. For approximately 2–4 sessions they are instructed to exercise to tolerance: "Do the exercise until pain, weakness, or fatigue cause you to want to stop. You decide when to stop." That defines the baseline. Next, set quotas for each exercise, starting at approximately 70–80 percent of baseline to ensure trials at levels demonstrated to be currently within the patient's performance range. Define quota increment rates; usually one repetition each session works well enough. This can be accelerated or decelerated based on clinical judgment, *but should be defined prior to quota trials.* Increment rates can also be adjusted upward or downward, depending on therapist observations and judgment. These changes should not be dictated solely by patient complaints of pain but on the basis of therapist judgment as to what the patient can presently achieve. Quotas are both floors and ceilings: to be reached but not exceeded. Target endpoints should be defined at the outset, again on the basis of medical prudence and patient post-treatment time scheduling issues. The objectives of exercising are more than physiologic conditioning. They are also to help the patient—and his or her family—learn that it is safe to move. In effect, it is a learning or teaching mode for the patient's whole system.

SOCIAL FEEDBACK

Those working with the patient, as well as those residing with him or her, need to be helped to understand that improvement will come from appropriately paced use, not from guarding or overprotection. The complaint of pain per se should not be seen as a signal to reinstitute previously unhelpful guarding and activity limitation.

Social and Vocational Implications

It is essential to direct major attention to what the patient will be doing following treatment. If he or she is in the labor force and destined to return to employment, care should be exercised to determine what vocational objectives are contemplated and the extent to which those objectives fit appropriately with the post-treatment activity level, as well as with patient talents and deficiencies. Special effort should be made wherever possible to facilitate graduated reentry into work until confidence of patient, coworkers, and employer has been established.

When pain problems arise from tissue injury, most chronic pain patients are found to have significant defects in their ability to be effectively well. The problems they have are endlessly varied: job instability, difficulties in relating to co-workers, deficiencies in establishing effective family and social support networks, histories of physical or sexual abuse, histories of alcohol or substance abuse, and marital discord. These are all encountered with great frequency, either singly or in various combinations. Such problems mean that being active and employed, or being identified as free from limitations of pain, will not inevitably lead to maintenance of treatment gains. Pain treatment programs cannot be all things to all people. It is important to recognize the power of these other problems to lead the patient back to chronic disability. How much can be done about these problems varies with resources and opportunity.

Conclusion

Chronic pain relating to tissue injury is a much greater problem than it needs to be in terms of human suffering, health care costs, disability maintenance costs, and lost productivity. A major reason for this is the persistent tendency to view pain solely from a medical model perspective. Application of the evaluation and treatment methods described here have been shown to reduce significantly the unneeded persistence of disability.

References

1. Andersson G, Svensson H, Oden A. The intensity of work recovery in low back pain. *Spine* 8:8, 880–884, 1983.
2. Fordyce W. *Behavioral methods in chronic pain and illness.* St. Louis, C.V. Mosby, 1976.
3. Fordyce W. Learning processes in pain. In: Sternbach R (Ed.), *The psychology of pain* (2d ed.). New York, Raven Press, 1986.
4. Fordyce W, Fowler R, et al. Operant conditioning in the treatment of chronic pain, *Arch Phys Med* 54:9:399–408, 1973.
5. Frenk H, Cannon T, Lewis J, Liebeskind J. Neural and neurochemical mechanisms of pain inhibition. In: Sternbach R (Ed.),*The psychology of pain* (2d ed.) New York, Raven Press, 1986, pp. 25–43.
6. Loeser JD. Perspectives on pain. In: *Proceedings of the first world conference on clinical pharmacology and therapeutics*, pp. 316–319, London, Macmillan, 1980.
7. Melzack R, Wall PD. The gate control theory of pain. *Science* 150:971–979, 1965.
8. Melzack R. Neurophysiology of pain. In: Sternbach R (Ed.), *The psychology of pain* (pp.1–26). New York, Raven Press, 1978.
9. Turner JT, Romano JM. Behavioral and psychological assessment of chronic pain patients. In: Loeser J, Egan K (Eds.), *Managing the chronic pain patient: Theory and practice at the University of Washington multidisciplinary pain center* (pp. 65–80). New York, Raven Press, 1989.

15

Progressive Neuromuscular Disorders

George H. Kraft, M.D.

The physician should be familiar with common neuromuscular disorders and their rehabilitative management. These disorders occur in both children and adults, and primarily constitute diseases of either peripheral nerve or skeletal muscle. Some neuromuscular disorders are self-limited and, being monophasic in character, may improve spontaneously. Examples of these disorders are Guillain-Barré syndrome and acute polymyositis. Self-limited disorders are physically treated by maintaining joint range of motion (ROM), prevention of decubitus ulcers, and by other types of supportive therapy during the period the disease is active.

This chapter discusses the progressive neuromuscular disorders. Many are hereditarily determined and their courses cannot be altered. Others are associated with various diseases (e.g., diabetic neuropathy) or are idiopathic in etiology (e.g., chronic inflammatory polyradiculoneuropathy).

At this point, it is useful to review the system of Mendelian inheritance. Rather than memorizing the pattern of inheritance, it is better to use pencil and paper to determine the three common possibilities of inheritance: autosomal dominant, sex-linked, and autosomal recessive. With Xs and Ys on paper, recall that for a patient to have a dominant disorder, one of the parents must also have that disorder. Conversely, an unaffected child cannot transmit an autosomal dominant disorder to any of his or her children. If one of the parents has the disorder, there is a 50–50 chance that one of the children will have the disorder, with no male or female preference.

Sex-linked disorders are similar except that if the defective gene is on the X chromosome (e.g., Duchenne muscular dystrophy), 50 percent of the male children will have the disease, and 50 percent of the females will be carriers (see Figure 15.1).

Autosomal recessive disorders are different in that usually neither of the parents of an affected child will have clinical manifestations of the disease. Both parents must have the defective recessive gene, but because the gene is recessive, the disease will not have been expressed in either of the parents. However, 25 percent of the children will have the disease and 50 percent will be carriers. In such a genetic milieu, consanguinity becomes an important determining factor.

Although the details are beyond the scope of this chapter, many new genetic tests are now available to determine a specific genetic defect and carrier status for a number of neuromuscular disorders.

Categories of Neuromuscular Diseases

The first comprehensive classification of neuromuscular diseases was published in 1968. Although a number of revisions have occurred since then, a major effort to update these diseases was begun in 1985. The final version is being prepared by an expert committee under the auspices of the World Health Organization, but an abbreviated (but still lengthy) version was prepared for the European Alliance of Muscular Dystrophy Associations in 1988 for use by those charitable bodies and lay organizations throughout the world that support muscle disease research. It is likely that the physician will encounter this classification, shown in modified form in Table 15.1. It is hoped that the physician will find the table useful for future reference.

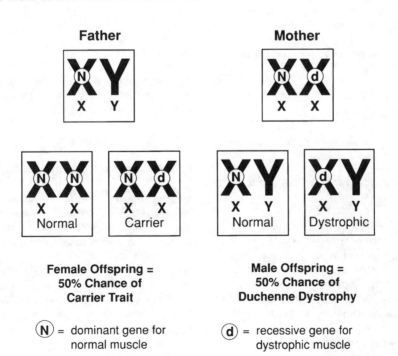

FIGURE 15.1. Methods of inheritance in Duchenne muscular dystrophy (sex-linked).

TABLE 15.1.

Classification of Neuromuscular Diseases

THE MOTOR NEURON DISEASES AND SPINAL MUSCULAR ATROPHIES (DISEASES INVOLVING ANTERIOR HORN CELLS AND MOTOR NUCLEI OF CRANIAL NERVES).

Infantile spinal muscular atrophy (acute or type 1—Werdnig-Hoffman disease)

Other inherited spinal muscular atrophies
Childhood form (type II)
Juvenile form (type III-Kugelberg-Welander)
Adult spinal muscular atrophy
Distal form
Scapuloperoneal form
X-linked bulbospinal neuropathy

Other Forms
Motor Neuron Diseases
Amyotrophic lateral sclerosis
Progressive muscular atrophy
Progressive bulbar palsy
Primary lateral sclerosis
Amyotrophy in hereditary ataxia
Familial motor neuron disease
Amyotrophic lateral sclerosis—Parkinsonism-dementia complex
Other

Other Forms
Unspecified

HEREDITARY AND IDIOPATHIC PERIPHERAL NEUROPATHY

Hereditary motor and sensory neuropathy (HMSN)

Type I—Peroneal muscular atrophy (Charcot-Marie-Tooth disease), hypertrophic type
Type II—Peroneal muscular atrophy, neuronal type
Type III—Hypertrophic interstitial neuropathy (Dejerine-Sottas disease) (recessive)
Roussy-Levy Syndrome

Amyloid neuropathy

Neuropathy in idiopathic porphyria

Refsum's disease (heredopathia atactica polyneuritiformis)

Neuropathy in inborn errors of metabolism

Neuropathy in association with hereditary ataxia

Neuropathy, hereditary, with liability to pressure palsy

Other inherited neuropathies

Idiopathic progressive polyneuropathy

Other forms

INFLAMMATORY, AUTOIMMUNE, AND TOXIC NEUROPATHIES

Acute postinfective polyneuropathy (Guillain-Barré syndrome)
Serum neuropathy
Shoulder girdle neuropathy

Polyneuropathy in connective tissue (collagen-vascular) disease (e.g., systemic lupus, rheumatoid arthritis, polyarteritis nodosa)

Diabetic polyneuropathy

Polyneuropathy in malignant disease

Polyneuropathy in other infective and inflammatory disorders (e.g., leprosy, diphtheria, mumps, mononucleosis, herpes zoster, AIDS, sarcoidosis, borreliosis)

Polyneuropathy in nutritional and metabolic disorders (e.g., vitamin B1, B2, B6, B12, vitamin E deficiency, alcoholism, heavy metal poisoning, acromegaly, hypothyroidism, hypoglycemia, uremia, critical illness)

Polyneuropathy due to drugs

TABLE 15.1. *(cont'd.)*

Polyneuropathy due to other toxic and environmental agents

Other inflammatory and toxic neuropathy

Unspecified

DISORDERS OF THE NEUROMUSCULAR JUNCTION

Myasthenia gravis
  Hereditary myasthenia gravis
  Neonatal myasthenia
  Drug- or toxin-induced myasthenia

Congenital or developmental myasthenia

Lambert-Eaton syndrome

Toxic Disorders
  Botulism
  Others

Other types

DISORDERS OF MUSCLE

Congenital muscular dystrophy
  Congenital muscular dystrophy
  Congenital muscular dystrophy with
    central nervous system involvement
    (Fukuyama type)

Morphologically defined congenital myopathy
  Central core disease
  Multicore disease
  Nemaline myopathy
  Myotubular (centronuclear) myopathy
  Fibre-type disproportion
  Other types

Muscular dystrophies
  Duchenne type
  Becker type
  Emery-Dreifuss type (scapuloperoneal
    muscular dystrophy)
  Fascioscapulohumeral type
  Limb-girdle muscular dystrophy
  Scapulohumeral type
  Pervifemoral type
  Autosomal recessive childhood
    dystrophy resembling

Duchenne/Becker
  Ocular type
  Oculopharyngeal type
  Distal type
  Other types

Myotonic disorders
  Dystrophia myotonica (myotonic
    dystrophy, Steinert's disease)
  Myotonica congenita
    Dominant type (Thomsen)
    Recessive type (Becker)
  Paramyotonica congenita
  Chondrodystrophic myotonica
    (Schwartz-Jampel
  Drug-induced myotonia
  Pseudomyotonia
  Neuromyotonia (continuous muscle
    fibre activity—Isaacs)
  Other types

Toxic myopathies
  Drug-induced myopathy
  Alcoholic myopathy
  Other toxic myopathies

Familial periodic paralysis
  Hypokalemic
  Hyperkalemic
  Normokalemic
  Myotonic periodic paralysis

Endocrine myopathies
  In hyperthyroidism
  In hypothyroidism
  In hypopituitarism
  In Cushing's disease
  In acromegaly
  In Addison's disease
  In hyper- and hypoparathyroidism
  In other forms of metabolic bone
    disease
  Other types

Inherited metabolic myopathies
  Glycogen storage disease of muscle
    Type I (von Gierke's disease)
    Type II (Pompe's disease—
      acid maltase deficiency)
    Type II (Cori-Forbes—debrancher
      enzyme deficiency)

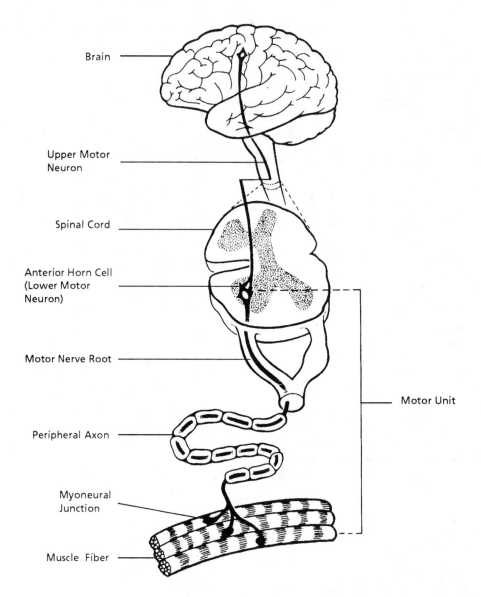

Brain

Upper Motor
Neuron

Spinal Cord

Anterior Horn Cell
(Lower Motor
Neuron)

Motor Nerve Root

Peripheral Axon

Myoneural
Junction

Muscle Fiber

Motor Unit

FIGURE 15.2. The motor unit, consisting of the anterior horn cell, motor nerve root, peripheral axon, myoneural junction and all muscle fibers innervated by the anterior horn cell.

The neuromuscular diseases discussed is this chapter are disorders of a component of the motor unit (Figure 15.2). They encompass disorders of the anterior horn cell, nerve root, peripheral nerve—either axon or myelin sheath—myoneural junction, or muscle.

In general, these disorders are categorized as diseases of either nerve, muscle, or the myoneural junction. Mechanical disorders of the nerve root (e.g., compression by herniated intervertebral disc) and purely sensory disorders are not

Type IV (Andersen-brancher enzyme deficiency)
Type V (McArdle-phosphorylase deficiency)
Type VII (Tarui-phophofructokinase deficiency)
Other types
Lipid storage myopathies
   Carnitine deficiency
   Carnitine palmityl transferase deficiency
   Other types
Myoadenylate deaminase deficiency
Mitochondrial myopathies
   Defects of mitochondrial substrate utilization
   Defects of the respiratory chain
   Defects of energy conservation and transduction
   Other types

Other metabolic myopathies
   Paroxysmal myoglobinuria
   Nutritional myopathy
   Amyloid myopathy

Inflammatory myopathies
   Infective myositis
     Viral myositis

Bacterial myositis
Fungal myositis
Parasitic myositis
Post-viral fatigue syndrome
Other types
Autoimmune myositides
   Dermatomyositis
   Polymyositis
   Polymyositis in association with collagen or connective tissue disease
   Inclusion body myositis
   Eosinophilic myositis
   Granulomatous myositis
   Myositis in sarcoidosis
   Polymyalgia rheumatica
   Other types

Other myopathies of uncertain etiology
   Localized myositis ossificans
   Traumatic lesions or infarction of muscle
   Compartment syndromes
   Volkmann's ischemic contracture
   Other types
   Progressive myositis ossificans
   Arthrogryposis multiplex congenita
   Progressive myosclerosis
   Other types

---

considered here, the former because they are a category of disorders secondary to spinal disease, the latter because muscle weakness is not a component.

Clinical Diagnosis of Neuromuscular Disorders

There are two basic differences between muscle and nerve diseases. Diseases of nerves—with the exception of anterior horn cell disease—generally affect both sensory and motor fibers, usually more markedly impairing sensation. Muscle diseases, on the other hand, are not associated with sensory loss. The second major difference is location; diseases of peripheral nerves tend to affect the distal portions of the longest nerves (i.e., the distal lower extremity) earliest and most severely, whereas muscle diseases have a predilection for proximal muscles.

On physical examination, the presence or absence of sensory deficit—especially in the feet—helps distinguish between these two major categories of disorders. The physician should also check for muscular weakness and atrophy, and note their distribution. Testing the deep tendon reflexes (DTRs) will help separate all types of motor unit diseases from other disorders. In both neuropathies and myopathies, DTRs are either absent or diminished.

A typical example of muscle disease is Duchenne muscular dystrophy, a disorder of male children inherited from the carrier mother (see Figure 15.1). Although these boys may have no apparent disease at birth, weakness becomes manifest within the first several years of life and they develop progressive weakness until, at approximately age 12, they become nonambulatory. The life span rarely extends beyond age 18–20, although with recent ventilatory support techniques, an increased life span may be possible. The defective gene has been determined and the missing gene product, dystrophin, identified. Today the definitive diagnosis of Duchenne dystrophy is the identification of an absence of dystrophin.

Myotonic dystrophy is a common dystrophic condition in adults. It is an autosomal dominant disorder; one of the parents must be affected in order to pass it on to a child. Some degree of mental retardation is reported to be common if the disorder is inherited from the mother. In addition to muscle weakness, its hallmark is the presence of myotonia (a sustained muscle contraction on percussion and the inability to release quickly) (Figure 15.3).

Another common adult-onset dystrophy is limb girdle muscular dystrophy, in which muscular weakness has a predilection for the pelvic and shoulder girdle region. This tends to be a difficult diagnosis to confirm because it is inherited in an autosomal recessive manner with neither of the parents manifesting the disease. It may be misdiagnosed as an unusual presentation of another type of dystrophy.

Facio-scapulo-humeral dystrophy is another type of adult-onset dystrophy. As the name implies, muscles most severely affected are in the face and proximal upper limbs. Many other muscle diseases are listed in Table 15.1.

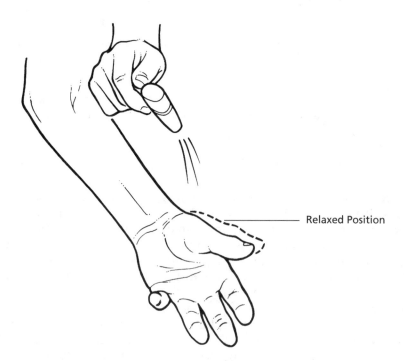

Relaxed Position

FIGURE 15.3. Percussion myotonia. Note the lack of relaxation of the thenar muscle following tapping the muscle with a reflex hammer.

Diseases of nerve can be divided into either hereditary or acquired neuropathies. The most common hereditary neuropathy is Charcot-Marie-Tooth disease, also known as hereditary motor-sensory neuropathy (HMSN I). This autosomal dominant disorder (one of the parents must have the disease) of the peripheral nerve primarily affects myelin. Clinical manifestations are distal motor and sensory loss. There is also a less common "axonal" type (HMSN II), which appears similar clinically but produces primary axonal loss. These two types of hereditary neuropathies can be distinguished by nerve conduction velocities (NCV), which are reduced in HMSN I, by electromyography (EMG), which shows denervation in HMSN II (see below and Chapter 4), and by nerve biopsy (see below).

Acquired neuropathies frequently can be associated with a variety of metabolic disease states. Diabetes is perhaps the most common, with several types of nerve dysfunction seen. Diabetic polyneuropathy is a peripheral neuropathy that fits the characteristic clinical picture of distal sensory and motor loss occurring most severely in the distal lower extremities. Many other medical disorders can produce changes in peripheral nerve (see Table 15.1).

In addition to hereditary and metabolic diseases, toxicity is a common cause of neuropathic dysfunction. The most common type is alcoholic neuropathy. Another major category of nerve disorders is the idiopathic neuropathies such as Guillain-Barré syndrome, an acquired idiopathic disorder which may not be progressive. The final major category is motor neuron disease (e.g., amyotrophic lateral sclerosis [ALS]), a relentlessly progressive degeneration of the anterior horn cells.

Laboratory Tests in the Diagnosis of Neuromuscular Disorders

Four major categories of tests are used in the diagnosis of diseases of nerve or muscle. It should be stressed that the initial diagnosis should be based on clinical and genetic information, using laboratory tests for confirmation.

These four categories are: (1) electrophysiologic, (2) biochemical, (3) genetic (DNA), and (4) structural. The most useful in the clinical setting are the electrophysiologic tests, because they differentiate normal from abnormal, and neurogenic diseases from myogenic disorders. The most common of these is EMG (see Chapter 4). This is a neurophysiologic test to determine whether the disease affects the anterior horn cell, nerve root, peripheral nerve myelin, peripheral nerve axon, myoneural junction, or muscle (see Figure 15.2). Not only does it identify the area of the motor unit affected, it also provides information about severity. Because this test can evaluate any major nerve or muscle in the body, it can provide information about the spatial presentation of the disease. It can be repeated easily and can therefore provide information about the temporal course.

Biochemical tests involve a number of simple to complex testing procedures of varying degrees of specificity. The most common is evaluation of the circulating creatine phosphokinase (CK) enzyme. This muscle enzyme is elevated in primary diseases of muscle, but not in diseases of nerve. The level can be extremely high in some acute inflammatory muscle diseases. Other more recent and sophisticated tests include that for dystrophin, the absence of which confirms the diagnosis of Duchenne muscular dystrophy.

DNA testing is now available for a number of genetically determined neuromuscular disorders, including Duchenne, Becker, and myotonic muscular dystrophy, Friedreich's ataxia, amyloid polyneuropathy, Kennedy disease, and Charcot-Marie-Tooth 1A disease.

Structural tests of various types represent the third category of laboratory studies. The most common are muscle and nerve biopsies. Typically, myopathies show small, irregular muscle fibers with centrally placed nuclei, often associated with fatty degeneration of muscle. On the other hand, nerve diseases show regions of grouped atrophy where groups of contiguous muscle fibers are hypertrophic, and other groups atrophic.

The peripheral nerve can also be biopsied and studied. Since nerve biopsy denervates the muscle or cutaneous sensory area innervated, typically only the sural nerve is biopsied for these studies. Newer methods of evaluating gross structural changes of muscle or nerve also include MRI employing short-term inversion recovery (STIR) sequences.

Rehabilitative Management

In considering a rational approach for creating substitutive rehabilitative strategies, the physician must have some idea of the natural history of the neuromuscular disorder and where along the natural course of progression the particular patient is at the time of intervention. The physician must be aware of and anticipate future changes so that function can be maintained as muscular strength declines. Patients with both nerve and muscle diseases may have difficulty ambulating, yet the mechanism of the gait dysfunction may be quite different and varying treatment strategies need to be employed. Throughout the rehabilitative planning stage, particular contraindications to a form of treatment must be kept in mind. For example, patients with severe sensory deficit may develop skin breakdown from the use of an insertable plastic ankle-foot orthosis (AFO); therefore, its use may not be indicated.

The rehabilitation of patients with progressive disorders is different from that of patients with nonprogressive disorders such as spinal cord injury, cerebrovascular accident (CVA), and amputation. The management of any progressive disorder requires assessment of the expected rate of progression and "overrehabilitation" treatment: providing somewhat more rehabilitation strategies than the patient needs at present will help to ensure long-term benefits. Thus the rehabilitation of patients with progressive neuromuscular disorders can be more difficult and is an ongoing process. Fortunately, however, a major problem that complicates the management of central nervous system disorders—bladder dysfunction—is rarely a problem in diseases of peripheral nerve.

Probably the most important rehabilitation intervention is the correction of joint contractures. Contractures of even several degrees can place the body in a disadvantageous position from the standpoint of efficiency. For example, if the center of gravity shifts behind the knee joint and anterior to the hip joint, the knee extensor muscles (quadriceps femoris), and hip extensor muscles need to be tonically activated during standing (Figure 15.4). This is very inefficient, fatiguing, and unlikely to be maintained by a patient with neuromuscular weakness.

Consequently, the most important physical intervention in a patient with

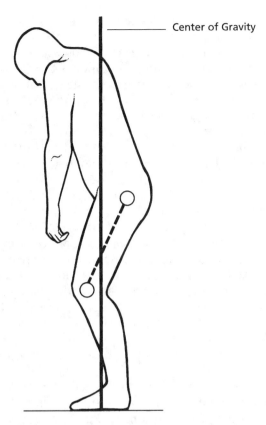

———————— Center of Gravity

FIGURE 15.4. Patient with severe hip and knee flexion contracture. Note that the center of gravity falls anterior to the hip joint and posterior to the knee joint, requiring constant hip extensor and quadriceps muscle activity for standing at rest.

any kind of weakness is to prevent or reverse flexion contractures. Correction is so vital that surgical release should be considered if conservative measures fail. There is one major exception: heel cord tightness and ankle flexion contracture is not an obvious treatment issue because a tight heel cord may stabilize the knee as weight is borne on the foot. The lever arm of the gastrocnemius and soleus muscles may "pull" the knee backward stabilizing the knee. Patients who have had surgical release of tight heel cords are sometimes no longer able to stand. Understanding the kinesiology of dysfunction is critical, and interventions must be planned that will foster function, not simply correct anatomic defects.

Because muscular weakness is a common denominator of diseases of nerve and muscle, and a major patient symptom, patients often ask about the benefits of exercise. In the early stage of myopathies, vigorous resistive exercise may produce some increase in strength. In the long term, however, exercise associated with an increase in serum CK may be either detrimental or have no effect. In our clinic, we prescribe exercise in such patients only with close physical monitoring of objective muscular strength and CK levels. We want to see an increase in and maintenance of strength as long as the exercise is continued. It is safe to say, however, that the use of exercise in progressive muscular disorders is still a procedure that must be monitored very closely and, at the present time, not considered of proven value.

The same caveats hold with regard to the use of exercise in peripheral nerve diseases. If there is a disuse atrophy component to the weakness, then that component can be reversed with exercise. The degree of disuse atrophy can be semi-quantitatively assessed by EMG to determine whether a given level of muscle strength is being produced by a few large, hypertrophied and overworking motor units or by many motor units not functioning at their full contractile capacity because of a component of disuse atrophy. Used in this way, the EMG can be a valuable adjunct to the development of an exercise program.

Lower limb function can be increased by the appropriate use of orthotics and other rehabilitation aids. AFOs can be used to correct dorsiflexion weakness and ankle instability. If knee stability is poor, it is important to use a lightweight articulating ankle (e.g., spring wire) AFO to reduce knee flexion movement on heel strike. Canes can be used to increase the base of support. Wheelchairs allow mobility when severe weakness is present. With each patient, however, the function lost needs to be evaluated and, with an understanding of kinesiologic principles involved, substitutive orthotic measures employed.

Because nerve diseases usually affect upper limbs less severely, functional orthotic aids are less often required. However, they are useful if hand function becomes severely impaired. In addition to orthotic management, attention should be given to respiratory support for severe myopathies and motor neuron diseases.

Finally, all patients with progressive neuromuscular diseases should be evaluated for vocational and psychological intervention. Young patients with slowly progressive weakness must be directed into employment situations that can be continued as their disease progresses. Psychologically, patients with progressive disease may be subject to depression, and coping skills need to be implemented.

In summary, there is much that rehabilitation has to offer patients with progressive neuromuscular diseases. For diseases that cannot be cured, rehabilitation strategies offer the only treatment currently available.

═══ Annotated Suggested Reading List

Dimitrijević, MR, Kakulas BA, Vrbová G (Eds.), *Recent achievements in restorative neurology: 2 progressive neuromuscular diseases.* Basel, S. Karger AG, 1986.
    An innovative approach to neuromuscular disease rehabilitation.
Fowler WM Jr. Rehabilitation management of muscular dystrophy and related disorders: II. Comprehensive care. *Arch Phys Med Rehab* 63:322–328, 1982.
    A summary of rehabilitation management of neuromuscular disorders.
Fowler WM Jr., Taylor M. Rehabilitation management of muscular dystrophy and related disorders: I. The role of exercise. *Arch Phys Med Rehab* 63:319–321, 1982.
    A good review of the role of exercise in neuromuscular disorders.
Kraft GH. Diseases of the motor unit. In: Rosse C, Clawson DK (Eds.), *The musculoskeletal system in health and disease.* Hagerstown, Harper & Row, 1980.
    An overview for medical students of this topic, and a practical approach to the diagnosis of neuromuscular diseases.
Kraft GH. Movement disorders. In: Basmajian JV, Kirby RL (Eds.), *Medical rehabilitation.* Baltimore, Williams & Wilkins, 1984.

A review of rehabilitation methods for movement disorders. Concise suggestions for various rehabilitation techniques in movement disorders.

Kraft GH. Peripheral neuropathies. In: Johnson EW (Ed.), *Practical electromyography* (2d ed). Baltimore, Williams & Wilkins, 1988.

A detailed review of peripheral neuropathies and the neurophysiologic approach to diagnosis.

Milner-Brown HS, Miller RG. Muscle strengthening through high-resistance weight training in patients with neuromuscular disorders. *Arch Phys Med Rehab* 69:14–19, 1988.

An interesting study, detailing a new approach to exercise in neuromuscular disorders.

Portwood MM, Wicks JJ, Lieberman JS, Duveneck MJ. Intellectual and cognitive function in adults with myotonic muscular dystrophy. *Arch Phys Med Rehab* 67:299–303, 1986.

Useful information for the comprehensive rehabilitation of myotonic dystrophy.

Young, RR, Delwaide PJ (Eds.), *Principles and practice of restorative neurology*. Stoneham, MA, Butterworth-Heinemann, 1993.

A contemporary review of the medical approach to the treatment of neurological disorders.

16

Rheumatic Disorders

Charles P. Moore, M.D.

The rheumatic disorders comprise a diverse group of disease processes that cause dysfunction of the musculoskeletal system. Arthritis is a common but not universal feature of these disorders, and is often the greatest cause of impairment. This chapter focuses on the principles of arthritis rehabilitation with emphasis on maintaining and maximizing function.

The term *arthritis* implies that inflammation is a primary part of the underlying pathology. In fact, the degree of inflammation varies from marked, in diseases such as rheumatoid arthritis, to minimal, in diseases such as osteoarthritis. Rehabilitation techniques will necessarily vary depending on the amount of inflammation and joint pathology, but the basic principles and goals of rehabilitation remain the same.

Goals of Rehabilitation

MAINTAIN COMFORT

Pain is the symptom that most frequently brings the patient to a physician. In some individuals, relief of pain is an adequate goal in itself. Rehabilitative techniques to relieve pain are a supplement to medical management, which often includes anti-inflammatory medications. Such medications alone frequently fail to adequately suppress pain. Pain medications, such as narcotics, are rarely indicated in the management of rheumatic disorders. Although rehabilitative approaches supplement medicinal treatment, their value in controlling pain is easily underestimated.

PREVENTION OR LIMITATION OF JOINT DESTRUCTION

The ensuing disease process often threatens the integrity of joint structures, including the cartilage, bone, synovium, fibrous capsule, and ligaments. The combination of deconditioned stabilizing muscles and overuse or misuse of joints further contributes to joint damage. If medical treatment is inadequate to halt the destructive forces, rehabilitative techniques may assist in limiting damage.

PRESERVATION AND MAINTENANCE OF FUNCTION

The goal of all arthritis management is preservation of function. Even if optimal management fails to prevent destruction and deformity, it is essential to assist the patient to the highest possible level of functioning consistent with the best control of the disease. With increasing impairment, patients may have to adapt to new ways of functioning in order to achieve an acceptable level of independence.

═══ Evaluation

Evaluation begins with a careful history that assesses the type of arthritis and its course to date. It is important to establish the amount and nature of pain and the patient's perception of functional limitations and capabilities. It is vital to understand the impact of the arthritis on specific aspects of activities of daily living (ADL), and vice versa. A questionnaire form that facilitates rapid assessment of functional abilities from the patient's perspective is shown in Table 16.1.

The physical examination together with the history will document the extent of joint involvement. In addition to the number and location of involved joints, attention is paid to the presence or absence as well as severity of inflammation, effusion, range of motion (ROM) limitations, muscle weakness and/or atrophy, and deformity. It is essential that the examiner observe the patient's mobility skills and upper extremity skills, including fine and gross motor coordination and reach. It is in the assessment of function involving multiple joints that the evaluator discovers the significance of disease activity in individual joints. More in-depth evaluations of mobility and ADL functions can be performed by physical and occupational therapists.

═══ Management

Rehabilitation management recognizes the inherent merit in applying the skills of individual disciplines in a team effort. In addition to the physician, the rehabilitation team may include a physical therapist, an occupational therapist, a social worker, a nurse, and a psychologist. The decision to involve only one or two members of the team as opposed to the entire team is based on the needs of the individual patient and can be made after the physician has performed his or her initial assessment.

One of the most common omissions in the management of rheumatic disorders is failure to recognize the influence of psychological and social factors on the course of the disease. Attending only to the physical aspects of the patient's problems limits the impact of rehabilitation, particularly in the most severely involved individuals. A vital task of the rehabilitation team is helping the patient adjust to the changes imposed by the disease.

REST

Rest has a long history in arthritis management. A specific daily period of complete rest is mandatory for many patients with inflammatory conditions, such as rheumatoid arthritis. During periods of severe inflammation, some patients benefit from complete bed rest for a period of several weeks or more. Such complete rest in the hospital setting has been documented to reduce inflammatory activity, particularly in the lower extremity joints, and is even associated with reduced erythrocyte sedimentation rate.

Prolonged rest unfortunately leads to generalized weakness, poor cardiovascular fitness, loss of bone mass, and potentially to reduced joint ROM, as described in Chapter 6. Clearly the benefits of bed rest must be weighed against the risks.

Complete rest of individual joints through casting or splinting predictably reduces inflammation during severe flareups. Such immobilization for less than one month does not lead to contracture, but is limited by patients' tolerance of casting or splinting major joints. Further, cartilage nutrition depends on joint compression, and complete immobilization may have some deleterious effects. Notwithstanding, when facing severe localized joint inflammation, consideration should be given to short periods of localized immobilization as a means of preventing rapid joint destruction.

MODALITIES

Application of heat or cold to increase comfort can facilitate an exercise program. Short periods of superficial heat, such as that produced by hot packs, paradoxically reduces the internal temperature of inflamed joints by reflex mechanisms. Pain and muscle spasm are also diminished.

Many patients begin their day with a hot shower or bath. This is probably the most practical day-to-day superficial heat modality for most patients. In addition to decreasing pain, such generalized application of superficial heat decreases joint stiffness. Deep heat application increases internal joint temperature. In the presence of inflammation, deep heat modalities are likely to increase pain and inflammation.

Ultrasound is a particularly effective means of delivering heat to deep joint structures and is especially useful for heating capsular and ligamentous collagen, thus enhancing ROM exercises in a condition such as frozen shoulder. Because such delivery of deep heat increases intraarticular temperature, ultrasound is contraindicated in acutely inflamed joints and must be used cautiously whenever joint inflammation is suspected. The same precaution applies to diathermy and microwave, although they penetrate tissue less effectively than ultrasound.

Some patients prefer cold modalities to heat, and cold application by ice pack or massage reduces pain and stiffness as well as muscle spasms. Cold application has been demonstrated to reduce joint inflammation in experimental arthritis and is therefore used preferentially by some experts during periods of intense inflammation.

RANGE OF MOTION EXERCISES

Loss of joint range is one of the most limiting features of arthritis, and a diligent daily program to maintain ROM can be critical to the maintenance of function. Unfortunately, exercises can easily incite increased inflammation and care must be taken to avoid this possibility. Even passive ranging has been documented to have this effect.

Complete rest until inflammation begins to subside may be prudent when treating severely inflamed joints. With decreasing inflammation, it is safe to advance to a program of passive ranging. Still later it is possible to progress to active assistive ranging, and finally to a program of active ROM.

It is important to keep in mind that even one motion through full range daily will serve to maintain joint range; therefore, several partial ranges followed by one full range may be adequate for inflamed joints. A more vigorous program is required if inflammation is well controlled and the goal is to regain lost range. Ceiling pulleys enhance an upper extremity ranging program by allowing the patient to more effectively range the shoulders.

It is important to remember that prolonged stretch distends and deforms collagen better than short duration, rapid stretch. Thus lying in the prone position reduces hip flexion contractures more effectively than does a program of repetitious ranging exercises designed to stretch the hip flexors.

A warm pool (92–94° Fahrenheit) is an excellent resource for maintaining and increasing ROM. The buoyancy and warmth of the water facilitates the ranging program, and the resistance of the water permits some muscle strengthening as well.

Increased pain, lasting more than 1 hr after any exercise, raises the question of a too vigorous program. Excess pain lasting greater than 2 hr after exercise clearly indicates an excessive program.

STRENGTHENING AND FITNESS EXERCISES

Atrophy and muscle weakness are common in arthritis and add significantly to total dysfunction. Unfortunately, the most functionally effective strengthening exercises are isotonic and isokinetic, both of which involve active movement against resistance. Such exercises tend to promote increased pain and inflammation and are only feasible if joint pathology is limited.

Isometric exercises (performed without joint movement) are usually tolerated even in severely affected joints. A maximum static muscle contraction lasting for a slow count of 6 to 10 (5–10 seconds) several times a day, while suboptimal, can help maintain strength. A program of isometric exercises utilizing large elastic bands and a partially inflated beach ball has been described by Swezey (2).

Decreased activity leads to compromised cardiovascular fitness. Dynamic, low-impact, low-resistance exercises should therefore be considered an important component of a balanced rehabilitation program. A well-designed pool program contributes to cardiovascular fitness, as well as to muscle strengthening and ranging. The stationary bicycle has also been used effectively in selected patients.

SPLINTING

Splinting and bracing are useful adjuncts in specific situations. Eliminating or limiting motion across joints can reduce pain and inflammation as well as stabilize joints weakened by damage to ligaments and other tissues. Unfortunately, there is no documented evidence that splinting prevents deformities. Therefore, the goals of splints are improved function, decreased pain and inflammation, and increased comfort.

Resting hand splints help control inflammation and can be used either at night or during periods of intense inflammation, intermittently during the day. These splints have the disadvantage of not permitting functional use of the hands while they are worn.

Functional splints can be fabricated to protect specific joints, such as the proximal interphalangeal joints and the first metacarpal phalangeal joints (Figure 16.1). One of the most useful splints is a functional wrist splint (Figure 16.1), which allows a good digital function while stabilizing the wrist. Occupational

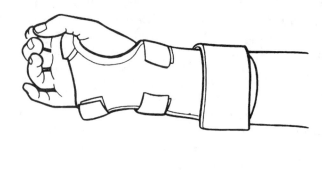

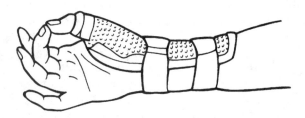

FIGURE 16.1. *Top:* Functional wrist splint. *Bottom:* Functional splint stabilizing the first metacarpalphalangeal and first carpometacarpal joints.

therapists with particular skills in upper extremity orthotics typically provide the necessary expertise for upper extremity splint fabrication.

Lower extremity orthotics require careful attention to the biomechanics of gait. The most successful intervention often involves the correct fitting of shoes. Care is taken to adequately stabilize the foot while also considering the extra space needed for comfort if deformities are present. Orthotic shoe inserts can provide additional support and comfort. Minimal alterations, such as a metatarsal bar or a cushioned sole insert, can have a dramatic impact. An orthotist skilled in lower extremity orthotics is essential in managing lower extremity instability and alignment problems.

ADAPTIVE AIDS

Assistive devices may improve function and protect joints during functional activities. Devices range from the very simple, such as large-handled eating utensils, to the expensive and complex, such as an electric mobility device.

Special chairs and elevated toilet seats are required by individuals who cannot rise from low seats. It is generally wise for physical therapists to evaluate and train a patient to use mobility aids in a therapeutic setting before such aids are prescribed for home use. Occupational therapists are experts in recommending devices to facilitate upper extremity function and assist in ADLs.

PATIENT EDUCATION

Education is the cornerstone of effective rehabilitation management (1). Effective education empowers the patient to take control of his or her life and adapt to a new and more appropriate lifestyle. It is the patient who must live with the arthritis, and it is only the patient who can balance his or her life in the fashion necessary to guarantee the best outcome.

Patients must know how much they can do, what they cannot do, and how to protect their joints during ADLs. Merely giving the patient a pamphlet or booklet is inadequate. Proper education must be viewed as a long-term process, with each member of the team providing appropriate information and answering questions as they arise. The best education occurs in the therapeutic setting while the patient is actually demonstrating newly learned skills. Reduction of fear and anxiety proceed from effective education.

The American Rheumatism Association has developed an excellent self-help course that is available in many communities at low cost. This program is an adjunct to services provided by rehabilitation professionals and does not substitute for necessary treatment.

Specific areas of education should include training in energy conservation and joint protection. Learning to plan and pace activities is critical in those individuals for whom fatigue or risk of further inflammatory flare-ups and pain are present. Learning to protect involved joints by techniques such as avoiding certain positions and using joints in positions of maximum stability can be vital in limiting further damage to joints.

References

1. Lorig K, Fries JF. *The arthritis health book*. Reading, MA, Addison-Wesley, 1986.
2. Swezey RL. *Arthritis: Rational therapy and rehabilitation*. Philadelphia, W.B. Saunders, 1978.

Suggested Reading List

Brattstrom M. *Joint protection and rehabilitation in chronic rheumatic disorders*. Frederick, MD, Aspen Publishers, 1987.

Ehrlich GE. *Total management of the arthritis patient*. Philadelphia, J.B. Lippincott, 1973.

Galloway MT, Jokl P. The role of exercise in the treatment of inflammatory arthritis. *Bulletin on the Rheumatic Diseases* 42 (1).

Goeppinger JP, Arthur MW, Baglioni AJ Jr, Brunk SE, Bruner CM. A re-examination of the effectiveness of self care education for persons with arthritis. *Arthritis Rheum* 32:706-716, 1989.

Hicks JE, Nicholas JJ, Swezey RL. *Handbook of rehabilitative rheumatology*. Atlanta, American Rheumatism Association, 1988.

McCarty DJ (Ed.). *Arthritis and allied conditions*. Philadelphia, Lea & Febiger, 1989.

Melvin JL. *Rheumatic disease in adults and children: Occupational therapy and rehabilitation* (3d ed.). Philadelphia, F.A. Davis, 1989.

17

Amputation Rehabilitation

Joseph M. Czerniecki, M.D.

Limb loss secondary to amputation is prevalent in the United States. It can have profound effects on physical functioning and psychological well-being. These effects can, however, be minimized with comprehensive rehabilitation, and in most instances, patients will be able to return to an effective ambulatory status and to lead rewarding and productive lives. It has been said that too often medicine views amputation as failure of medical care; rather it should be viewed as a reconstructive procedure that acts as a starting point for return to function.

Epidemiology

The number of amputees in the United States has been estimated at greater than 2 million. The National Center for Health Statistics (1983) estimated an annual incidence of 150,000 amputations, excluding Veterans Administration and public health hospitals. Of these, 35,000 were above knee level; 37,000 below the knee; 11,000 in the foot; and 35,000 involved the digits (2). A total of 118,000 amputations were therefore performed in the lower extremity. The disproportionate number of lower extremity amputations relates to the etiology of limb loss (Table 17.1).

The two major contributors to amputation secondary to medical disease are atherosclerotic vascular disease and diabetes. Approximately 70 percent of all lower extremity amputees have vascular disease, and of these, approximately 80 percent have diabetes. As a cause of amputation, vascular disease and diabetes have special implications because both processes are generalized multisystem disorders. Atherosclerosis involves not only the peripheral vascular system, but also the cardiovascular and cerebral vascular systems. Therefore, this population

TABLE 17.1.

Causes of Lower-Extremity Amputation

ETIOLOGY	PERCENT OF TOTAL AMPUTATIONS
Medical disease	70.3
Trauma	22.4
Tumor	4.5
Congenital	2.8

of amputees may exhibit a high incidence of myocardial infarction, congestive heart failure, angina, TIA, or stroke. This has major ramifications when considering rehabilitation of the dysvascular amputee. Additionally, diabetes affects the nervous system, causing polyneuropathy, and can also result in vision loss secondary to diabetic retinopathy. These factors can also complicate rehabilitation management.

There is a high mortality rate among individuals with amputations secondary to vascular disease and diabetes. The survival rate 3 years after a patient's first amputation is only 61 percent. In addition to an increased mortality, there is a much greater incidence of amputation of the contralateral limb. In diabetics there is an 11.9 percent incidence of secondary amputation within 1 year; 17.8 percent after 2 years; 27.2 percent after 3 years; and 44.3 percent after 4 years. Amputation is therefore the result of a generalized pathological process that results in a high incidence of mortality, as well as a risk of further amputation in the contralateral lower extremity.

Etiology

The increased risk of amputation in the diabetic is related to a number of variables, including limb ischemia, neuropathic changes, and increased risk of infection (Figure 17.1). Diabetics have an accelerated rate of atherosclerosis. While the distribution of the atherosclerosis is similar to that of nondiabetics, medium-sized arteries tend to be affected as well as larger vessels. In addition to the large-vessel atherosclerosis, the diabetic is also subject to a microangiopathy affecting the small arterioles and capillaries. There is considerable controversy as to whether this contributes to the increased risk of amputation; however, it is felt that it does increase the risk of small-vessel thrombosis, secondary to either trauma or infection. The end result of ischemia may be tissue necrosis and gangrene, leading to amputation.

Impaired motor and sensory function in the distal lower extremities predisposes the diabetic to the development of skin ulcers, which may become secondarily infected. Diabetic polyneuropathy affects sensory, motor, and autonomic nerves in a symmetric "glove and stocking" distribution, with earliest involvement in the sensory system. With an insensate foot, the patient is often unaware of recurring or acute tissue injury, and is therefore unable to prevent or respond to damage occurring to his or her foot. In addition to sensory impairment, the motor component of the neuropathy causes weakness and atrophy of the intrinsic muscles in the foot, leading to an unbalanced pull by the long extensors and flexors of the toes, and resulting in the typical claw toe deformity. This deformi-

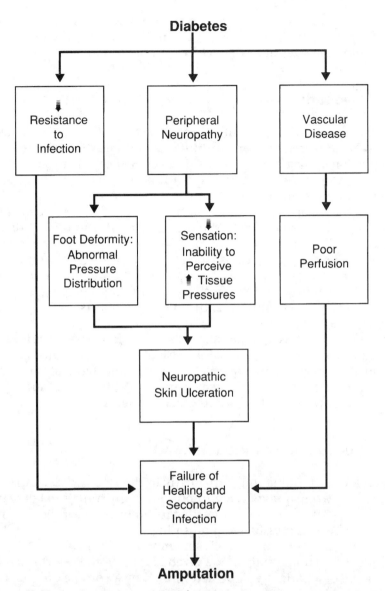

FIGURE 17.1. Diabetes is a common risk factor for amputation. The associated peripheral neuropathy, vascular disease, and reduced resistance to infection can lead to skin ulceration, tissue necrosis, and gangrene, which may necessitate amputation.

ty can progress to the point where there is subluxation of the metatarsal–phalangeal joints, and prominence of the metatarsal–phalangeal joints on the plantar surface and proximal interphalangeal joints dorsally. The prominence of these bony areas, combined with reduced sensation, is likely to produce ulceration. The impairment of autonomic outflow decreases sudomotor function, causing dry skin and fissuring.

The diabetic has an increased susceptibility to infection because polymorphonuclear leukocyte function is impaired. Therefore, once an opening in the skin has occurred, either through neuropathic ulceration or fissuring, an entry point is provided to allow bacteria into the subdermal tissues. Infection can then occur, leading to impaired healing, cellulitis, osteomyelitis, or sepsis. These factors may ultimately result in the need for amputation.

Prevention

With the use of appropriate preventive measures, the high risk of limb loss in the diabetic can be decreased. In some institutions, preventive programs led to a 50 percent reduction in major amputations. The key element in any prevention program is education. This can be done through specialized clinics and with preprinted educational materials.

To reduce the risk factors for atherosclerosis, the patient should be instructed to stop smoking, cholesterol levels should be checked, appropriate dietary recommendations should be made, and optimum management of hypertension should occur. The second aspect of the prevention program should relate to general foot care. The patient should be educated thoroughly about techniques that prevent tissue injury, and an effective nail and foot care program should be instituted by a physician, nurse practitioner, or podiatrist experienced in the management of the diabetic foot.

If foot deformities develop, specialized footwear, footwear modifications, and orthotics may be necessary to reduce the risk of neuropathic ulceration. These recommendations should be made by a podiatrist or rehabilitation medicine specialist. In some instances, an orthopedic surgeon's opinion regarding a surgical approach to the correction of deformities may be necessary.

Selection of Amputation Level

Amputation level determination, particularly in the elderly dysvascular patient, is complex. The two major goals are to minimize any functional deficit resulting from amputation while at the same time to remove all necrotic and/or infected tissue and achieve successful wound healing.

As a general rule, the more distally an amputation is performed, the greater the subsequent functional status. At a given amputation level, the actual functional outcome of a patient will be determined by a complex interaction of a number of variables. Therefore, the preoperative evaluation must include an assessment of the patient's cognitive, intellectual, and perceptual function, visual function, cardiopulmonary function, musculoskeletal status, and neuromuscular status. This assessment, combined with a knowledge of the necessary functional requirements for successful prosthetic use, will allow one to make a reasonable determination of the amputation level that will lead to the best functional outcome.

In the dysvascular patient, the more proximal the amputation is performed, the greater the likelihood of wound healing. To optimize function and achieve the greatest likelihood of wound healing, the surgeon must perform the amputation at the most distal level compatible with wound healing. The likelihood of wound healing after amputation is dependent on the patient's general nutritional status, the presence of concurrent major medical conditions, the local circulation to the skin at the time of the amputation, the surgical technique, and the quality of postoperative wound care. Skin circulation can be evaluated clinically on the basis of limb temperature and the location of a temperature transition from warm to cool as the hand is moved in a proximal to distal direction over the lower extremity, as well as the presence of chronic hair loss and other cutaneous changes. The clinical evaluation is likely to be successful when performed by a surgeon with extensive experience in amputation management; however, more objective and sensitive means of predicting wound healing have been developed to augment the bedside examination. These include segmental blood pressures and transcutaneous partial pressures of oxygen (TCPO$_2$). Vascular surgery can sometimes be used to improve perfusion, and thereby alter the level at which successful wound healing may occur. This may be critically important in the patient where the preservation of a distal amputation level is essential to the maintenance of function.

SEGMENTAL BLOOD PRESSURES

The magnitude of the systolic arterial blood pressure can be determined using a Doppler device over superficial arteries at many locations. The ankle-arm index is a ratio of the systolic pressure in either the dorsalis pedis or posterior tibial arteries of the foot over the brachial artery systolic pressure. A number of studies suggest that healing is correlated with an adequate absolute pressure, or an adequate ankle-arm index. This technique has some limitations with the diabetic patient because calcific changes in the vessel wall are common and lead to erroneously high pressures.

TRANSCUTANEOUS PARTIAL PRESSURES OF OXYGEN

The measurement of transcutaneous partial pressures of oxygen (TCPO$_2$) is a relatively new technique used to evaluate skin blood flow is through the use of transcutaneous partial pressures of oxygen (TCPO$_2$). An electrode is placed on the skin of the lower extremity in standard locations. Oxygen transpired through the skin causes a voltage change, which is measured by a computer. The amount of oxygen transpired through the skin depends not only on the oxygen saturation of the blood, but also on the local perfusion to the skin and the amount of oxygen metabolized in the skin. The results of early studies suggest TCPO$_2$ measurements may be useful in the prediction of successful healing at various amputation levels.

Common Amputation Levels of the Lower Extremity

PARTIAL FOOT AMPUTATIONS

Recently there has been a resurgence of interest in preserving the foot by doing partial foot amputations rather than performing the amputation above the level of the ankle; therefore, there has been a increasing number of digit and ray amputations. For conditions where pathologic involvement is limited to the digits, the amputation of single toes through the level of the metatarso-phalangeal joint is a reasonable procedure (see Figure 17.2). If the level of pathology extends proximally to the level of the metatarso-phalangeal joints, the amputation may be extended to include a portion of the ray. These amputations, if healed, provide little functional deficit and require only minor modifications to footwear. Their advantage compared to more proximal amputations is that the proprioceptive and neuromuscular function about the foot and ankle remains intact.

Moving proximally, the next most common level of amputation is the transmetatarsal amputation. This procedure is often performed on the diabetic patient when there is evidence of toe deformities that cause the patient to be at increased risk for further development of neuropathic ulceration, or when there is necrosis of a number of digits. Little function is gained by preserving the remaining digits. This amputation can be carried out at any point along the length of the metatarsals, provided that there is adequate plantar skin and soft tissue to allow a long plantar flap. This amputation is generally viewed favorably because it preserves neuromuscular function about the foot and ankle. There may be a need

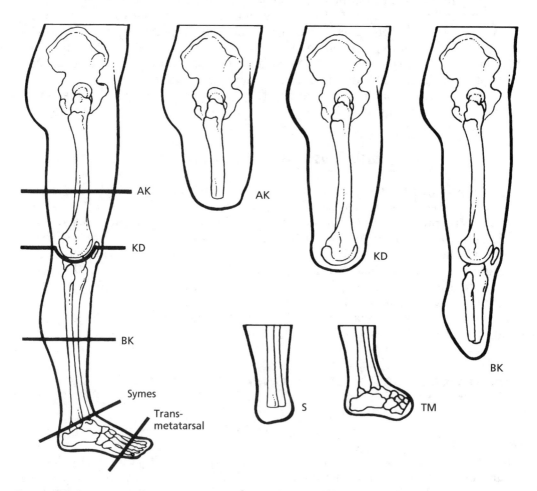

FIGURE 17.2. Common lower-extremity amputation levels.

for some simple modifications to footwear after this procedure, which may include a custom-molded insole or a spring steel plate in the sole of the shoe, with a rocker bottom adaptation.

The Lisfranc amputation is carried out through the tarsometatarsal junction, whereas the Chopart amputation is performed through the more proximal intertarsal region—commonly at the talonavicular and calcaneo-cuboid junctions. The deformity that results from these amputations is typically an equino-varus deformity, and is the result of two factors: The resection of the attachments of the dorsiflexors of the foot leaves an unbalanced foot overpowered by the plantar flexing musculature, and the deformity is caused by loss of the distal bony portion of the longitudinal arch of the foot. These two amputation levels are held in poor regard at this time due to the risk of having a painful weight-bearing residual limb, plus an increased risk of developing skin ulcerations on the plantar surface resulting from the abnormal pressure distribution on the plantar aspect of the foot remnant.

The prosthetic management of this amputation level is variable. In some patients, management similar to that of the transmetatarsal amputation works well: a custom-molded in-shoe orthotic with a spring steel plate in the sole of the shoe and rocker bottom modification to the shoe. For amputees who experience discomfort or blistering, there are numerous modifications of the Chopart prosthesis, which extend it proximally to include a shank segment; this minimizes shear forces applied to the residual limb.

SYMES AMPUTATION

The Symes amputation is performed through the ankle joint. The tips of the medial and lateral malleoli are resected to the level of the talotibial articulation and the plantar heel pad that normally exists under the calcaneus is brought up to cover the distal surface of the residual limb. There are a number of benefits to this level of amputation. The patient has an end-bearing residual limb that can be used for short-distance ambulation in the house without a prosthetic device. The length of the residual limb provides greater proprioceptive feedback, and there is also a reduced metabolic energy demand at this amputation level compared to higher levels. The disadvantage of this amputation level is that it leaves a somewhat bulbous-shaped ankle that lacks the normal contours of the intact lower extremity. The Symes amputation represents a choice between the functional and the cosmetic needs of the patient.

BELOW-KNEE (BK) AMPUTATION

The BK amputation should be performed at three-fourths of the length from the knee joint to the musculotendinous junction of the gastrocnemius, or at least 19 cm below the knee. It is common, however, that in the dysvascular amputee the residual limb may need to be shorter than this recommended level. The fibula is shortened approximately one-half inch less than the tibial remnant; the anterior distal aspect of the tibia should be beveled and rounded to avoid sharp bony prominences underlying the skin and subcutaneous elements. The long posterior musculo-cutaneous flap of the gastrocnemius soleus is attached to the periosteum of the tibia and fascia of the muscles of the anterior and lateral compartment. In all cases, the preservation of the knee joint leads to a more functional end result for the patient, and even a very short BK amputation should be chosen before extending the amputation through the knee or above it. There are many prosthetic options for this amputation level, including many types of suspensions and prosthetic socket designs, as well as prosthetic interfaces between the socket and skin, and prosthetic foot designs. BK amputation is a highly successful amputation level, and there are many choices of components to enhance function.

THROUGH-THE-KNEE AMPUTATION

There has been a resurgence of interest in the knee disarticulation level amputation in some centers. The advantages of this amputation level relative to the above-knee amputation are that there is a longer residual limb, and therefore a more powerful movement arm for controlling the prosthetic limb, and it is an end-bearing residual limb that provides greater proprioceptive feedback. The reluctance to perform this procedure in some centers is based on the fact that the cutaneous flap required for this procedure is long and often tenuous in the patient with poor vascular perfusion. This leads to a higher than normal requirement for revision. Also, the residual limb is bulbous in appearance because of the widened femoral condyles, and it is therefore difficult to cosmetically incorporate into the socket. Recent improvements in prosthetic components have led to an enhancement of function. This amputation level is particularly useful in the traumatic amputee where the below-knee segment cannot be salvaged.

ABOVE-KNEE AMPUTATION (AK)

Amputation above the knee (AK) ideally should be performed approximately 3 inches above the joint line because it will maximize the length of the residual limb and at the same time leave enough space for the prosthetic knee. The advantages of the long residual limb are, once again, increased preservation of muscle power and greater surface area for distribution of forces.

HIP DISARTICULATION AMPUTATION

This relatively uncommon level of amputation can occur secondarily to underlying vascular disease, tumor, or trauma. This amputation is carried out through the hip joint. The muscular remnants of the hip musculature are used to cover and protect the underlying bony prominences of the os coxae. This level of amputation results in a major functional deficit for the patient. Patients often do not pursue the use of a prosthesis because of greater speed and ease of ambulation on the remaining lower extremity with two forearm crutches. However, prosthetic components are available for this amputation level and provide both a cosmetic and functional lower extremity for short-distance ambulation.

Rehabilitation Management of the Lower Extremity Amputee

The optimum management of the lower extremity amputee requires a team approach, involving the skills of prosthetists, physical therapists, occupational therapists, social workers, vocational counselors, and psychologists. An integrated and comprehensive approach to patient management is essential for achieving both immediate and long-term success.

PRE-AMPUTATION REHABILITATION

Many patients who have a limb at risk for amputation spend considerable time on medical or surgical wards to heal infected foot ulcers or deal with the management of trauma or revascularization procedures. During this time, there is a significant risk of deconditioning and development of contractures, particularly in the elderly individual. It is therefore imperative at this phase that a maintenance program of physical therapy be instituted to prevent contracture and to maintain joint range of motion (ROM), muscle strength, and cardiopulmonary endurance.

Once the decision has been made to amputate, it is important that the patient be educated as to what to anticipate during the operative and postoperative phases. In many amputation centers, audiovisual presentations have been developed. Amputee support groups also can be used to help the patient deal with some of the psychological consequences and stress that surround the pending amputation.

EARLY POSTOPERATIVE MANAGEMENT

The major goals during the early postoperative phase of rehabilitation are to continue the strengthening and endurance program, continue the psychological support of the amputee, ensure wound healing and stump maturation, and effectively manage pain.

Wound healing and stump maturation are integral to the long-term effective functioning of the amputee. There are many different techniques used during this phase to enhance the likelihood and rate of healing and maturation. The advantages and disadvantages of these techniques are reviewed here.

Soft Dressing with External Elastic Compression

The traditional postsurgical management of the amputee has been with a soft dressing (Figure 17.3C), which may or may not have external compression by an elastic ace bandage or stump shrinker. The ace bandage is applied in a figure-of-eight wrap, with graded pressure applied distally to proximally. It is important in this type of dressing that no circumferential proximal compression occur because the resultant tourniquet effect will increase swelling and may delay or prevent wound healing. The extensive use of staff resources makes this technique infeasible in most settings, and teaching patients to use this procedure effectively is difficult.

The stump shrinker is an elastic device, pulled onto the residual limb, that provides external compression through the elastic quality of the material. Use

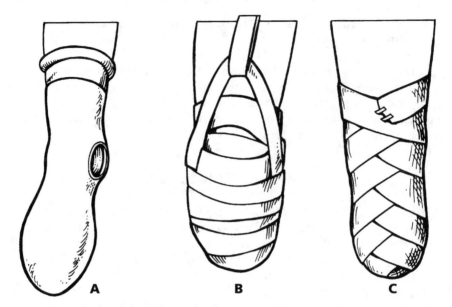

FIGURE 17.3. Methods of postoperative wound care include: (A) rigid dressing; (B) removable rigid dressing; (C) elastic ace wrap.

of the shrinker avoids the potential problems of either a tourniquet effect or lack of uniform pressure application, which may occur with the elastic bandage. The stump shrinker, however, only comes in a limited number of sizes, and the amount of compression depends on the volume of the stump in relation to the size of the shrinker. It is therefore difficult to control the magnitude of pressure applied. Variations in the shape of the residual limb will create inconsistency in the externally applied pressure as well. In the early postoperative phase, the application of the stump shrinker may cause traction forces across the incision and subsequent wound disruption. Once wound healing is complete, this is a safe and effective means of controlling stump volume.

Jobst Air Splint

An air splint is a double-walled plastic device that is placed over the residual limb of either the above- or below-knee amputee. The splint is filled with air to a fixed pressure. The pressure is typically lower while the patient is in bed, and is increased in standing to allow a certain amount of weight bearing. This system, although having some benefit in terms of accessibility of the wound postoperatively, has several disadvantages: it is hot, and fluid accumulation due to perspiration may interfere with stump healing. Air splints are also notoriously problematic in terms of frequency of puncture. The air splint extends across the knee in the below-knee amputee and forces the patient to walk with a fully extended knee.

Rigid Dressings

A plaster cast is applied immediately after skin closure in the operating room. This technique, termed *the immediate postoperative prosthesis* (IPOP), was initially used in conjunction with the application of a temporary prosthetic pylon and foot. Using this technique, the amputee began some early weight bearing on the day after amputation. Because of an increased rate of failure of healing and need for revision—especially in the dysvascular population—this technique has been modified to what is termed an *early postoperative prosthesis* (EPOP), in which ambulation is delayed from 10 to 21 days postoperatively. During this time, prior to the initiation of weight bearing, the rigid dressing is simply termed the *immediate postoperative rigid dressing* (IPRD) (Figure 17.3A).

An IPRD enhances wound healing by preventing edema and mechanical trauma to the healing incision. It also prevents the development of knee-flexion contractures because the knee is rigidly immobilized in near full extension. It is also thought to reduce the incidence of phantom limb pain and cause a more rapid rate of stump maturation. The overall effect is to accelerate the rate of rehabilitation, shorten hospital stay, and decrease mortality. This technique is limited because there is no means to accelerate shrinkage of the residual limb between cast changes, which occur at 1–2 week intervals. As the residual limb shrinks, there may be "pistoning" within the rigid dressing, causing mechanical trauma to the incision. When ambulation is initiated with this type of dressing, the knee is immobilized in near full extension, resulting in gait abnormalities that may be difficult to change once the prosthesis is provided. Finally, the rigid dressing is fixed to the limb, preventing assessment of the effect of ambulation on the integrity of the wound.

A postoperative protocol using a removable rigid dressing has been developed to address these limitations (Figure 17.3B). This rigid dressing extends only to the level of the knee. It has the advantages of the IPRD in immobilizing and protecting the tissues, and accelerating the rate of maturation, but does not immobilize the knee. When the patient is able to begin gait training, the effect of ambulation and the integrity of the residual limb can be easily evaluated by removal of the rigid dressing. The knee is free to flex during ambulation and a more normal gait pattern can be developed.

LATE POSTOPERATIVE MANAGEMENT

The late postoperative period begins only 3 weeks after amputation. At this point, the usual below-knee dysvascular amputee has healed the residual limb to the point that weight bearing can be initiated while wearing a removable rigid dressing. The patient begins standing with 40 pounds of weight bearing for short periods, followed by a reevaluation of the residual limb by removal of the rigid dressing. The amount of weight bearing is determined by a scale placed underneath the amputee's rigid dressing and pylon system during standing. Weight bearing is increased quickly to 40 pounds during ambulation using the parallel bars, progressing in 20-pound increments to the patient's full body weight. As the patient's balance and gait improve, he/she begins walking outside the parallel bars using two forearm crutches.

Usually at about 5–6 weeks post-amputation, there has been considerable shrinkage and maturation of the residual limb, and the patient is typically ready for an interim prosthesis. The residual limb will continue to shrink and shape over the ensuing 3–6 months, at which time a permanent prosthesis will be provided. In reality, all prostheses are somewhat temporary and will need to be replaced due to deterioration in fit or mechanical breakdown. The selection of prosthetic components for each amputation level is complex and takes into account many variables. At the below-knee amputation level, the process of choosing prosthetic components must include an evaluation of the patient's cardiopulmonary status, body weight, vocational and avocational interests, length of the residual limb, and whether the residual limb has special characteristics, such as split thickness skin grafts, scar tissue, or neuromata. The prosthetic prescription includes the following major categories: suspension, prosthetic socket design, interface between the prosthetic socket and the residual limb, shank characteristics, and prosthetic ankle–foot characteristics. The choice of components is often made in conjunction with the prosthetist who will manufacture the limb.

Another major focus of the rehabilitation process at this time is continuation of education in management and hygiene of the residual limb and care of the prosthesis. The volume of the residual limb gradually decreases after the patient begins to ambulate. The reduction in volume must be accommodated by an increase in the thickness (ply) of socks that are worn while using the prosthesis. If this is not done appropriately, it will lead to discomfort and an increased risk of skin breakdown. This is particularly true in the patient who has an insensate residual limb.

Patients are provided a home exercise program to maintain and increase the strength of their lower extremity musculature. The most important muscle groups for using a prosthesis are the hip extensor and hip abductor groups, both at the below-knee and above-knee amputation levels. The preservation of ROM after discharge from the hospital is essential, as hip and knee flexion contractures can occur from prolonged sitting. One of the simplest ways to avoid these contractures is to have the patient lie prone twice a day for 20 min.

Effective long-term care of the amputee requires follow-up by an individual experienced in prosthetic care: either a rehabilitation medicine physician or a prosthetist. Careful follow-up of these patients allows one to anticipate problems in prosthetic fit before it causes skin breakdown and the possible need for surgical revision. This is also an ideal opportunity to evaluate and reinforce appropriate care of the intact lower extremity, therefore preventing further amputation.

Outcome of Lower-Extremity Amputation

FUNCTIONAL OUTCOME

The functional outcome after lower-extremity amputation is based on many variables other than the amputation itself. The patient population tends to be elderly with concurrent medical diseases, all of which complicate the interpretation of any functional change resulting from amputation. Age as an isolated variable is not critical to the outcome. In a follow-up study of 116 lower-extremity amputees older than 65, Steinberg et al. (3) reported that, at a mean time of 22 months after amputation, 73 percent of the below-knee amputees and 33 percent of the bilateral below-knee amputees were full-time users of their prosthesis.

A retrospective evaluation of functional outcome after amputation was reported by Kegel et al. (1), who administered a detailed questionnaire to 134 amputees ranging in age from childhood to the ninth decade. This study demonstrated that most amputees need to make some adaptations to maintain function, and that full preoperative function is not restored. In this population, only 1 percent of the unilateral below-knee amputees did not walk, while 19 percent of the above-knee amputees and 35 percent of the bilateral amputees did not walk. However, 45 percent of both the unilateral below-knee and above-knee amputees felt they walked as much as a normal person.

Employment is significantly impacted by an amputation, especially if the patient's job demands a significant amount of standing, walking, or walking over complex surfaces. In Kegel's study, only 60 percent of patients who were of employment age returned to some type of employment, and of those, only 22 percent were employed in their pre-amputation occupation. The use of vocational rehabilitation services is important in order to understand the functional demands of the patient's employment prior to amputation, and whether the post-amputation function is compatible with a return to this employment. Simple adaptations to the job often can be made, or, if return is not possible, retraining may be required to achieve employment in a more sedentary occupation.

Sexual activity is also affected by amputation. There is a reduction of sexual activity in both men and women after lower-extremity amputation; this reduction is greater in amputees at the above-knee level than at more distal levels of amputation. The decrease in sexual function was greater in unmarried amputees than in married ones, and by their report was related to impairment of both body image and sense of masculinity or femininity more than to physical limitations.

PSYCHOLOGICAL EFFECTS

The psychological reaction to the loss of a limb is complex, and also somewhat unique to the individual. It depends on age, chronicity of disease prior to amputation, time since amputation, and the importance of physical appearance to the patient's psychological well-being. The young traumatic amputee is said to undergo acute psychological distress in the early postoperative period, involving feelings of anxiety, resentment, and defiance. This is followed by fairly rapid adjustment. In contrast to the traumatic amputee who has little time to come to grips with the prospect of limb loss, the elderly dysvascular amputee often has had a prolonged period of illness with the limb being painful and dysfunctional. In the early postoperative period, the elderly amputee may actually be relieved to have had the amputation. Subsequently, the reality of potential loss of independence may lead to a sense of hopelessness and despair. These feelings may be amplified during the rehabilitative process, especially as discharge from the hospital approaches.

The amputee patient population as a group has been described in a number of studies as manifesting little in the way of extended psychologic distress. Yet, when examined in more detail by psychologic testing or by structured interviews, a high incidence of depression is seen; the frequency of such depression may be as high as 30–35 percent. The clinician caring for the amputee must be sensitive to subtle affective responses that may suggest its presence. In fact, it is recommended that amputees participate in a peer support group to allow effective role modeling and emotional support. If this is not available, short-term individual psychologic intervention may be useful.

═══ Complications

Pain is a significant problem in many lower-extremity amputees. After the early postoperative period, the differential diagnosis of post-amputation pain can include phantom limb pain, neuroma, referred pain from proximal sources, ischemia, mechanical irritation from the prosthetic socket, deep vein thrombosis, and infection. The evaluation of post-amputation pain requires a careful history and physical examination, as well as laboratory investigations.

PHANTOM LIMB PAIN

Phantom limb pain is defined as pain after amputation which is in the distribution of the amputated limb segment. This pain may have many characteristics; aching, burning, stabbing, or electrical sensations may occur. It is important to differentiate phantom limb pain from phantom limb sensation, in which the amputee has the perception that the limb is still present, and in some situations can move and position the amputated segment of the limb. The painful phantom occurs in as many as 90 percent of all amputees and is a major functional impairment in about 10 percent of these. The etiology of phantom limb pain is not well established. It is felt by most to be the result of deafferentation and the loss of sensory input. It commonly occurs in the same distribution as the pre-morbid amputation pain, and there is an association between the severity and duration of pre-amputation pain and the likelihood of developing post-amputation phantom limb pain. Phantom limb pain typically decreases somewhat in the first 6 months to 1 year after amputation. If the pain persists beyond this time, there is little likelihood that it will ever spontaneously resolve.

The treatment of phantom limb pain is sometimes difficult and requires an evaluation of behavioral and psychologic aspects of the patient in addition to other possible sources of pain. Agents specifically shown to be effective in phantom limb pain include the anticonvulsant family of medication, in particular Tegretol and Clonazepam. Other agents shown to have some utility include Elavil, propranolol, and, more recently, Mexilitine, an oral lidocaine-like medication.

NEUROMATA

Neuromas are said to occur any time a peripheral nerve is cut. Axonal sprouts and buds appear at the cut end of the nerve, with proliferation of myelin sheaths and Schwann cells. These become symptomatic when their location subjects them to mechanical trauma from a prosthesis or other external source. Typically the pain is an electrical sensation that radiates in the distribution of the peripheral nerve where the neuroma is located. This diagnosis can be confirmed by careful palpation of the residual limb and a knowledge of the common peripheral nerve distributions at each amputation level. If local palpation over the cut end of a nerve identifies a nodule with the appropriate sensory experience, a neuroma is likely to be the source of the discomfort. Management of this problem primarily revolves around the selection of an appropriate prosthetic socket and interface material, designed to minimize mechanical trauma to the neuroma. If pain persists despite optimum prosthetic management, the residual limb may have to be revised, the neuroma excised, and the sectioned nerves relocated to an area that will be less likely traumatized.

MECHANICAL IRRITATION

Probably the most common source of discomfort in the amputee's residual limb is mechanical irritation from an ill-fitting prosthetic socket. The cause of this discomfort can be due to abnormal alignment of the prosthesis or to abnormalities in the fit of the prosthetic socket. If this occurs, the patient's prosthetist should evaluate the problem and make necessary modifications to the prosthesis. It is common for an amputee's residual limb to change shape over many years and for new prosthetic sockets to be required.

ISCHEMIA

The most common cause of amputation is vascular disease, and an amputee remains subject to the progression of atherosclerotic vascular disease. This may lead to intermittent claudication or rest pain. If the patient's symptoms are compatible with this possibility, a vascular workup must be pursued with appropriate referral to vascular surgery for evaluation.

DEEP VEIN THROMBOSIS

DVT is a very common sequela of amputation, particularly in the early postoperative period. It is difficult to make the diagnosis due to the postoperative changes of swelling and discomfort in the residual limb. One must be keenly aware of its possibility and should readily use laboratory tests such as venous Doppler studies or venography as needed.

References

1. Kegel B, Carpenter ML, Burgess EM. Functional capabilities of lower extremity amputees. *Arch Phys Med Rehab* 59:109–120, 1978.
2. Rutkow IM. Orthopedic operations in the United States, 1979 through 1983. *J Bone Joint Surg* 65A:716–719, 1986.
3. Steinberg FV, Sunwoo I, Roettger RF. Prosthetic rehabilitation of geriatric amputee patients: A follow-up study. *Arch Phys Med Rehab* 66:742–745, 1985.

Annotated Suggested Reading List

Burgess EM, Matsen FA. Determining amputation levels in peripheral vascular disease. *J Bone Joint Surg* 63A:1493–1497, 1981.
   A review article that discusses the relative merits of each of the noninvasive tech-

niques for determining the likelihood of healing an amputation.

Levin MD, O'Neil LW. *The diabetic foot* (4th Ed). St. Louis, C.V. Mosby, 1988.

An excellent up-to-date reference dealing with many aspects of the diabetic foot, including the pathological changes, the etiology of these problems, prevention of foot injury, and management of neuropathic ulceration.

Malone JM, Moore W, Leal JM, Childers SJ. Rehabilitation for lower extremity amputation. *Arch Surg* 116:93–98, 1981.

This review discusses team management of the amputee and its importance in minimizing costs of patient care as well as enhancing functional outcome.

Moore, WS, Malone JN. *Lower extremity amputation* . Philadelphia, W.B. Saunders, 1989.

A textbook that deals with many aspects of lower-extremity amputation, including selection of level, surgical techniques, postoperative management, new prosthetic approaches, and phantom pain. The chapter on phantom pain is one of the most succinct and useful guides available on management.

Saunders GT. *Lower limb amputation: A guide to rehabilitation*. Philadelphia, F.A. Davis Co., 1986.

Although this book has information that deals with the breadth of amputation management, its major utility is in the rehabilitation approach and the evaluation of pathological gaits that arise from problems with prosthetic fit.

Wagner FW. The diabetic foot. *Orthopedics* 10:163–172, 1987.

A review article on evaluation of the diabetic foot and also prevention and management of neuropathic ulceration.

The Rehabilitation of Children and the Elderly

18

Principles of Pediatric Rehabilitation

Ross M. Hays, M.D., and Linda J. Michaud, M.D.

Approximately 10–15 percent of children in the United States have some form of chronic disease. Ten percent of this group, or 1 percent of all children in the United States, have a significant disability that interferes with life on a daily basis. At the turn of the century, infectious disease was the principal threat to health in the young; with current immunization practices and antibiotic availability, chronic diseases and injuries have replaced acute illnesses as the major cause of mortality and morbidity for children in this country. Physical disability differs in children and adults even when the underlying diagnosis is the same. The most significant difference is the child's dynamic state of development. The adult who acquires a disability suffers a loss of independence; the child who has or acquires a disability suffers loss in his or her *potential* to achieve independence.

══ Epidemiology

The demography of chronic disease and disability in childhood is dependent on incidence, geographic variation and migration, survival rates, and trends in the size of birth cohorts. The number of children with chronic childhood diseases has increased significantly in recent decades. There is good reason, however, to expect that the marked increase in these numbers experienced in the last generation of medical care will not continue at the rates most recently observed. This can be more easily understood by briefly examining each of these four determinants of the demography of chronic disability in childhood.

Many complicated and interdependent factors are involved in the changes in

215

the incidence of chronic pediatric disability. When Gortmaker and Sappenfield (3) reviewed 11 common childhood chronic diseases in 1981, they concluded that there is little evidence to suggest that significant changes in the incidence of chronic disease in childhood will occur in the near future. There are geographic variations in the incidence and prevalence of pediatric disability. For example, the major cause of acquired disability in childhood—injury—has wide geographic variation within the United States. Pediatric injury mortality rates (an indirect indicator of morbidity) are three times greater in Alaska (35/100,000/year) than in Massachusetts (11/100,000/year). Infection, environmental teratogens, and poor access to prenatal care are all related to different social, economic, and physical environments. Massive migrations of groups could have significant impact on the numbers of children with chronic disease and disability; however, it is extremely unlikely that any such migrations will occur in the United States in the near future.

The survival of children with chronic diseases has increased dramatically in the last generation of medical care. A sevenfold increase in the survival to age 21 among children with cystic fibrosis occurred between the 1940s and the mid-1970s. There has also been a twofold or greater increase in the survival for children with leukemia and congenital heart disease. Advances in trauma care systems and intensive care unit technology have been associated with increased survival of children who have sustained severe neurotrauma. When incidence of a disorder is constant and the chance of survival to adulthood reaches 100 percent, the childhood prevalence rate equals the incidence rate. Overall estimates of prevalence indicate that more than 80 percent of the maximum prevalence for the 11 most chronic diseases in children from birth to 20 years has already been achieved. The number of children in the birth cohort is the overwhelmingly dominant factor in the equation used to predict the numbers of children with chronic disease and disability. U.S. census reports suggest that the birth cohort will reach 4.0 million in the early 1990s and then decrease; the nadir will occur around the year 2000 and then will very gradually rise again until the year 2040.

There is little data, then, to indicate that a significant change should be expected in the incidence of common chronic diseases. The past generation has seen both a marked increase in the survival of children with chronic disease and disability and a similar rise in the birth cohort during the "baby boom." A decline in the birth cohort, little change in the incidence, a near-ceiling limit achieved in survival, and no change in migration is likely to result in little net increase in the observed numbers of children with chronic disability.

The demographic trends describing the future numbers of children with chronic disease and disability must be interpreted in the light of a continuing and appropriate demand for optimal quality of life for all individuals. This is reflected in recent and ongoing legislation associated with the rights and needs of people with handicaps. The future direction of pediatric rehabilitation will not be dictated by rapidly increasing numbers of children with handicaps, but by the challenge to improve the level of function of this population.

Habilitation is the term applied to the process that facilitates the development of function in children with congenital disabilities, or with disabilities acquired at an early age. *Rehabilitation* is the process of restoration of function, and is applicable to children who have lost previously acquired functions secondary to injury or illness. This distinction blurs when one considers that development takes place across multiple areas that affect physical, emotional, and social functioning. Some areas of function can be restored in children and adolescents who acquire a disability, but others are often lost.

Children with both congenital and acquired disability may be managed in either an inpatient or an outpatient setting, but the larger category of admissions to pediatric inpatient rehabilitation centers is for children with acquired conditions. Children who have experienced severe changes in their level of function are most likely to be managed on an inpatient basis. In general, children with congenital disabilities are more likely to be managed in the outpatient setting of a hospital, rehabilitation center, a school, or the home.

The goal of pediatric rehabilitation is to optimize the child's quality of life. A useful concept in dealing with conditions that are permanently disabling and have their onset in childhood was developed by Williams (13) in 1985. This measure is now referred to as the quality adjusted life year (QALY). Quality of life is affected by physical, emotional, and social functioning in the child as well as the adult. QALY incorporates considerations both of the impact of the disability on the individual's quality of life and the life expectancy. For a given increase in function associated with an improvement in the patient's quality of life that may result from provision of rehabilitation services, the youngest may be expected to gain the most.

Principles of Evaluation

The purpose of the evaluation in pediatric rehabilitation is primarily to assess those functions necessary to guide intervention. The history and physical examination are frequently supplemented by standardized assessments of motor, communication, perceptual, and cognitive function.

HISTORY

Developmental history is related to functional history in the child. Developmental data should include the age of accomplishment of developmental milestones in motor, language, adaptive, and social areas, and information should be obtained regarding skills that were achieved and subsequently lost. When early development was not normal, an attempt should be made to differentiate general delay in development from delay in a specific area of development, such as language or motor. Whether development was delayed or otherwise quantitatively abnormal should also be distinguished. Unlike adults, the child may be expected to be dependent at different stages of development for some or all of his or her functional activities.

In assessing mobility, the child's preferred mode of locomotion should be identified, as well as the highest level possible. Information regarding the level of independence in self-care activities should be assessed. A distinction should be made between those activities the child is capable of completing independently and those he or she actually does complete, and an attempt should be made to determine reasons for any discrepancies.

The child's social function is typically centered around his or her family and school. Information should be obtained regarding other members of the child's family. The availability of extended family support may influence the ability to meet any increased demands that the child's disability may have made on the family. An effort should be made to estimate the level of family stress and to ascertain whether problems related to the child's disability have contributed to this stress.

Outside of the family, school is the major social environment for a child. It is also the environment in which most rehabilitation interventions—including physical, occupational, and speech therapies—will be provided for children with disabilities. For children with acquired disabilities, a history of school performance prior to the injury or illness may be helpful in the identification of premorbid abilities, aptitudes, and deficits. A prevocational history should be elicited from adolescents with disabilities. Vocational interests, academic and other skills, and the expectations of both the adolescent and his or her parents regarding potential employment should be assessed.

PHYSICAL EXAMINATION

All children require a complete physical examination. In pediatric rehabilitation, most abnormalities are noted when examining the musculoskeletal and neurologic systems. Certain elements of the general pediatric examination are found to be abnormal with sufficient frequency to warrant mention. Growth parameters should be noted on standardized charts. The skin must be examined for integrity, particularly over the bony prominences and insensate areas, and a search should be made for neurocutaneous lesions. The cardiac examination may be abnormal in children with congenital syndromes, especially those that involve a limb deficiency. Restrictive pulmonary disease is frequently encountered in children with later-stage neuromuscular disorders. Evaluation of the Tanner stage of development is frequently helpful with regard to prediction of further growth and psychosocial assessment.

The musculoskeletal evaluation includes an assessment of the spine and extremities for symmetry, presence of deformity, and range of motion (ROM). Normal physiologic limitations in the ROM in children should be appreciated so that they may be differentiated from deformity; for example, a lack of complete hip and knee extension is normal in the newborn, and decreased femoral anteversion and physiologic bowing which results in the appearance of increased knee varus is normal for the toddler.

Some differences from the neurologic examination of the adult should be noted. Deep tendon reflexes may be absent, and reflexes that are pathological in the adult, such as the Babinski sign and grasp reflex, may be present in a normal infant. Postural reflex assessment receives more emphasis in the pediatric examination. Persistence of primitive reflexes or a failure of more advanced postural reflexes to appear when expected should be noted. Sensory testing is guided by the child's ability to cooperate with the evaluation. Pain sensation can sometimes be assessed even in the infant by the response to pinprick. Response to pinprick can, however, be misleading in the young child with myelodysplasia or spinal cord injury: a response to the stimulus may represent purely reflex mediated activity in those children. Useful information in the older child may be obtained by assessment of tactile, temperature, proprioceptive, and vibratory sensation, as well as of higher integrative sensory functions, such as stereognosis, two-point discrimination, and graphesthesia. Some clues regarding sensory function in younger children can be inferred through the history and through observation of the child's motor skills.

Muscle tone, bulk, strength, and symmetry are assessed when evaluating motor function. Formal manual muscle testing to grade strength is of limited utility in young children due to their inability to cooperate with the testing. Observations of posture and spontaneous movement are often helpful in detecting the presence and distribution of weakness. An inability to isolate volitional movement out of flexion or extension synergies should be detected, as well as the use of substitutions or "trick" movements. The presence of fasciculations or a tremor should be noted. Balance and coordination are assessed in relation to a child's age.

An understanding of the normal development of gait is a prerequisite to the ability to evaluate abnormalities of ambulation in children. Cadence, step length, duration of single-limb stance, and the ratio of pelvic span to ankle spread are determinants by which the maturity of a child's gait can be assessed. In children who are unable to ambulate, the quality of rolling and crawling and the child's preferred mode of locomotion should be assessed. The ability of the child to assume and maintain various positions appropriate to his or her level of development should be evaluated. Assessment of higher levels of balance and coordination may be helpful, particularly when evaluating children with milder deficits.

DEVELOPMENTAL/FUNCTIONAL ASSESSMENT

Standardized assessments are very commonly used in pediatric rehabilitation to determine a child's development in comparison to same-age children or to the child's own previous performance. Standard developmental screening tools are most useful when it is not clear whether the child's development grossly deviates from normal. Assessments specifically focusing on a particular aspect of development are more commonly used in pediatric rehabilitation. These domain-specific evaluations are more sensitive to changes in the child's status. They are typically performed by pediatric physical and occupational therapists, speech pathologists, and psychologists. Assessment of cognitive abilities in children may include tests of intellectual ability, academic performance, and neuropsychological function.

Vision and hearing should be screened in all children, and must be evaluated with particular care in children with cerebral palsy and acquired brain injury. Awareness of any sensory impairment is critical in the implementation of rehabilitation and education programs. The ability to drive a power wheelchair safely or to use a particular augmentative communication device requires adequate vision. Programs directed toward increasing language and cognitive skills may need to be modified to accommodate sensory impairment.

Frequent reevaluation is important in pediatric rehabilitation to modify interventions in a timely manner. Changes in function may occur in children with physical disabilities as a result of the natural history of their condition, the effects of growth and development, or secondary complications. For example, a progressive decline in ambulation skills is the expected course in Duchenne muscular dystrophy. In cerebral palsy, a decline in ambulation skills or decrease in endurance may be associated with more rigorous mobility requirements in adolescence or with secondary complications in the musculoskeletal system, such as increased contractures with growth spurts. In adolescents with spinal cord injury or myelodysplasia, changes in ambulation may represent the first clinical symptoms of treatable complications of the central nervous system, such as hydromyelia, syrinx formation, and tethering of the spinal cord.

Principles of Management

The major objective in pediatric rehabilitation is to facilitate independent function. Function is promoted in the areas of mobility, self-care, communication, perceptual-cognitive, and emotional and social development. In each of these areas, efforts are initially directed toward assisting the child to accomplish skills independently when possible. When necessary, prescription of equipment or modifications to the environment may provide the child with greater independence. Prescriptions for therapy programs, adaptive equipment, prostheses, and orthoses should include consideration of the child's ongoing growth and development.

MOBILITY

As the child develops motor skills, he or she is also actively engaged in exploring the environment. In the process of normal motor development, the child encounters a variety of stimuli that promote both language and social development. The child with delayed, abnormal, or lost motor skills may need assistance in achieving his or her maximum level of independent mobility. Many children with physical disabilities are able to ambulate if provided with therapeutic exercise programs, orthoses, and/or additional gait aids (walkers or crutches). For some, ambulation may be limited to short distances within the home or school, and wheelchair mobility may be indicated for longer distances. For others, minimal bracing may allow unlimited community ambulation. A manual or power wheelchair can provide functional mobility for children who cannot ambulate at all.

Safe transportation should be provided for children with physical disabilities. These children often outgrow approved child restraint systems without having developed adequate head and trunk control to be safely restrained with standard lap and shoulder seat belts. Alternative restraint systems, which have passed dynamic crash tests, are necessary for them.

COMMUNICATION

Children with physical disabilities may demonstrate discrepancies between receptive and expressive language; receptive skills may be relatively appropriate for age but speech may be less intelligible due to oral motor dysfunction. Augmentative communication devices are often appropriate for these children. Options range from the simpler "yes–no" communication board to computerized aids with speech synthesis or printed output.

GENERAL HEALTH MAINTENANCE

Issues of general health maintenance are important for all children, but there are special considerations related to the general health care for children with disabilities. While routine childhood immunizations are generally indicated, deferment of pertussis immunization is recommended for children with certain neurologic disorders, particularly those associated with seizures or neurologic deterioration. While not routinely recommended for children, influenza and pneumococcal vaccine are indicated for those with chronic respiratory problems related to neuromuscular disease or upper cervical spinal cord injury. Variations in energy expenditure and nutritional requirements reflect alterations in body composition related to the child's diagnosis. Weight control is especially important in children with mobility limitations, as the level of independence in ambulation or transfers may be severely compromised by the increased energy requirements imposed by obesity. Dental care may need to be specialized.

Increasing attention is being directed toward the needs of older adolescents with physical disabilities and their families during the process of transition from pediatric to adult primary care. Patients and their families may hesitate to transfer from the multidisciplinary pediatric clinics to the adult care system. Families may fear that the adult clinic lacks the expertise to properly address the problems related to their young person's "developmental" disorder. Transfer of care to an adult facility is perhaps less difficult for young adults with acquired disabilities than for those with congenital disabilities because the adult system is more likely to offer specialized services for the more common acquired disabilities, such as those due to spinal cord and brain injuries. Adolescent and young adult patients with physical disabilities should be educated about their medical needs throughout childhood in order for them to be able to advocate for their own healthcare needs in adulthood.

EDUCATION

Education has been defined by Roos, in Haring's (4) textbook *Behavior of Exceptional Children,* as "the process whereby an individual is helped to develop new behavior or to apply existing behavior, so as to equip him to cope more effectively with his total environment." This definition would also serve as a reasonable description of rehabilitation. Interchangeability of these definitions highlights the overlap in the goals of rehabilitation and education programs for children with disabilities. The Education for All Handicapped Children Act, Public Law 94-142 of 1975 (now re-enacted as Public Law 101-476, the Individuals with Disabilities Education Act: I.D.E.A.) mandates provision of appropriate educational programs for children with disabilities. This law requires that special education services be provided in the least restrictive environment consistent with the child's disability. Provision of an individualized education program (IEP) is required for each child with a handicap. Special services provided as part of the education plan must include physical and occupational therapies if relevant to the educational goals. Other supportive services to assist the child with communicative, cognitive or sensory deficits, and/or behavioral and emotional difficulties are also mandated. The Education for the Handicapped Act Amendments of 1986 (P.L. 99-457) address the needs of infants and toddlers with disabilities. Federal funds are authorized to provide financial assistance to states for community-based health, developmental, educational, and social services for children with special needs from birth until they are eligible for school-based services at age 3. Provision of an individualized family service plan is required for each family served.

VOCATIONAL

Vocational outcome is one measure of the effectiveness of medical, therapeutic, and educational interventions for children with disabilities. When the onset of disability occurs during childhood or adolescence, there is a risk of loss of an entire lifetime of potential productivity with enormous personal, social, and economic costs. Independent vocational function should therefore be a major goal of the provision of rehabilitative services.

Common Childhood Disabilities

CEREBRAL PALSY

Cerebral palsy (CP), defined as a disorder of motor control due to an injury or abnormality affecting the immature brain, is the most common condition associated with childhood disability. The incidence is 2 per 1,000 live births. Spastic, athetoid, ataxic, hypotonic, or mixed patterns of motor disability may be present. There may be severe involvement of all four extremities (quadriplegia); involvement primarily of the lower extremities with upper extremity deficits only present to a lesser degree (diplegia); involvement of an upper and lower extremity on the same side of the body (hemiplegia); or, rarely, involvement of a single extremity (monoplegia). The type of motor disability depends of the site of insult to the developing brain; spasticity results from involvement of deep white matter and cortex; athetosis is associated with damage to the basal ganglia. The severity is variable. The etiologies are diverse and can be divided into prenatal, perinatal, and postnatal factors. An example of prenatal etiology is congenital infection. Perinatal causes are associated with any period of anoxia or brain injury associated with labor and delivery. Postnatal etiologies include any insult to the brain in the early period of childhood, including neoplasia, trauma, or anoxic injuries to the central nervous system. The etiology of CP remains unclear in many cases (14).

While the prevalence of cerebral palsy remains stable, there have been changes in the incidence of the types of cerebral palsy that reflect changes in common etiologic factors. There has been a reduction in pure athetoid cerebral palsy during the past generation of medical care, primarily due to a decrease in the incidence of hemolytic anemia, hyperbilirubinemia, and kernicterus. This is a result of the practice of immunizing Rh-negative mothers and the clinical advances in the treatment of infants with hyperbilirubinemia. Hypoxia is now the most common factor associated with athetosis in CP. In contrast, there has been an increase in spastic diplegic cerebral palsy associated with the increased survival of premature infants, who are predisposed to insults involving the periventricular vasculature of the immature brain.

The problem of motor control accounts for many of the functional deficits. Associated problems include poor oral motor control, feeding problems, gastroesophageal reflux, seizure disorders, sensory impairments, and secondary orthopedic deformities. Although children with CP can have impaired, average, or superior intellect, there is a higher incidence of cognitive dysfunction and communication deficits in this population. The clinical course of CP is nonprogressive, although clinical manifestations may change with normal growth and development.

MENINGOMYELOCELE

Meningomyelocele is the second most common congenital cause of pediatric disability. Its incidence is slightly less than 1 per 1,000 live births in the United States. The cause is unknown, but appears to be multifactorial and includes a polygenetic inheritance pattern and environmental factors. The defect results from failure of neural tube closure in the developing embryo at the end of the fourth week of gestation. Hydrocephalus associated with the Arnold-Chiari Malformation is present in over 90 percent of affected children. Medical management issues are related to the neurologic level of the neural tube lesion. Forty five percent of the lesions occur at the L-5/S-1 levels, whereas 92 percent will occur at L-2 and below. Less than one-third will have completely flaccid paralysis below the level of the lesion; the remainder will have a combination of flaccid paraplegia, spasticity, and occasionally some spared voluntary activity. Virtually all children with lesions above L-2 will be wheelchair users. Approximately 50 percent of children with spared L-3 innervation will walk in childhood, and 20 percent will walk independently as adults. With L-4-5 sparing, nearly 100 percent of children will ambulate in childhood, but a lesser number will have independent ambulation in adulthood. The majority of patients with intact innervation to S-1 will be independent ambulators in adulthood.

All children with meningomyelocele have neurogenic bowel and bladder. Bowel management is of tremendous significance to the child's self-esteem and socialization. Management of the neurogenic bladder is imperative in order to prevent secondary damage to the upper urinary tract and the life-threatening complications of infection and renal failure. The survival rate for children born with meningomyelocele in the 1950s was less than 10 percent; it is now greater than 90 percent. Diagnosis is now often made prenatally and adjustments made to labor and delivery in order to minimize additional damage to the infant. Current medical management in the newborn period includes early surgical management of the open neural tube defect and ventriculoperitoneal shunting to reduce hydrocephalus. Continued aggressive management designed to prevent secondary complications associated with the urinary tract have dramatically decreased the incidence of morbidity and mortality associated with renal failure. The most common cause of death for children with meningomyelocele at this time is central ventilatory dysfunction. This complication is associated with the Arnold-Chiari malformation and abnormalities at the level of the brain stem.

Nearly 100 percent of these children will suffer skin breakdown associated with insensate skin. Maximum education and intervention should be provided to the child and his or her family to prevent the occurrence and the secondary complications of decubiti.

If the most efficient form of mobility for an affected child is independent ambulation, considerable effort should be directed to the provision of appropriate orthotics, orthopedic surgery, and therapy to maintain this skill. Wheelchair prescription is required if the child's functional needs will best be met with augmentative mobility.

The first large cohort of patients with spina bifida surviving with modern medical management is just now entering adulthood. Early studies directed toward evaluating the clinical needs of this population suggest that they have a high incidence of late neurologic complications, ongoing musculoskeletal complications, an unacceptably high rate of skin breakdown, and significant psychological, social, and vocational needs.

NEUROMUSCULAR DISORDERS

Neuromuscular disorders commonly encountered in children differ from those typically seen in adults. This is true for each level of the motor unit. The most common form of anterior horn cell disease in the pediatric age group is spinal muscular atrophy. Peripheral neuropathies are relatively rare in childhood and are more likely to be inherited. Some are caused by inborn errors of metabolism affecting myelin, such as metachromatic leukodystrophy and Krabbe's disease; others are associated with hereditary dysfunction of myelin (e.g., Charcot-Marie-Tooth disease or Déjérine Sottas interstitial neuritis). Peripheral neuropathy may also be acquired in childhood, as in the case of inflammatory polyneuropathy or Guillain-Barré syndrome, or following toxic exposure to chemotherapeutic agents and heavy metals. The more commonly seen disorders of the neuromuscular junction in children are myasthenia gravis and infantile botulism. Myopathic processes presenting in the pediatric age group include inherited muscular dystrophies, myotonic dystrophy, congenital myopathies, and inflammatory myopathies.

The most common muscle disease in childhood is Duchenne muscular dystrophy, an X-linked recessive genetic condition. This single-gene defect results in a deficiency of the muscle protein dystrophin and subsequent progressive deterioration of skeletal muscle. Affected boys characteristically have histories of delayed motor development; proximal weakness becomes apparent by the age of 3 to 4 years. Early manifestations of this weakness classically include the presence of a Gower's sign, in which the hands are used to "walk-up" the thighs to assume a standing position. Diagnosis is aided by the finding of a marked elevation in the serum creatine kinase, cDNA gene probe to identify the abnormality at the gene locus, characteristic abnormalities in the muscle biopsy and specific histochemical assay to document the absence of dystrophin. Weakness is inexorably progressive. The period of ambulation may be prolonged with aggressive physical therapy, orthopedic surgical intervention, and the use of orthoses. Recent trials with prednisone have had encouraging results, with slowing in the rates of decline in strength and function. Loss of the ability to ambulate and complete dependence on a wheelchair usually occur before 12 years of age. The patient's course may be complicated in the later stages of the disease by scoliosis, decreasing pulmonary function, and cardiac involvement. Approximately one-third of boys with Duchenne muscular dystrophy have intellectual impairment. Death usually occurs in the late teens or early in the third decade from respiratory compromise. Assisted ventilation in the end stage may prolong life, but in the face of continuing irreversible disease, decisions regarding its use must be considered on an individual basis.

Spinal muscular atrophy (SMA) describes a group of genetic, primarily autosomal recessive, disorders characterized by degeneration of the anterior horn cells. Classification systems vary; one useful system suggests the division into three major types. SMA-Type I is the acute infantile syndrome, Werdnig-Hoffman disease; SMA-Type II is an early-onset chronic childhood form; and SMA-Type III, or Kugelberg-Welander disease, has a later onset. Infants with SMA-Type I may present shortly after birth or within the first 6 months of life with respiratory distress and feeding difficulties. Weakness is generalized and symmetric; there is limited development of motor function, with affected infants typically never sitting independently. Death usually occurs secondary to respiratory compromise by 2 years of age. At the other end of the spectrum of severity, SMA-Type III is usually clinically detected between the ages of 5 and 15 years. Proximal weakness occurs initially, with more distal involvement later in the course of the disease. Progression is highly variable, with some patients remaining ambulatory for decades and others losing the ability to walk by age 20. The majority of affected children have the intermediate form. The age at onset is variable and overlaps with the age at onset of SMA-Type I. Delayed motor development is characteristic; while some children will develop the ability to sit and stand independently, most will maintain these skills only briefly and will be dependent on a wheelchair for mobility by 2 or 3 years of age. Bracing and physical therapy may prolong ambulation briefly. Life span is extremely variable, but death usually occurs as a consequence of pulmonary complications. There is no intrinsic intellectual impairment associated with spinal muscular atrophy.

LIMB DEFICIENCIES

An absence of part or all of an extremity in childhood may be due to congenital deficiency or acquired amputation. Over two-thirds of the children with limb deficiency have congenital lesions. The most common congenital limb deficiency (25 percent of the entire group) is the below-elbow transverse defect. Among children with acquired amputation, lower-extremity amputation is more common. For unknown reasons, left-sided congenital lesions predominate, and boys are more affected than girls. The etiology is unknown in over 90 percent of children with congenital limb deficiency. These deficiencies may be associated with inherited syndromes of multiple malformations. Those involving the radius have been associated with congenital heart disease, blood dyscrasias, and vertebral anomalies. Trauma accounts for 70 percent of acquired amputation and malignancy is responsible for most of the remaining 30 percent.

Prostheses are provided to children with limb deficiencies to accommodate function. Provision of the initial upper-extremity prosthesis has generally been recommended at the age at which the child is able to sit. There is a trend toward earlier prescription, and some clinicians provide prostheses for children as young as 3–4 months of age. The initial upper-extremity prostheses are passive devices that allow the infant to hold large objects, support weight bearing, and provide some sensory feedback. Cable activation of a prehensile terminal device is introduced at age 18–24 months, when the ability to learn to operate the device has developed. For children with above-elbow deficiencies, the elbow joint is activated at approximately 3 years of age. Consideration in selection of prostheses for children should include growth potential, durability, comfort, weight, and cosmesis. The devices should be as simple as possible in construction and in their operating requirements. One exception is the provision of myoelectric prostheses. In certain selected cases, upper-extremity prostheses with electrically powered terminal devices and/or elbow joints are used. Recommendations for myoelectric prostheses are based on the functional needs of the child and the user's ability to adapt to the prostheses rather than on age alone.

Not all children with congenital or acquired amputations will benefit from prosthetic devices. There are high rates of rejection of prostheses, particularly at the extremes of residual limb length. Children with very distal amputations are usually more functional using their residual hand or foot than a prosthesis. Excessively high energy requirements may be required for the use of prostheses by children with short lower-extremity amputations. Prostheses provided for some proximal upper-extremity amputations may be so cumbersome that they offer only a minimal functional advantage. It is important to note that children born with only one usable upper extremity will generally become completely independent in all aspects of self-care without a prosthesis. Children born with an absence of both upper extremities can be expected to be independent in most aspects of their self-care by using their feet.

Surprisingly, children with these deficiencies require very little formal therapy. The adaptive nature of the developing child encourages them to teach themselves one-handed or no-handed techniques. If a prosthesis improves the child's function, it will usually be accepted. Upper-extremity prostheses are rejected at a high rate, both for functional and cosmetic reasons; in contrast, lower-extremity prostheses are so functionally useful in gait that they are nearly always accepted. Most children with limb deficiencies who become successful prosthesis users learn to use them without extensive periods of training in physical and occupational therapy.

SPINAL CORD INJURY (SCI)

Spinal cord injury (SCI) most often occurs in adolescents and young adults between the ages of 15 and 25 years. When SCI occurs in young children, the results are frequently more devastating. Several developmental anatomic and biomechanical differences in the immature spine predispose the upper cervical spine to the most severe injuries in younger children. These include increased ligamentous and joint capsule laxity, incomplete ossification of the vertebrae, immature shape of the vertebral bodies, and incomplete muscular development. All of these contribute to increased mobility in the developing upper cervical spine. The mass of the infant's head is proportionally higher than in the adult, and the fulcrum of flexion-extension of the cervical spine is higher, with a gradual shift from the C2-3 level in the infant to C5-6 level in the adult spine. These developmental factors result in a higher proportion of quadriplegia in young children with SCI. With high cervical cord lesions, the child may be dependent on mechanical ventilation.

Management of the neurogenic bladder is critical to avoid renal damage. A child with paraplegia may be expected to perform intermittent catheterization independently at approximately 5 years of age. Neurogenic bowel retraining and regulation is generally accomplished without great difficulty in younger patients. Injury during adolescence, when bone metabolism is very active, may be complicated by immobilization hypercalcemia. This problem should be suspected in teenagers with SCI who present with lethargy, anorexia, nausea, headache, polyuria, and polydipsia. Heterotopic ossification and deep vein thrombosis following SCI occur less frequently in children than in adults.

PEDIATRIC BRAIN INJURY

One million children sustain head trauma annually. Traumatic brain injury is the most prevalent cause of acquired disability in childhood and is presently the most common diagnosis leading to inpatient pediatric rehabilitation. Etiologies in children are, in order of frequency: falls, motor vehicle accidents, pedestrian accidents, bicycle injuries, and sports injuries. Child abuse is a common cause of serious brain injury among children less than 2 years of age. While motor vehicles do not account for the majority of all brain injuries in children, they are the major cause of severe brain injury. Severity of injury for children is greatest under 2 years and over 14 years of age. These extremes may be associated with the mechanisms of child abuse and motor vehicle accidents, respectively. The frequency and severity of pediatric brain injury in children is higher in boys than girls.

Neurologic sequelae depend on the location and severity of the brain injury and the age of the child. Motor dysfunction reflects the site(s) of involvement in the motor pathways, and may result in spasticity, ataxia, and/or extraneous movements that impair the child's mobility and self-care. Visual disturbances include deficits in acuity, visual fields, and perception. Hearing deficits are especially associated with fractures of the temporal bone. Conductive hearing losses are associated with longitudinal fractures, whereas sensorineural losses are associated more frequently with transverse fractures. Expressive language disorders following brain injury in children may include dysarthria and aphasia. Receptive language deficits may be related to hearing loss or auditory perceptual problems.

Cognitive problems following traumatic brain injury typically include deficits in attention, concentration, memory, information processing and performance speed, cognitive flexibility, abstract problem-solving skills, and judgment. These deficits may persist even when intellectual function and academic performance test results are within normal ranges. These cognitive difficulties have obvious educational implications. Evidence of such deficits may not be detected initially following injury, but may become more apparent with time. For example, a child injured as a toddler will not demonstrate difficulty with tasks requiring abstract problem solving until demands are placed on him or her to participate in these activities in early elementary school. Changes in personality and behavior may also follow traumatic brain injury in childhood. Decreased frustration tolerance, poor anger control, and increased aggressiveness and hyperactivity have been observed to follow even mild brain injury in children. While the sequelae of moderate and severe brain injury in childhood is most likely to warrant referral to pediatric rehabilitation, the effects of even minor injury may be more significant than is generally appreciated. Subtle neuropsychological and neurobehavioral changes may impair the child's ability to function in school sufficiently to warrant special education intervention.

It is not clear that outcome following brain injury is either better or worse for children than for adults. Physiologic differences exist between the child's and the adult's brain in parameters that include cerebral metabolic rate and mechanisms regulating cerebral blood flow. Skull compliance, cerebral water content, and extent of myelination vary with age and degree of brain development. Some of these factors increase, and others decrease, the likelihood of recovery of function in children.

══════ Suggested Reading

1. Brook MH. *A clinician's view of neuromuscular diseases* (2d ed.). Baltimore, Williams & Wilkins, 1986.
   This reference offers very readable, clinically oriented descriptions of neuromuscular diseases affecting both adults and children. The chapter on symptoms and signs of neuromuscular disease provides an excellent discussion of clinical clues useful in evaluation of pediatric patients with these disorders, with an emphasis on functional evaluation.
2. Downey JA, Low NL (Eds.). *The child with disabling illness: Principles of rehabilitation* (2d ed.). New York, Raven Press, 1982.
   Disorders of the neuromuscular and musculoskeletal systems and chronic medical illnesses that occur in childhood are covered comprehensively. Management is discussed with an emphasis on promoting the development of the child's residual capacities to minimize the impact of these disease processes on development and function.
3. Gortmaker SL, Sappenfield W. Chronic childhood disorders: Prevalence and impact. *Pediatric Clinics of North America* 31:3–18, 1981.
   This comprehensive study examines the epidemiologic trends for chronic childhood diseases, including some estimates of future prevalence based on incidence, survival, geographic distribution, and birth rates.
4. Haring NG, Smith J. The profoundly handicapped. In: Haring NG (Ed.), *Behavior of exceptional children* (2d ed.). Columbus, Charles E. Merrill Publishing, 1978:241.
   Roos' definition of education is cited in the chapter on education of the profoundly handicapped in this introductory special education text. This definition is applicable to any level of education and is descriptive of rehabilitation as well.
5. Jaffe KM (Ed.). Pediatric head injury. *Journal of Head Trauma Rehabilitation* 1(4), 1986.
   Traumatic brain injury in childhood is the topic of this issue, which includes relatively brief but comprehensive articles that provide a good introduction to the subject. Epidemiology and prevention, sequelae, and rehabilitative management of brain injuries are reviewed with an emphasis on aspects particulary relevant to pediatrics.
6. Molnar GE (Ed.). *Pediatric rehabilitation* (2d Ed.). Baltimore, Williams & Wilkins, 1992.

Fundamentals of diagnosis and management in pediatric rehabilitation are present-ed in the first part of this text. The second part describes specific applications of rehabilitative interventions to the common disabling conditions of childhood.

7. Setoguchi Y, Rosenfelder R (Eds.). *The limb deficient child.* Springfield, IL, Charles C. Thomas, 1982.
   Etiology, classification, and management of congenital limb deficiencies and ampu-tations acquired in childhood are described. The chapters on basic principles of pros-thetics and prosthetics for the upper and lower extremities provide a good introduc-tion to the subject of prosthetic components appropriate for use with children.

8. Shurtleff DB (Ed.). *Myelodysplasias and exstrophies: Significance, prevention, and treat-ment.* Orlando, FL, Grune & Stratton, 1986.
   This text carefully examines embryology, incidence, prevention, and management of children with neural tube defects. The text is comprehensive with over 1,200 ref-erences.

9. Sutherland DH. *Gait disorders in childhood and adolescence.* Baltimore, Williams & Wilkins, 1984.
   The development of normal gait is described. Methods for studying gait in children are presented, and gait disorders commonly seen in pediatrics discussed.

10. Taft LT (Ed.). Cerebral palsy. *Pediatric Annals* 15(3), 1986.
    This entire issue is devoted to providing a broad review of the subject of cerebral palsy. Articles are well-written with numerous references on etiology, diagnosis, and man-agement, including one specifically addressing rehabilitation strategies.

11. Waller AE, Baker SP, Szocka A. Childhood injury deaths: National analysis and geo-graphic variations. *Am J Public Health* 79:310–315, 1989.
    Significant geographic variations in the United States in rates and causes of fatal child-hood injuries were demonstrated in this study. While morbidity was not assessed, there are implications of this study that are relevant to the epidemiology of childhood disability caused by injury.

12. Wilberger JE. *Spinal cord injuries in children.* Mount Kisco, NY, Futura Publishing, 1986.
    This book offers an overview of the problems unique to spinal cord injury in children, and comprehensively covers acute medical, surgical, and rehabilitative management issues. In the chapter on rehabilitation, function to be expected at each level of injury is outlined and emphasis is appropriately placed on the goals of spinal cord injury rehabilitation as they specifically apply to children.

13. Williams A. Economics of coronary artery bypass grafting. *Br Med J* 291:326–329, 1985.
    The concept of combining life expectancy and quality of life into the quality adjust-ed life year (QALY) is presented. This concept has significant potential for generaliz-ability to the field of pediatric rehabilitation.

14. Kuban K, Leviton A. Medical progress: Cerebral palsy. *New Eng J Med* 330:188–195, 1994.
    This is a current review of the etiology, epidemiology, and classification terminology of cerebral palsy.

19

Principles of Geriatric Rehabilitation

Marvin M. Brooke, M.D.

The term *geriatric rehabilitation* refers to the systematic use of therapy and other interventions to restore individuals 65 years of age or older to their former functional status, or to maximize function if some impairments cannot be completely overcome. It is important to separate the normal changes of aging from those decreases in functional abilities (impairments) due to disease, to unrecognized, and sometimes multiple, chronic conditions, and/or to disuse. It is not uncommon for an elderly patient to have one or more chronic conditions that have gradually progressed to the point where they limit function, but have not been addressed by either the patient or physician. The combination of some decline in function due to age with one or more chronic conditions may make the impairment from a single illness more severe than would otherwise be expected.

Three types of evidence should make us aware that declines in function do not necessarily occur with aging, and may be prevented by activity and rehabilitation intervention. First, many elderly individuals remain highly functional, and may perform at a level above younger persons. Second, there are wide variations within the elderly population; this variability usually exceeds the decline documented, on average, with advancing years. Third, most functional measures that have been shown to decline with age have also been shown to be maintained despite age if individuals remain active and practice those skills.

Demographics

The geriatric population is defined as those individuals 65 years of age and older. This population is increasing dramatically. At the turn of the century, approximately 4 percent of Americans were 65 or older (8). In 1966, this had increased to 9.4 percent, and it should reach 13.1 percent by the year 2000 (United States National Center for Health Statistics). This percentage is increasing because many more Americans reach age 65 than die, adding nearly 2,000 older people to the population every day. The current life expectancy of 85 years is increasing steadily with improved prevention and treatment of illnesses. Recent declines in mortality (e.g., from better treatment of hypertension) may increase this decline even further.

Some define the age of 75 as the age at which geriatric medicine begins. This population, sometimes called the "older-old," have proportionally more illnesses, disability, and care needs. It is estimated that, by the year 2000, half of the elderly (age 65+) will be age 75+ or more years of age. In the future, the elderly will include increasing numbers of individuals who have survived disabling illnesses and injuries due to improvements in both acute and rehabilitation care.

Demographics of Disability

The elderly have proportionally more illnesses that result in some functional impairment and, as a result, have more functional limitations and require more assistance for independent living (Table 19.1).

There has been a significant increase in the percentage of older persons who are residing in the community rather than in a nursing home, but who have health-related difficulties in one or more personal-care areas. In 1984, 23 percent of older persons residing in the community had deficits in one or more self-care activities, including bathing, dressing, eating, transferring, walking, or toileting. Twenty-seven percent had difficulty with one or more home-management activities, such as meal preparation, shopping, money management, house cleaning, or telephone use. The percentage of functional impairments increases at more rapid rates as people become older. At age 85 , for example, approximately one-half the population residing in the community needs assistance in one or more personal-care or homemaking activities. There are thus a significant number of older individuals residing in the community who require assis-

TABLE 19.1.

Percentage of Americans 65 or More Years of Age with Health Problems That Commonly Have Functional Impairments (1)

Arthritis	48 percent
Hypertension	30 percent
Heart Disease	30 percent
Hearing Impairments	29 percent
"Orthopedic"	17 percent
Cataracts	14 percent
Other Visual	10 percent
Diabetes Mellitus	10 percent
Tinnitus	9 percent

tance from family, friends, or caregivers—often at significant expense to themselves and society (1). The percentage who needed functional assistance (as measured by the U.S. National Center for Health and Statistics) increased dramatically with age (8), as shown in Table 19.2.

The proportion of older Americans in nursing homes is increasing each year and increases with age among the elderly population. In 1985, 5 percent of the elderly—or 1.3 million individuals—were institutionalized in nursing homes (Table 19.3).

══ Mechanisms of Aging

No agreed-upon theory explains all of the changes seen with aging. Changes occur in molecules, cells, and organ systems ; these decrease both organ system functional reserves and homeostatic controls. It is not known exactly which of the observed decrements in function control are the initial cause of aging, or which result from some other more fundamental cause.

MOLECULES

Several changes occur at the molecular level (7). A free radical is a molecular subgroup with an unpaired electron that are produced briefly during metabolic reactions; it is highly unstable and therefore a potent oxidizing agent. One theory of aging is that these free radicals combine with and deactivate essential molecules, such as DNA and regulatory proteins, with progressive damage building up over the years. This is the theoretical basis of feeding antioxidants to animals, which in some cases led humans to increased longevity; however, the results from such studies are conflicting. Aldehydes, which are produced in oxidation reactions, can form cross-linkages in collagen and other large molecules, decreasing flexibility and the transport of nutrients and waste products. Finally, another result of oxidation is the deposition of insoluble lipofuscin in cells, which may interfere with their function.

TABLE 19.2.
The Percentage of Americans Needing Functional Assistance By Age (8)

AGE	PERCENT NEEDING ASSISTANCE
18–44	1
45–64	3
65–74	7
75–84	16
85+	39

TABLE 19.3.
Percentage of Americans 65 Years of Age or Older in Nursing Homes (1)

AGE	PERCENT IN NURSING HOMES
65–74	1 percent
75–84	6 percent
85+	22 percent

Cells

There has been much speculation about changes at the cellular level that result in a decrease in function with age. Environmental damage could occur as a cumulative effect of various toxins and radiation; for example, from solar gamma rays which could damage important genes. Increased errors in protein synthesis could be caused by some species having fewer redundant messages in their DNA so that, as the years go by and errors increase, there is less backup of undamaged DNA to produce normal proteins. In a similar way, the age-related increase in stability of the DNA double helix requires more energy to separate its strands and allow genetic information to be transcribed. The fact that human fibroblasts can reproduce only a finite number of times in vitro supports a theory that there is a programmed genetic signal limiting the reproduction of the cells. One could propose an analogy to planned obsolescence in mechanical systems, and suggest that expected failures in cells and organs due to problems in reproduction and repair result in an expected failure of organ function.

Organ System

Changes in organ systems have also been studied as fundamental causes of aging. Age-related changes in the immune system decrease the capacity to fight infections and increase the tendency to form antibodies that fight one's own tissues, resulting in autoimmune diseases. In a similar way, some propose that predictable timed pacemakers of neuroendocrine function cause multiple other organ systems to age.

There is as yet no single, unified theory of aging. It appears likely that such a complex phenomenon may be based on both genetically influenced events and nongenetic or environmental events. This would better explain the observed phenomenon of differential aging; that is, different people age at differing rates. Most would agree that the rate of aging is affected by genetic, environmental, lifestyle, disease, and psychological factors.

═══ Normal Physiologic Changes of Aging Organ Systems

It is important to understand the normal physiologic changes in the different organ systems with increasing age so that one can:

1. separate disease processes from normal aging;
2. appropriately plan rehabilitation; and
3. prevent functional decline.

The older individual will normally function well despite a decrease in organ system capacity until illness or changed functional requirements lead to a functional deficit or problem. Medical interventions may produce additional stress on some organ systems; for example, an exercise program for the stroke patient may exceed his or her cardiovascular capacity. Progressive decreases in organ system functions with age occur in three broad categories and are as follows:

1. decreased reserve capacity, such as a decrease in maximum heart rate with exercise or decreased speed of learning new information;
2. decrease in homeostatic control, such as the reflexes that prevent orthostatic hypotension, dehydration, and hyperthermia; and
3. decreased ability to respond to change and stress, such as new living situations, extremes of temperature, exertion, or fever.

Together these changes mean that the older person is more likely to have problems with disease and injury, and needs more careful monitoring and therapeutic intervention.

Cardiovascular System

Two recent changes in our understanding of normal aging in the cardiovascular system point out previous misconceptions and problems with methodology in research. It was previously felt that cardiac output progressively declined after age 20, at approximately 1 percent per year. It now appears, however, that if one excludes biases due to unrecognized cardiovascular disease, such as atherosclerotic coronary artery disease, cardiac output may not decrease significantly with advancing age. There is a decrease in the maximum heart rate, even though the resting heart rate does not change. The maximum oxygen consumption decreases, resulting in reduction in exercise capacity.

Physically active older people have much smaller decreases in maximum aerobic capacity and may actually have higher capacities than younger, sedentary persons. Endurance training is highly effective in the elderly. Walking becomes more effective for aerobic conditioning with increasing age because it requires a larger percentage of exercise capacity. It is obviously important to monitor exercising older subjects for symptoms of cardiovascular disease, as well as excessive challenge to their fluid, temperature, and blood pressure homeostasis. Subjects are often monitored in order to keep their exercise heart rate well below 75 percent of maximum (the maximum heart rate is approximated at 220 minus the age; or 185 minus 70 percent of the age) and to avoid a change of more than 20 in heart rate or blood pressure.

There has been a dramatic change in the acceptance of blood pressure elevation with advancing age. Even though average blood pressure does increase with age, an elevated blood pressure is now known to be a risk factor for cerebrovascular and cardiovascular disease. The current recommendation is that blood pressure of 140mm Hg systolic or 90mm Hg diastolic should be treated; treatment at this level decreases the incidence of stroke by 50 percent (2). Because up to 40 percent of the elderly may have elevated blood pressures by these standards, high blood pressures should not be overlooked or accepted as a normal part of aging. Another well-documented change with age is a decreased sensitivity of the baroreceptor system that results in a failure of heart rate to increase when rising from the supine position and leads to orthostatic hypotension. Compounding this problem are decreases in renin, angiotensin II, and vasopressin. The elderly are more sensitive to orthostatic changes and more likely to have carotid sinus, cough, and micturition syncope.

Pulmonary System

There is a well-documented decrease in pulmonary reserve capacity with age (2). The maximum ventilation decreases approximately 60 percent from age 20 to age 70, with a corresponding decrease in vital capacity, total lung capacity, forced expiratory volume, and respiratory reserve. Decreases also occur in the elastic properties of the lungs, compliance of the thoracic wall, and arterial oxygen pressure. The elderly are more vulnerable to injury from hypoxia as a result of this mild decrease in oxygen pressure, which is compounded by a decreased homeostatic ability to compensate for changes, and an increase in breathing disorders during sleep.

Finally, the elderly have a higher incidence of pneumonia, due not only to difficulty with immunologic disease, but also to a high incidence of diseases, such as chronic obstructive pulmonary disease, aspiration and swallowing disorders, and decreased levels of consciousness (2). There are two encouraging pieces of information, however. First, the maximum oxygen consumption can be improved significantly with training at any age, increasing the reserve for stress and illness. Much of the decline in function could probably be changed by a greater emphasis on activity in the elderly. Second, much of the decline in pulmonary function is due to the cumulative effects of pollutants, cigarette smoking, and respiratory infections. Lung functions may also be improved by improving the environment, lifestyle, and the treatment of acute illnesses. It is therefore very important to maintain the maximum respiratory function and to continue exercise programs in the elderly.

Nervous System

A decrease in performance occurs in many areas of the nervous system with increasing age, when one looks at the average performance of groups of individuals. This generalization should, however, be interpreted with some caution. There is a tremendous amount of variability within the elderly group, and many of the neurologic functions that can be measured are maintained fairly well with practice and activity. Many studies have been subject to biases, unless the same group of individuals has been studied carefully for many decades. The multiple disease, sensory, and environmental factors seen in the elderly may impair their performance on tests. In general, those young individuals who performed and adjusted well among their peers tend to preserve their rank and remain bright and well-adjusted older individuals.

SPEED OF PERFORMANCE

The speed of performance of tasks in general declines with age, although some activities only show a mild decline (5). For example, the speed of performing simple aimed movements decreases approximately 10 percent from age 20 to age 70. For tasks involving more central processing or cognitive function, such as choosing which button to push depending on which light comes on, the time increases approximately 25 percent in the same age range. The increase in response time may be 50 percent or more for more complex cognitive processes as when the response button is on the opposite side from the stimulus (5). Discrete discontinuous tasks, such as responding with a break between tasks, are performed better than continuous tasks in which each response is followed immediately by another stimulus. When older subjects are given adequate time, however, they can often compensate and be as accurate as younger subjects. For very highly complex tasks, however, their compensation with increased time becomes less effective and more errors occur.

The practical consequences of these changes are seen in the workplace. The elderly tend to retire, not only from strenuous jobs, but also from lighter jobs that require rapid continuous activity, such as an assembly line. Older workers are more commonly injured by moving objects or falls, whereas younger workers are more often injured due to inexperience or poor impulse control. Motor vehicle accidents in the elderly are more commonly due to difficulty in responding to rapidly changing and multiple stimuli, whereas younger drivers may take more risks.

MEMORY AND LEARNING

On average, older subjects can recall a 6- or 7-digit number immediately after hearing it as well as younger subjects. When the number of items is increased, however, the elderly do less well, probably due to difficulty transferring all of the material from short-term to intermediate-term memory and to "less strength of the memory trace" itself (5). The "strength" of the trace can be increased by repetition, and, indeed, older subjects who have learned material do not forget it more rapidly than younger people. This difficulty in storing information, more than retaining information in long-term memory, may explain many of the difficulties with problem solving and other complex tasks.

This has several implications for learning in the elderly. Compensatory strategies, such as note-taking and allowing more time, are obvious interventions that will work *if* the older subject adopts these new skills. Another successful strategy is the "guided discovery method," in which the person being trained is given just enough information to allow him or her to discover alone how to perform the task or solve the problem. This active involvement appears to facilitate registration in long-term memory, and allowing enough time to discover the solution compensates for decreased speed of processing.

There are documented changes in the sensory and perceptual systems with age (5). Again, it is important to be aware that such changes may be the result of disease, injury, or inactivity; and that there is wide variation in the performance of the elderly, such that many exceed the average performance for younger subjects. A decreased flexibility of the lens of eye means that focusing on near objects is more difficult. There is also an increase in yellow pigment in the eye, some decrease in acuity, a slight decrease in the visual field, some color loss, and increased vulnerability to glare. Tests of the efficiency of functional visual tasks, however, may surpass that of many young subjects. It is also true that we do not know how much effect training may have on visual skills. Many common eye problems severely interfere with function; the elderly have a greater incidence of cataracts, macular diseases, glaucoma, and retinal, vascular, and corneal diseases.

The decrease in hearing—especially of the higher frequencies—usually is not of great functional significance in the elderly. In general, although sensitivity to higher frequencies decreases with age, the functional range necessary for understanding speech is well preserved. The loss of high-frequency hearing may be caused by a combination of environmental noise damage, trauma, infection, and drug-induced damage. The importance of prevention is therefore obvious in the elderly. Treatment is also important, since hearing aids can often effectively overcome these difficulties if combined with appropriate training and counseling.

Decreases in peripheral sensory functions, such as touch and position sense, are more difficult to study. It does appear that joint position sense decreases with age. This may be due as much to cumulative effects of subclinical neuropathy, dietary problems, and trauma as to age itself. Most of the peripheral sensory modalities do decline with age. One result of this is a difficulty with balance. There is also a decline in the speed of motor activities, although this can be prevented or improved with activity and practice. The elderly generally show decreases in coordination, balance, and proprioception, so that tasks such as standing on one foot with the eyes closed or in the dark may be difficult.

There are some irreversible causes of dementia in the elderly, such as Alzheimer's disease, multi-infarct dementia, and other degenerative diseases. However, a large number of treatable causes of dementia often go unrecognized because they are not looked for. Drug reactions and overprescription are common causes. Depression, metabolic disturbances, and the cumulative effects of mild problems, such as dehydration, malnutrition, and sleep disorders, should be sought. Other reversible causes of dementia include fever, infection, cardiovascular disorders, brain disorders, pain, sensory deprivation, and alcohol and drug abuse. Treatable causes compounding sensory deficits such as vision and secondary complications such as dehydration must be diagnosed and treated.

Musculoskeletal System

Aging is accompanied by a decline in the number of motor units, a decrease in the mass of muscles, and a decrease in fiber size and cellular components. A decreased work capacity of about 50 percent occurs from age 20 to age 70. Maximum power output decreases more rapidly, while muscle strength is preserved somewhat through middle age, and muscle endurance remains stable, perhaps due to an increase in Type II fibers.

Degenerative joint disease—osteoarthritis—is very common and is usually diagnosed as a disease when related symptoms and disability occur. Cartilage changes in weight-bearing joints are in essence universal in the elderly, due to molecular changes in cartilage and its resulting breakdown, which exposes bone. This problem is exacerbated by the repeated stresses of weight bearing, especially by abnormal stresses such as trauma or congenital deformity. Even though the majority of the elderly have degenerative changes and even x-ray abnormalities, significant symptoms and functional disability occur in about half of the elderly (1).

===== Other Systems

The immune system becomes less efficient in fighting infection, which is compounded by problems such as diabetes and skin breakdown. Older patients may experience less pain, fever, or rapid response to an infection. In addition to the skin becoming thinner and drier, the nails become thicker and less able to heal due to decreased circulation. It is critical that older individuals perform proper skin care, avoid pressure sores, and perform foot care, including cleaning, inspection, trimming, and fitting of socks and shoes.

In addition to decreases in taste and smell, there are changes in the gastrointestinal tract, including decreased secretion of saliva and intestinal motility. The incidence of hiatal hernia increases, and may lead to esophagitis or aspiration. Glucose tolerance also diminishes. While liver function is usually maintained, there is a decrease in kidney function. Both should be watched carefully in the older patient given potentially toxic medications.

===== Psychological and Social Function

Although basic needs for emotional and social esteem and relationship support do not change with age, there is a decrease in the older person's ability to change and maintain his or her lifestyle. Not only do older people gradually lose friends and relatives due to illness and death, but our current society has disrupted the nuclear family support system. Important areas to evaluate in elderly patients therefore include previous lifestyle, present family and friend support, role within these relationships, present living situation, and leisure time activities. Educational, cultural, and religious factors may be extremely important in assessing their overall stability and functions. Economic resources are often limited. It is often true, however, that families are happy to have their older relative live with them and that the older person may perform a very useful function within changed social settings. Architectural barriers, of course, should be eliminated if at all possible. The importance of injury prevention cannot be overemphasized. Maintaining familiar surroundings may well improve cognitive and functional abilities of the older person. Sexual needs continue in old age and function may be preserved, but is frequently not addressed by clinicians. Often, by reviewing all of these different factors, the older person at risk for problems may be identified and injury or illness prevented.

As mentioned above, exercise can maintain or reverse some of the decreases in function associated with age, and especially with disuse. It is important to maintain realistic functional goals because exercise is specific and most helpful when clearly directed toward a goal that is understood and desired by the patient. Also, precautions as discussed above should be followed. In addition to cardiovascular precautions, body temperature, fluid status, and risks of injury should be considered. Frequent rest periods are often important to allow cooling down and supplemental fluid intake. Patients should obviously be evaluated before an exercise program is begun, should have specific programs prescribed, and should be monitored by a physician.

===== **Rehabilitation of the Elderly**

The relevant data should be assembled before developing and prescribing a rehabilitation program. The history should include functional, cognitive, psychosocial, and environmental factors. The examination should focus on the predicted organ system changes and risks, as well as emphasizing the mental status examination and functional evaluation. It is often helpful to observe the patient in the home or during therapy, as well as to administer standardized tests, such as the Mini Mental Status Exam, the Blessed Information Memory and Test, and the Geriatric Depression Scale. Other diagnoses and impairments should be evaluated, including hearing, vision, sensory deprivation, fatigue, sleep, nutrition, continence, pain, musculoskeletal, and balance problems. Often, a trial of interventions at a slow pace with careful monitoring for side effects and functional gains is the best way to confirm the usefulness of an initial treatment plan.

===== **Identification of Rehabilitation Goals**

Several principles should be kept in mind when identifying rehabilitation goals after the relevant data have been accumulated; these are shown in Table 19.4.

The rehabilitation program will be most appropriate for the individual and most effective if it is built on a careful assessment of specific problems (for example, poor hygiene); focused on concrete functions (ability to transfer to and from the bathtub) and oriented toward realistic goals (safe, daily bathing). Some of the most important goals are independence in bowel, bladder, self-care, and mobility functions. Family and other social support is critical, yet often overlooked. Important goals should be to reduce the demands on the family. Physical assistance may not be as important as emotional, behavioral, verbal, nocturnal, and time demands—all of which are very wearing over time. A key to success is selecting goals with the involvement of the patient and family, which are appropriate for the individual's setting and which try to return to premorbid functions and environments. It is also important to attempt to decrease further declines, accidents, and inappropriate health care utilization.

TABLE 19.4.

Ideal Rehabilitation Goals for the Elderly

1. Functional, problem, and goal-oriented;
2. Independence in bowel, bladder, self-care, and mobility;
3. Reduce level of emotional, behavioral, verbal, nocturnal, and time demands on the family;
4. Return to premorbid functions and environment;
5. Appropriate for environment and support;
6. Agreed to by patient and family;
7. Decrease the functional impact of physiologic aging and deconditioning;
8. Prevent accidents; and
9. Decrease health care use.

An appropriate assessment by a physician specializing in physical medicine and rehabilitation will include psychological and social aspects of care. In addition to looking for problems such as depression and alcohol abuse, the overall function of the patient and his/her support system should be considered. It is important to consider the patient, the family, and caregivers who need to adjust to losses as opposed to letting their fears and issues impact on the patient. A role model and problem-oriented, goal-directed approach can help patient and family. Keeping the older person in their own environment and support system helps their function and adjustment. Respite care, support services, and family/friend involvement need to be specifically arranged and scheduled to be most effective. Motivation of caregivers and families must be attended to. In nursing facilities, the nursing aides really provide the care with few rewards, so social and gift reinforcers may be very necessary. At times, creative alternative settings such as group homes can meet the needs better than traditional options. Patients and families should be encouraged to call on multiple resources such as the local Alzheimer's Association, ombudsman for the elderly, or nursing homes, association of retired persons, social organizations, and special geriatric and rehabilitation programs.

It is extremely important to examine the feasibility of rehabilitation goals on an individual basis (Table 19.5). Associated problems, lack of stability in the current status, and unrealistic goals may make a program unsuccessful. Goals should take into account the individual's premorbid abilities, emotional status, and motivation. Deciding on a goal of daily bathing may be inappropriate, for example, if multiple sclerosis makes water immersion unsafe, the person's strength is declining so it will not be a long-lasting accomplishment, or the person did not see the value of bathing daily before their illness. It is likewise very important that patients be aware of their deficits. If goals can be developed with the individual, and presented in a way that is acceptable to both their own personal goal and style and level of motivation, then cooperation will increase significantly. Again, it is important to decide on goals that are appropriate for the person's environment and level of support. If, for example, the bathtub is not available to the individual more than twice a week because there is no family support in case of a fall, this may be an unrealistic goal. Selecting an unrealistic or unobtainable goal may have a deleterious effect on patient and family motiva-

TABLE 19.5.

Examination of the Feasibility of Rehabilitation Goals on an Individual Basis

1. Associated problems;
2. Stability of status;
3. Premorbid abilities, emotional status, and motivation;
4. Awareness of deficits;
5. Personal goals and style;
6. Environment and support;
7. Limitation on predictive ability for one individual; and
8. Feasibility determined by outcome measures that often have idiosyncratic degrees of importance for different observers, caregivers, or family members.

tion and compliance. It is much more important to individualize and be practical about goal setting than to base one's goals on the literature or some standardized formulae. Most of the literature is based on group studies or abstract theories that have a very limited ability to predict individual function. Much of the literature on rehabilitation is based on outcome measures which, although often valid and reliable, may not have validity or be acceptable to patients, family members, or caretakers. For example, the ability to dress oneself independently may not be as important if the family has great time demands and can more quickly do most of the dressing themselves.

Due to the frequency and difficulty of cognitive impairment, the identification of cognitive assets and disabilities deserves special attention (Table 19.6). Because cognitive deficits are often overlooked by patients and families—not to mention health-care providers—it is often helpful to have a standardized assessment to identify deficits. It is also important to obtain information from the patient and family about particular strengths and assets that may allow the patient to perform better than expected. This is very commonly the ability to use previously learned skills or cognitive aids. It is also important to carefully analyze the tasks that we are asking our patients to perform. Often, by observing a patient or working closely with the therapists who do a more detailed analysis of tasks, we may identify problems, see patient responses that lead to solutions, or find ways of modifying a small step in the overall task.

Some individuals perform better on verbal tasks as opposed to pictorial or gesture described tasks. Previous memory skills may be more easily used than a memory method unfamiliar to the patient. For example, if a patient has always used grocery lists on a small piece of paper, tasks may be written down and posted at appropriate places. It is helpful to decide which tasks need to be retrained, which tasks can be circumvented by changing the environment or having others perform the task, and which tasks can be compensated for by relying on other maintained abilities. It is very important to have good team communication due to:

1. the complex nature of cognitive deficits and tasks that need to be performed;
2. the benefits of a careful assessment and working with specialized team members; and
3. the importance of modifying the rehabilitation program as training proceeds.

TABLE 19.6.

Identification of Cognitive Strengths and Weaknesses

1. Detailed analysis of tasks and patient responses;
2. Verbal, written, pictorial, gesture or physical input, manipulation, and expression;
3. Old similar memory skills;
4. Retraining, circumventing, or compensating for deficits; and
5. Team communication, assessment, and modification of program.

TABLE 19.7.

Design of Compensatory Strategies That Capitalize on Cognitive Strengths

1. General principles, not rigid step-by-step methodologies;
2. Task subset analysis and treatment in steps or "chains";
3. Simplification and slow changes "start slow and go slow";
4. Teach principles and self-instruction strategies that may generalize;
5. Compensation with opposite hemisphere, other intact skills, or combination of abilities, aids, and assistance;
6. Practice correctly, immediate feedback, praise and remind one of the importance to the ultimate goal of increased independence;
7. Memory disorders and new learning deficits: aids, mnemonics, imaginal techniques, repetition or written, picture, or physical cues;
8. Visual perceptual disorders: scanning, environmental or assistive device changes;
9. Reduced attention span: shorter, more frequent quiet sessions;
10. Group, social, and environment support;
11. Addition or multiplication of effects of more than one strategy applied;
12. Behavior modification, self-monitoring strategies.

Our understanding of cognitive strengths and weaknesses as well as individual motivation and performance levels is usually very limited. We should therefore obtain all the assistance we can, and realize that a rehabilitation program cannot be set in concrete without a need for modification as it is being carried out.

It is very helpful to try to design compensatory strategies that capitalize on an individual's cognitive strengths (Table 19.7). The program will be most successful if the patient and family agree to the goals, if it is individualized and modified as the program progresses. For example, it will be more helpful to instruct a patient how to ask for directions in order to find his or her way around a new building than to memorize a path through the building they are currently residing in. Several different theories of training should be kept in mind. Often it is helpful to analyze a task in various small steps and then train the person to achieve each step before combining the steps together into a chain for the overall task. It is also very helpful to simplify and make very slow changes in an older patient's activities. Not only is it helpful to teach principles, but it is also very helpful if patients can learn strategies to give themselves instructions, which then generalize. For example, verbally rehearsing the instructions or compensatory strategies may be helpful as a patient carries out tasks. It is often helpful to analyze compensatory strengths based on what we know about the person's neurologic deficits or intact neurological structures. For example, if a patient with a right brain infarction has difficulty with diagrams or maps, it may be more helpful to use verbal or written instructions that depend on the intact left hemisphere.

From the beginning, it is extremely important to train with correct procedures so that instructions are consistent and do not train a task in differing ways that add to confusion. Positive reinforcement in the form of verbal or social praise is very helpful, as is giving very specific immediate feedback and reminding the individual of the importance of the overall goal. Often it is helpful to have a verbal or pictorial representation of the desired goal, such as walking to the movie theatre. The detailed strategies to compensate for various cognitive deficits are beyond the scope of this chapter. One should be aware that there are many different approaches to a memory deficit, such as verbal or pictorial aids, mnemonics or physical cues provided in the environment. It has been shown that patients with difficulty recognizing items in one visual field can be taught to scan to one side and can also be helped by assistive devices, such as a highly visible tag. Often the attention span is reduced, but this can be improved by having short sessions and more frequent treatments with rest periods in between. The emotional support and interindividual communication, which can be provided by group or social settings, can be a very important aid to difficult task accomplishments. Since there are no guaranteed approaches to such complex problems, it may be helpful to try to accomplish the same task with multiple approaches and strategies that add to one another. Finally, it is helpful to keep the overall realistic goals of the program in mind and to teach a patient, as much as possible, to monitor their own performance and maintain their rehabilitation program independently in the future.

REFERENCES

1. American Association of Retired Persons: A profile of older persons. AARP, Washington D.C., 1986.
2. Borhani NO. Prevalence and prognostic significance of hypertension in the elderly. *J Am Geriatr Soc* 34:112–114, 1986.
3. Carotenuto R, Bullock J. *Physical assessment of the gerontologic client*. Philadelphia, F.A. Davis, 1981.
4. Gwither LP. *Care of Alzheimer's: A manual for nursing home staff*. American Public Health Care Association and Alzheimer's Disease and Related Disorders Association, 1985.
5. Katzman R, Terry R. Normal aging of the nervous system. In Katzman R, Terry R (Eds.), *The neurology of aging*. Philadelphia, F.A. Davis, 1983, pp. 15-50.
6. Rosenthal M. Geriatrics: An updated bibliography. *J Am Geriatr Soc* 37:894–910, 1989.
7. Schneider EL, Reed JD Jr. Life extension. *N Engl J Med* 312:1159-1168, 1985.
8. U.S. National Center for Health Statistics, Washington, D.C., 1986.
9. Williams TF. *Rehabilitation in the aging* . New York, Raven, 1984.

Recommended Reading

American Association of Retired Persons. A profile of older persons. AARP Washington D.C., 1986. U.S. National Center for Health Statistics, Washington, D.C., 1986.
This reference is a useful collection of medical and functional problems pertinent to rehabilitation of the elderly.
Carotenuto R, Bullock. *Physical assessment of the gerontologic client*. Philadelphia, F.A. Davis, 1981.
A good text about all aspects of evaluation.
Felsenthal G, Steinberg FU. *Rehabilitation of the aging and older adult*. Baltimore, Williams and Wilkins, 1993.
Gwither LP. *Care of Alzheimer's: A manual for nursing home staff*. American Public Health Care Association and Alzheimer's Disease and Related Disorders Association, 1985.
Practical information about caring for the cognitively impaired elderly patient.

Mace N, Rabins P. *The 36-hour day: A family guide to caring for persons with Alzheimer's disease, related dementing illnesses, and memory loss in later life.* Baltimore, Johns Hopkins Press, 1991

Rosenthal M. Geriatrics: An updated bibliography. *J Am Geriatr Soc* 37:894-910, 1989.
    A comprehensive bibliography by subject heading with several hundred references.

Schneider EL, Reed JD Jr. Life extension. *N Engl J Med* 312:1159-1168, 1985.
    A good review of current theories about molecular and cellular aging.

Psychosocical and Vocational Aspects of Disability

20

Psychological Adjustment to Disability

David R. Patterson, Ph.D.

The onset of disability or chronic disease usually results in significant change for most people, and their psychological well-being will depend on their ability to adapt to these transitions. Although such change can be source of stress and far-reaching disruption, there is still ample room for providing optimism to patients with even the most stressing of disabilities and chronic diseases. The application of psychology to the area of adjustment to such maladies is still at a relatively early stage. Before discussing how various behavioral and emotional problems can be addressed in this population, it will be necessary first to address some of the myths and outdated conceptualizations that have been applied to people with disabilities and chronic disease.

═════ Misleading Models

Every theory in science has a range of convenience. Specifically, a given scientific theory will be able to explain some phenomena better than others. The same notion applies to psychological aspects of disability. Some models will provide useful formulations that will enable patients to move quickly through rehabilitation, while others will actually steer clinicians away from effective approaches. The disease-medical model, in which symptoms are treated by attacking an underlying pathogen, offers a conceptualization that does not apply to the process of rehabilitation. Whereas this approach may be useful in the diagnosis and treatment of many medical conditions such as viral infections, it falls dreadfully short when it comes to determining why a patient does not appear motivated to participate in his or her rehabilitation (4). Similarly, a popular contention is that people adjusting to disability will go through an orderly series of psychological stages (e.g., denial, anger, grief, and so on). However, recent reviews of the literature on spinal cord injury indicate that there are no good data to demonstrate that any order of stages exists for the adjustment to this form of trauma. It appears that people's reactions to disability vary based on their unique individual histories. Another clinical myth is the assumption that there is a particular personality type associated with any type of chronic disease or disability, particularly one that can be changed to facilitate rehabilitation. Research fails to provide any evidence that unitary personality types are associated with patients faced with medical disorders (10). Finally, the idea that people do not respond well to any form of medical rehabilitation because of a deficit in their motivation represents another erroneous conceptualization that is bound to frustrate the practitioner as well as the patient.

═══ Applicable Models

COGNITIVELY-BASED THEORIES

Cognitively-based theories of behavior change treat an individual's thought processes as behaviors that can be changed with a resulting positive impact on associated emotions. Some of the more recent popular cognitive theories that have a potential application to people with disabilities include learned helplessness, self-efficacy, and locus of control.

Proponents of the learned helplessness theory would argue that the onset of a disease or disability creates a state of learned helplessness in a person which leads him or her to take a more passive stance toward life events (9). Self-efficacy theory refers to the degree to which people feel that they are able to master one of life's tribulations before even approaching a particular event (1). Since people in the early stages of disease or disability often lose part of their physical or cognitive capacity to act on the environment, a decrease in their sense of self-efficacy is an understandable outcome. Similarly, the locus of control theory hypothesizes that people vary in the degree to which they perceive themselves as the source of control over life's circumstances, or whether they see what happens to them as caused by external forces out of their control (8). All of these theories would predict that people have a shift in their cognition early in the course of a disability such that they feel less in control of their lives. The goal of rehabilitation is consequently to restore a greater sense of control or self-efficacy during this phase of recovery.

BEHAVIORAL APPROACHES

One of the most popular approaches to the psychological assessment and management of disabilities is couched in learning theory. Of particular use is operant conditioning, the process by which voluntary actions are strengthened by the reinforcer that follows them. Learning theorists argue that the onset of a disability involves an immediate, dramatic decrease in the output of behaviors by the disabled individual. Because patients are no longer able to perform those behaviors for which they were once frequently reinforced, they undergo a crisis period and potentially show a number of psychological symptoms. During this crisis phase, the losses patients have suffered (e.g., relationships or jobs) may lead them to view both their disability and the ensuing process of rehabilitation as a form of punishment. As a response to this perceived punishment, patients may verbally or physically strike out at staff, withdraw into fantasy, or enter a period of mindless inactivation. According to this model, treatment is based on extinguishing disability-inappropriate behaviors and strengthening those behaviors that patients will find rewarding even with their particular disability.

It should be emphasized that the cognitive and learning theories do not offer the only useful conceptualizations for understanding the process of rehabilitation. However, of the theories available in the fields of psychology and psychiatry (e.g., psychodynamic systems, etc.), these two have a range of convenience that is particularly applicable to the process of recovering from a disability.

═══ Frequent Psychological Problems

DEPRESSION

The label *clinical depression* is one that is unfortunately applied too frequently and capriciously to people with disabilities. A popular belief, for example, is that anyone who sustains a spinal cord injury will become depressed. To the contrary, in a recent review, Roberta Trieschmann concluded that "spinal cord injury does not necessarily lead to depressive reactions in most people soon after onset, and the absence of depression does not imply denial of injury or poor adjustment to disability" (10). Prior to 1940, life expectancy after this type of trauma was greatly shortened, and depressive reactions were justifiably anticipated. However, as improved medical treatment and rehabilitation have resulted in life spans approximating those of the general population, the incidence of depression in this population has decreased dramatically.

It is important to distinguish depression from normal grief, since there are definite treatments for the former. Some of the main criteria for depression listed in the *Diagnostic and Statistical Manual,* third edition, of the American Psychiatric Association include dysphoric mood, loss of pleasure, poor appetite, insomnia, psychomotor agitation or retardation, loss of energy, problems with thinking, and recurrent thoughts of death or suicide (3). Most of these symptoms have to be present nearly every day for a period of at least two weeks for a diagnosis of major depression to be made. Antidepressant pharmacological interventions and cognitively-based psychotherapies have both been found useful for treating most people suffering from depressive disorders (5).

GRIEF

Grief, as differentiated from depression, is a more frequent, naturally occurring, and less problematic sequela of a disability or chronic disease. Learning theorists regard grief as a result of the patient's loss of reinforcers; treatment involves allowing him or her to gain access to reinforcing activities as expeditiously as possible. Cognitive therapists would regard the treatment of grief as enhancing the patient's self-efficacy and degree of control over the environment. A comprehensive process of rehabilitation will automatically provide the patient with psychological benefits from both theoretical standpoints. It is important that the staff, as well as the patient, understand that the process of grieving is, by definition, temporary and will usually dissipate on its own.

SUICIDE

Although the literature on suicide in populations with chronic disease and disability is somewhat equivocal, the rate for people with disabilities does not appear to vary dramatically from that of the population as a whole. It is not uncommon to encounter suicidal ideation in people who are early in the course of a new disability or disease. In the vast majority of cases, such ideation will *not* represent serious intent and can be regarded as an expected component of the crisis phase of disability described by Fordyce (4). However, such verbalizations should never be taken lightly. The clinician can clarify intent with a few simple questions, such as asking patients if they are truly serious or if they have a plan for harming themselves. Formal psychiatric intervention is certainly warranted if patients remain adamant and serious about their suicidal intent, if they have a prior history of attempts, or if they have a history of depression.

AGITATION/AGGRESSION

From a learning theorist's perspective, many patients may react to new disabilities as if they are being punished and may respond toward the staff with agitated or aggressive behavior. The ideal intervention is to ignore these behaviors, with the understanding that failing to reinforce them with attention will extinguish them with time. According to this theory, such behaviors can be expected to occur with some frequency in patients who are in crisis after a disability; however, they should also resolve on their own as the natural process of adjustment unfolds. If staff become involved in a cycle of conflict with the patient, aggression and agitation can be exacerbated. At the same time, however, whereas verbally abusive behavior can often be ignored, the physically combative or escape responses of patients with brain injury may require physical restraints or behavioral and/or pharmacologic interventions.

DENIAL

The more current literature in the area of disability minimizes denial as a problem during rehabilitation. Whereas denial was once considered a stance that would hinder rehabilitation and recovery, it is now often regarded as a patient's expression of hope. For example, a patient who has an intractable disease may repeatedly claim that he or she is going to be cured nonetheless. Although it is important that at some point patients receive accurate information about their disease and particularly if they ask for it, it is also important that the clinician not feel compelled to repeatedly "bludgeon the patient with the truth." Patients with spinal cord injuries who claim that they will someday walk again, and are repeatedly corrected by the staff, usually come to resent what they perceive as the discouraging attitude of the health-care workers. As long as the patient is showing disability-appropriate behaviors, that is, learning new behaviors consistent with his or her disability, no particular concern needs to be applied to such verbalizations. If patients are failing to perform health-related behaviors because of a process of denial, these behaviors can be identified and strengthened without necessarily confronting the patient's defenses.

Specific Interventions

REHABILITATION

A comprehensive, multimodal rehabilitation program provides the most effective treatment for most of the psychological problems discussed. From a cognitive standpoint, participation in therapies increases a patient's sense of self-efficacy and mastery over his or her environment. Behaviorally, patients are learning disability-appropriate behaviors and are discouraged from participating in behaviors that will no longer promote satisfaction with their current level of ability. Within the rehabilitation setting, psychological interventions are consequently often geared toward maximizing performance in the various therapies.

BEHAVIORAL INTERVENTIONS

Operant-based behavioral interventions have been frequently cited in the literature as useful in the management of people with disabilities. The sequence for setting up an operant-based behavior change project includes the following:

1. pinpointing the behavior to be increased or decreased;
2. defining measurable units of behavior;
3. recording the rate and occurrence of a given behavior;
4. identifying effective reinforcers;
5. specifying a scheduled reinforcement; and
6. trying out the program.

A useful guide to the identification of reinforcers involves using the Premack principle, which states that of two behaviors observed, the more frequent behavior can be served as a reinforcer for the less frequently occurring behavior. For example, if a patient is observed to enjoy taking frequent naps, his or her rest periods can be used as a reinforcer for a less frequent behavior, such as attending therapy sessions (7).

FAMILIES

It is wise to involve families as strong participants in the rehabilitation process for several reasons. First, regardless of how well patients learn rehabilitation, they will be required to generalize those behaviors outside of the hospital setting, and in a setting where family support or reinforcement will be crucial. Second, a concerned family is also often extremely helpful in resolving disputes between the patient and the rehabilitation staff regarding the course and nature of rehabilitation. It is also most likely that the patient will turn to his or her family for social support, and this will often be a more effective psychological intervention than any type of psychotherapy the staff can provide.

Conferences with the patient and family are particularly useful in facilitating the acceptance of disability-appropriate behaviors. It is important to emphasize, however, that such conferences are frequently conducted without the active participation of the patient and/or the family (10). Specifically, physicians often run the conferences in a didactic style in which family and patients are forced into a passive role. In most cases it is preferable to allow the patient or family to begin a conference with questions or concerns they may have, particularly if they are angry about any issues.

Summary

Recent developments in the application of psychology to disability and chronic disease have made it easier for us to help patients adjust to the changes in their lives as a result of these unfortunate occurrences. Patients and clinicians alike must often shed erroneous models of adaptation to disability for which there has not been adequate scientific justification. It is apparent that stage theories, personality types, conceptualizations that view motivation as being an internal trait of the patient, and a disease model are of little or no use in helping people through this process. On the other hand, some of the more recent cognitive and behavioral-based theories of psychology can be particularly useful with this population.

Many of the psychological problems frequently seen in people with disabilities will often dissipate on their own because they are a function of the temporary phase of adjustment to a change in physical status. A comprehensive rehabilitation program is particularly effective in alleviating such problems. Rehabilitation programs teach patients autonomy, renew their sense of self-efficacy, and increase disability-appropriate behaviors. If patients have difficulty complying with the standard rehabilitation program, it is often useful to apply specific behavioral interventions to enhance performance (e.g., rewarding performance with rest or attention). The clinician will be well-advised to include family members in rehabilitation during most instances. The more the entire rehabilitation team becomes adept at applying the psychological principles discussed above, the better the patient's physical rehabilitation will be. Equally important, as rehabilitation staffs increasingly apply accurate models for adjustment to disability, we can be optimistic that the emotional recovery of this group will be facilitated.

Annotated Suggested Reading List

Bandura A. Self-efficacy: Toward a unifying theory of behavioral change. *Psych Rev* 84:191–215, 1977.

The first comprehensive discussion of self-efficacy as a concept of behavior change available in the literature.

Bowe F. *Handicapping America: Barriers to disabled people.* New York, Harper & Row, 1978.
A view of coping with society from an author with a disability.

The diagnostic and statistical manual of mental disorders (3d ed.). Washington, D.C., The American Psychiatric Association, 1987
Provides the criteria of differentiating between a major depression and other mood disorders that may be seen in patients with disability.

Fordyce WE. Psychological assessment and management. In: Kottke FK, Stillwell GK, Lehmann JL (Eds.), *Krusen's handbook of physical medicine and rehabilitation.* Philadelphia, W.B. Saunders, 1982.
A revised version of the classic text on applying learning theory to the process of rehabilitation.

Hollon S, Beck AT. Research on cognitive therapies. In: SL Garfield, AE Bergin (Eds.), *Handbook of psychotherapy and behavioral change.* New York, John Wiley and Sons, 1987.
Provides a review of various treatments for depression.

Marinnelli RP, Dell Orto AE (Eds.). *The psychological and social impact of physical disability.* New York, Springer, 1977.
This collection of articles discusses such issues as societal attitudes, personality functioning, and sexuality.

Premack D. Toward empirical behavior laws: I. Positive reinforcement. *Psych Rev* 66:219–233, 1959.
Premack's principle, that a more frequently occurring behavior can be used to reinforce a less frequent one, is discussed in this article.

Rotter J. Generalized expectancies for internal versus external locus of control. *Psychological Monographs: General Application* 80:1–28, 1966.
A discussion of the locus of control theory.

Seligman M. *Helplessness: On depression, development and death.* San Francisco, W.H. Freeman and Company, 1975.
A book discussing the application of the learned helplessness theory of depression.

Trieschmann RB. *Spinal cord injuries: Psychological, social and vocational rehabilitation* (2d ed.). New York, Demos Publications, 1988.
A comprehensive discussion of the psychological rehabilitation of people with spinal cord injuries.

21

Social Support and Community Resources

Jay M. Uomoto, Ph.D., Elissa Barron, M.S.W., and Norma Cole, M.S.W.

Introduction

The concept of commmunity support for patients with disabilities is rather broad in scope and often poorly defined. At the very least, the term *support* is a multi-dimensional variable as reported in the psychological literature. However the concept is defined, the general finding is that social-community support for patients with acute or chronic illness is a positive influencing factor toward the restoration of physical, psychological, and social well-being. While a large knowledge base for this idea exists in the mental health arena, fewer studies have been reported to apply this knowledge to patients with disabilities. What follows is an attempt to apply these concepts to the areas of chronic disease and disabilities.

The Process of Social-Community Support in Rehabilitation

The process by which support systems change and reorganize after the onset of a disability is illustrated in Figure 21.1. For the most part, by adulthood individuals tend to have established a routine of social and community connectedness that includes independence in carrying out vocational tasks and activities of daily living (ADL), engaging in recreational pursuits, and maintaining interpersonal contacts. With the onset of a disability (e.g., spinal cord injury, traumatic

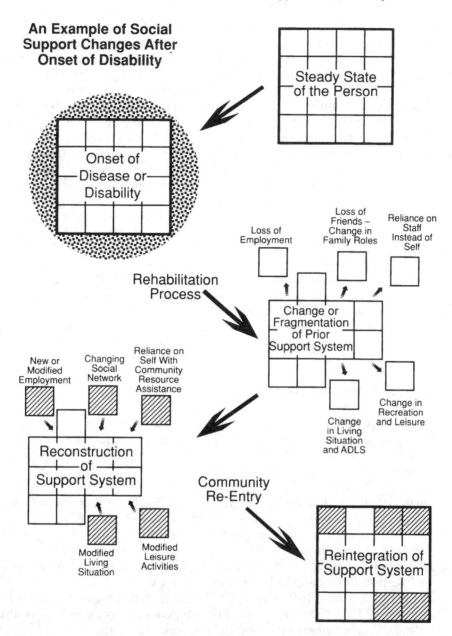

FIGURE 21.1. A chronology of social changes after disability onset.

brain injury, multiple sclerosis, limb amputation secondary to an industrial accident), this support system can radically change for the individual. Early in the rehabilitation process, roles can change in the family, the patient may not be residing at home but rather on an acute rehabilitation unit, and, depending on the nature and scope of the disability, a person's independence in ADL may be impaired. The patient's network of friends may shrink. This often happens, for example, in traumatic brain injury where in addition to physical changes, the personality changes that may occur tend to alienate friendship ties. Much of rehabilitation is spent in therapies of various sorts, with less time devoted to recreational activities, let alone pleasant ones. The physical disability may also limit a patient's access to predisease/disability leisure activities. In short, there is a fragmentation of the support system after the onset of a disability.

Throughout the duration of rehabilitation it is the task of professional staff to assist the patient in reconstructing this support system. Before discharge from an acute rehabilitation unit, for example, patients should be counseled and resources mobilized to prepare them for community reentry. Far too often the patient's social support and community reentry needs are given secondary consideration, yet the patient's success in maintaining treatment gains may rest upon these aspects. Modifications of work, social, and family environments may be addressed by rehabilitation staff before formal discharge from inpatient or outpatient services. Assisting the patient to seek appropriate social outlets may be needed in modifying or replacing the preinjury/disease network. New sources of recreation or leisure activities may need to be generated and encouraged on reentry to the community. In the ideal case, what became fragmented after disability onset is reintegrated, with modifications over the ensuing months and years. This process of reintegration will likely involve the collaborative effort of the interdisciplinary team, across treatment and resources settings, and with the involvement of family and other significant individuals in the patient's social network.

Types of Support and Resources

A variety of support resources are available in urban as well as some rural settings. It may require creative thinking and problem solving to link patients to such resources. In linking patients to resources, it is important to take into consideration:

1. their specific psychosocial needs (as perceived by staff, patient, and family);
2. the timing within which patients should be linked with resources (e.g., a patient may be more accepting of independent living options at a later time rather than immediately);
3. which resources are feasible (from a logistical, economic, and environmental point of view) to utilize; and
4. the match between interpersonal-social style (e.g., gregarious individual with self-initiative versus an isolative-dependent person who has difficulty self-initiating activity) and the services to be used.

Given these conditions, three types of resources and one warning can be stated.

TANGIBLE RESOURCES

A number of social-community services provide instrumental help in terms of equipment needs, home care, chore services, legal advice, and other forms of more "hands-on" assistance. These are delineated more specifically below. An example is the use of community home health agency to provide basic nursing care to a high-level quadriplegic. Financial counseling and agencies are other examples of tangible support. In other cases, mobilizing reliable and accessible family members and friends can be useful to provide help with instrumental tasks.

EMOTIONAL RESOURCES

Many patients with disabilities experience difficulties in adjusting to the physical, emotional, interpersonal, and social changes that occur after onset. They may or may not be open to referrals for counseling or support group opportunities. Family, friends, and religious organization resources often provide informal social support. There is a growing body of literature on the stress-buffering effect of social support. Naturally occurring emotional resources can provide needed support. A problem can occur, however, when the emotional needs of the patient exceed the supportive help that family or friends can provide. In this regard, another body of knowledge is accumulating in the caregiver burden arena. In brief, significant others can be highly burdened by the task of caregiving over the duration of rehabilitation and throughout the care of the patient. This sometimes results in increased family stress and interpersonal conflict. Rehabilitation professionals are therefore cautioned against expecting more from the naturally occurring support system than can be delivered. Careful psychosocial and behavioral assessment is thus a critical part of patient's rehabilitation program.

PERSONAL COPING

Individuals have their own set of coping abilities for life stressors. Each patient with a disability may cope differently, depending on his or her own history. Some cope by denying the existence of limitations, whereas others use cognitive self-management strategies to help put their life stressors into perspective. There is no particular set of most effective personal coping strategies; rather, coping must be assessed and enhanced given the person–situation match. For example, it may be very effective and necessary to minimize in one's mind the impact of disability as an initial coping mechanism immediately after spinal cord injury; later on, it may be more adaptive to utilize cognitive self-statement/perspective-taking strategies as a means of managing daily stressors. A psychologist, social worker, or other counselor may be best suited to assess the personal coping styles of patients and to provide further counseling to both patients and their significant others.

MISCARRIED HELP

It seems reaonsable that family members, close ties of the patient, and other well-meaning individuals would appropriate choices from which to elicit social support. Although this is more often the case than not, in some situations the support given can be a problem in and of itself. That is, miscarried attempts to be of assistance can be counterproductive to the physical and psychosocial welfare of the patient. Family members can become overinvolved in the responsibilities at home. Initially this may lessen the burden for the patient, yet in the long run this form of miscarried help can lead to decreased independence in functional activities. Other family members can, for example, overprotect the patient from learning on a trial-and-error basis, thus making it difficult for the him or her to be independent in new environments or settings (such as living alone in an apartment or handling an interpersonal rift without the aid of others). Rehabilitation professionals must also be careful in trying to balance assistance with appropriate latitude for the patient to have success as well as failure experiences. In sum, it is important for staff to be aware of well-meaning efforts by persons in the patient's support network that may lead to counterproductive outcomes, and not readily assume that "more support is better." Turning this situation around can be difficult and usually involves educating family members or significant others about ways they can promote independence and reframe their miscarried efforts as a "good start" and that the next step involves "letting go" to a certain extent.

Linking Patients with Resources

Social problems and needs can be relatively easy to identify; however, the more challenging task is knowing how to connect needs with appropriate resources. Utilizing the expertise of professionals trained in the management of chronic disease and disability is likely to be the most productive and efficient means of linking patients/clients with those services that will be beneficial. Currently, most hospitals and a select number of medical clinics employ bachelor's or master's level social workers and/or discharge planners who are skilled in this area.

The role of the social worker in the medical setting is multifaceted and includes the following: discharge planning, advocacy, patient and family education, psychosocial assessment and intervention, and referral to and coordination of community resources. Physicians or other rehabilitation professionals who identify a problem or need can contact the social work department of the hospital and request that their patient/client be seen. In hospitals or clinics where social workers and discharge planners are not readily available, nursing staff are frequently aware of community resources and the method by which such sources may be contacted. Public health nurses frequently perform this function in smaller, more remote communities and can be an excellent resource when services are being explored in these areas. It often requires creative discharge planning to link patients in rural regions to needed resources.

When the professional expertise of social workers, discharge planners, public health nurses, and so forth are not accessible or cannot be utilized due to the community size or locale, physicians and rehabilitation nurses may need to perform the linkage role between patient and community resources. To effectively carry out this task, the following points should be considered.

1. Many communities develop a resource guide that lists all available social service organization and groups for a particular catchment area. Such materials can often be purchased through the United Way or a similar organization.

2. If no resource guide exists in the community you are working in, the Yellow Pages of the local telephone directory list numerous social service agencies by category. The Blue Pages list governmental offices/organizations. Several telephone calls and a systematic record of appropriate or good resources should be kept on hand for future reference.
3. Frequently, if an agency or organization cannot be of assistance, it will be able to refer you to the appropriate referral source.
4. If presented with the name and telephone number of a referral agency, patients and families can often contact the various referral sources on their own. Whether or not the patient/family is capable of making this contact is largely dependent on their level of psychosocial functioning and their level of acceptance of the illness and/or disability.

The actual linkage of patients to resources tends to be very straightforward and elementary. Knowing which resource provides the best fit between need and service is a more difficult task, and often involves time-consuming investigation. However, once the clinician has worked with a particular population for a period of time, these resources will become familiar and easier to access.

═══ Specific Resources

Following a careful assessment of the patient's psychosocial situation, including the nature of the illness or disability, prognosis, family support network, economic/financial considerations, vocational options, and accessibility to resources, the social worker or discharge planner will assess the available community resources and make appropriate referrals. The skillful linkage with community resources will enable the individual to function at the highest level of independence possible. These community resources may often make the difference between independent lifestyle and the need for placement in a facility or institution. As is the case in the mental health field, placement and long-term functioning in the least restrictive environment is a goal to which rehabilitation professionals direct their efforts.

The following outlines community resources available to assist chronically ill or disabled patients.

FINANCIAL ASSISTANCE PROGRAMS

A number of programs are operated by federal and state governments to provide some level of financial assistance for low-income clients with disabilities. There are strict eligibility guidelines for all programs. These are generally administered through the Social Security Administration (e.g., Social Security Disability Insurance and Supplemental Security Income) or through the state's social, health, or family services departments (e.g., Medicaid, public assistance, rent and energy subsidies).

FOOD AND NUTRITIONAL PROGRAMS

A wide variety of services are available in the community to assist with meeting the patient's nutritional needs, including meal sites at senior activity centers, schools, churches, food banks, home-delivered groceries, home-delivered meals, nutritional counseling, and classes. Government-sponsored food stamp programs are available to the low-income client.

HOME HEALTH CARE

Many agencies provide services that allow patients with chronic illnesses and disabilities to remain in their own homes, with intermittent visits or full-time care. A wide range of services are offered, including visiting nurses, nurses' aides, personal caregivers who can provide assistance with activities of daily living (ADL), social workers, occupational therapists, physical therapists, speech therapists, respiratory therapy and equipment services, nutritional therapy, and equipment. Home health-care providers offer a safety net to the individual and can link the patient to other resources as needed.

ADULT DAY PROGRAMS

These programs often have a sliding-fee schedule and are located in churches, community centers, medical facilities, and privately owned facilities. They provide daily or weekly programs in productive, supervised settings. Some services offered include occupational therapy, physical therapy, speech therapy, recreational activities, medical monitoring, counseling services, vocational rehabilitation services, and social activities. These programs can provide respite for caregivers in a structured setting.

CHORE SERVICES

Help with household chores can be essential to the patient who is no longer able to drive, shop for groceries, do the laundry, cook meals, or perform similar housekeeping tasks. State-sponsored chore assistance is available for low-income individuals. Additionally, many community agencies and volunteer programs can provide chore assistance for a minimal fee.

HOUSING RESOURCES

A careful evaluation of the patient's financial situation, medical condition, and support network will determine the type of housing referrals and recommendations that are needed. A wide variety of options are available for housing, including retirement and nursing facilities, group homes, adult foster homes, subsidized apartments, and rent subsidies. Also, a number of community agencies can provide assistance with home repair and modifications.

MENTAL HEALTH SERVICES

A wide range of services are offered through local community mental health centers, including case management; crisis/emergency counseling and outreach; drug and alcohol assessment and counseling; vocational programs; parenting classes; and individual, group, and family therapy. Services are often available on a sliding-fee scale. Many centers will accept medical coupons. Additionally, a range of counseling services are available through family service agencies, churches and synagogues, and private practitioners.

SUPPORT GROUPS

Numerous support, education, and advocacy groups can provide a setting for patients, families, and caregivers to share feelings about illness and disability. Opportunities are available to sort through issues of grief, resentment, frustration, and anger in a supportive atmosphere. Educational presentations and advocacy for client's rights can be a positive and constructive outcome of the group support.

TRANSPORTATION

The lack of affordable, accessible, and convenient transportation often presents the disabled individual from interacting with the community. The social worker, acting as a discharge planner, can refer the client to agencies that can provide reduced fees for bus and taxi rides, ride-sharing programs, and low-cost van services.

REFERRAL SERVICES

Many cities have telephone information and referral services that can provide the health-care professional further help in locating appropriate community resources. These services often are offered as a part of a 24-hour crisis intervention line. Another way to obtain appropriate referrals for services of a mental health nature can by through local or state psychological, social work, or psychiatric associations. Such offices usually maintain a listing of private practitioners or agencies for specific kinds of problems and locales.

NATIONAL ORGANIZATIONS

A number of organizations provide referral, information, and advocacy assistance on a national level. They often provide toll-free telephone access and maintain numerous listings and resources that are available at the state, city, and county level. They also can assist in matching resources to the particular problems at hand, as well as providing educational materials aimed at patients, family members, and professionals. A list of some of the major national organizations relevant to chronic disease and disability follows.

===== **Conclusions**

It is important to consider social support and community resources as a vital part of any treatment program. Rehabilitation is seen here as not ceasing at the point of discharge but rather continuing in the community, perhaps with less reliance on professional intervention and more involvement of naturally occurring and community-based supports.

Underlying the need for support is the goal for patients to continue to improve their daily functioning and maintain treatment gains after formal rehabilitation. In this regard, Meichenbaum and Turk (1987) have aptly summarized 10 principles to assist in obtaining and maintaining treatment adherence. We feel these principles apply to the patient with chronic disease or disability who reenters the community and needs to be cared for by health-care professionals. They find the following techniques to be critical.

1. *Anticipate nonadherence.* Professionals need to plan ahead for the high possibility of patients not following through with recommendations and referrals.
2. *Consider the prescribed self-care regimen from the patient's perspective.* Too often we may recommend ideas and strategies that are simply not understood or acceptable from the patient's point of view. Alternative means of framing maintenance programs and follow-up with community resources may need to occur long before the patient leaves formal rehabilitation work.
3. *Foster a collaborative relationship based on negotiation.* Referrals will be better heard and acted upon if a basic relationship exists between professional and patient in which the latter is included in the decision making.
4. *Be patient-oriented.* It is important to assess the patient's view of his or her disease, its prognosis, and expectations for follow-up with community resources in order to discover potential problems with the process of community reentry. All referrals made and communications about linking patients to resources should be clearly understood from the patient's perspective.
5. *Customize treatment.* Those referrals and resources, be it natural supports or community agencies, should match well with the patient's beliefs, expectations, and needs.
6. *Enlist family support.* Successful community reentry may require family input to assist the patient to recognize the need for follow-up, and for patients to feel they do not have to mobilize help on their own.
7. *Provide a system of continuity and accessibility.* Clear communication, reduction of ambiguity in feedback, and an open stance to patient feedback and desires will assist in the transition back to community life.
8. *Make use of other health-care providers and personnel as well as community resources.* As stated above, a psychological sense of community perceived by the patient is important to normalize as much as possible his or her longer-term adjustment to chronic disease and disability.
9. *Repeat everything.* It is not enough to give a patient a referral and hope that a connection will be made in the future. Repetition of information, and walking through the steps of linking the patient to a resource, can only expedite the process.

10. *Don't give up.* While this may sound trite, it is true that much creative problem solving and brainstorming may be required to coordinate and link appropriate resources for the patient in the community. The process may indeed require a few iterations before the correct match is found between patient and resource, though in the long term it will likely benefit the patient's quality of life in coping with chronic disease or disability.

Recommended Reading

Callahan D. Families as caregivers: The limits of morality. *Arch Phys Med Rehabil,*69:323–328, 1988.

This article discusses the ethics of family members acting as caregivers for patients with disabilities. Psychological and moral dilemmas that confront caregivers are delineated. The heroic duties of family members providing care to the disabled is reinforced by the larger culture that rewards heroic effort. An argument is made for a cultural change in attitude toward heroic family efforts, rather than simply improving the social services that are available in the community.

Cohen S, Wills TA. Stress, social support, and the buffering hypothesis. *Psych Bull* 98:310–357, 1985.

The authors in this review article describe numerous research findings that provide evidence for buffering effects of social support on psychological stress experienced by the individual.

Levesque, JD. Assessing the foreseeable risks in discharge planning. *Social Work Health Care* 13:49–63, 1988.

The difficulties in finding an appropriate discharge plan for a brain-injured patient with significant cognitive impairment is discussed in the article. There is a tension between the needs of the patient and the ability of the discharging institution to find appropriate community resources. The paper is intended to be a practical guide from the perspective of the hospital's duties, with consideration being given to the potential risks to the patient.

Lezak MD. Brain damage is a family affair. *J Clin Exp Neuropsych,* 10:111–123, 1988.

Dr. Lezak delineates some of the most common cognitive, physical, and behavioral sequelae after traumatic brain injury, and very practically discusses the impact these problems have on the family system. The article can be used as good reading material for family members themselves.

Meichenbaum D, Turk DC. *Facilitating treatment adherence: A practitioner's guidebook.* New York, Plenum Press, 1987.

This is an important text that combines a balanced assessment of the research on treatment compliance, as well as provides practical clinical information about facilitating treatment adherence. The approach taken by these authors is primarily from a behavioral point of view. Any health-care professional who works with difficult to manage patients can benefit from the principles outlined in this book.

Pitzele SK. *We are not alone: Learning to live with chronic illness.* New York, Workman Publishing, 1985.

This book was written as a self-help guide for spouses and family members who must deal with a person with chronic disability in the home. It is a combination of practical help and information about typical reactions by family members in such situations.

National Organizations for Chronic Disease and Disability

CHRONIC DISEASE

AIDS Medical Foundation
230 Park Avenue, Room 1266
New York, NY 10169
212-949-9411

American Cancer Society
777 Third Avenue
New York, NY 10017

American Diabetes Association
505 Eighth Avenue
New York, NY 10038

American Heart Association
7320 Greenville Avenue
Dallas, TX 75231
214-750-7300

American Kidney Fund
P. O. Box 975
Washington, DC 20044

American Lung Association
1740 Broadway
New York, NY 10019

American Red Cross
17th and D Streets, NW
Washington, DC 20006
202-734-8300

Arthritis Foundation
3400 Peachtree Road NE
Atlanta, GA 30326

Emphysema Association
P. O. Box 66
Fort Meyers, FL 33902

Leukemia Society of America
Public Education and Information
800 Second Avenue
New York, NY 10017

National Cancer Information Service
    Hotline
1-800-638-6694

National Kidney Foundation
Two Park Avenue
New York, NY 10016

U.S. Public Health Service
Public Affairs Office
Hubert H. Humphrey Building
Room 724-H
200 Independence Ave., SW
Washington, DC 20201

DISABILITY AND REHABILITATION

Alzheimer's Disease and Related
    Disorders Association
70 East Lake Street, Suite 600
Chicago, IL 60601
1-800-621-0379

American Coalition of Citizens with
    Disabilities
1200 15th St., NW
Suite 201
Washington, DC 20005

American Geriatric Society
10 Columbus Circle
New York, NY 10019

American Parkinson's Disease
    Foundation
116 John Street
New York, NY 10038
212-732-9550

Amyotrophic Lateral Sclerosis
    Association
185 Madison Avenue, Suite 1001
P. O. Box 2130
New York, NY 10016

Disabled American Veterans
3725 Alexandria Pike
Cold Springs, KY 41076

Epilepsy Foundation of America
4351 Barden Drive
Suite 406
Landover, MD 20785

Information Center for Individuals
  with Disabilities
20 Park Plaza, Room 330
Boston, MA 02116
617-727-5540

Multiple Sclerosis Society National
  Headquarters
733 Third Avenue
New York, NY 10017
212-986-3240

Muscular Dystrophy Association
  National Office
810 Seventh Avenue
New York, NY 10019

Myasthenia Gravis Foundation, Inc.
7-11 South Broadway, Suite 304
White Plains, NY 10601

National Association for Hearing and
  Speech Action
10801 Rockville Pike
Rockville, MD 20852
1-800-638-8255

National Head Injury Foundation
1776 Massachusetts Ave., N.W.
Suite 100
Washington, DC 20036-1904
202-296-6443

National Institute on Aging
National Institutes of Health
Building 31, Room 5C35
Bethesda, MD 20205
301-496-1752

National Paraplegia Foundation
333 North Michigan Avenue
Chicago, IL 60601

National Rehabilitation Association
633 South Washington Street
Alexandria, VA 22314

National Rehabilitation Information
  Center
4407 Eighth Street, NE
Washington, DC 20017-2299
1-800-34NARIC

National Spinal Cord Injury
  Assocation
149 California Street
Newton, MA 02158

Paralyzed Veterans of America
801 Eighteenth Street, NW
Washington, DC 20006
202-872-1300

22

Vocational Aspects of Rehabilitation

Rochelle V. Habeck, Ph.D., Michael J. Leahy, Ph.D., and Barry Goldstein, M.D., Ph.D.

This chapter is a general overview of contemporary vocational rehabilitation for individuals with chronic disease and disability. It includes a brief description of the development and organizational structure of the field, the service process and resources used, and the implications of vocational issues for physicians.

Recent estimates in this country indicate that approximately 40 million individuals have some type of physical or mental impairment that significantly affects life activities. While considered a highly heterogeneous population, these individuals face common obstacles and barriers following disability in relation to attainment of their individual vocational, independent living, and quality of life aspirations. An estimated 14 percent, or 27 million individuals in the adult working age population, have disabilities (4), and over 10 million of these adults with physical or mental impairments could probably benefit from vocational rehabilitation services (6). One of the most compelling facts underscoring the need for continued vocational services and enhanced opportunities is that 62 percent of people with disabilities are currently outside the labor force and between 56–75 percent are denied access to various aspects of community life (4).

While there is no question that the personal loss associated with disability (e.g., career disruption, income loss, psychological, social, and family impact) is of predominant importance, the impact on society and business (e.g., lost productivity, income benefit costs) of not adequately addressing these human and economic costs provides a compelling rationale for the provision of vocational services to individuals with disabilities. A fundamental premise that underlies rehabilitation efforts has been that successful vocational outcome as defined by job stability and satisfaction provides a basis for satisfactory life adjustment, personal independence, economic self–sufficiency, and opportunities in most areas of life.

As is true with many other problems that people with disabilities encounter, vocational handicaps result from unique interactions of factors related to the individual, the impairing condition, its functional consequence, and the external environments in which the individual functions. The World Health Organization has thus differentiated the following concepts:

1. impairment—as evidence of a physiologic, psychological, or anatomic loss or abnormality resulting from disease or injury;
2. disability—as a restriction on or lack of ability to perform an activity in the normal range due to impairment; and
3. handicap—as a disadvantage that limits fulfillment of normal roles due to consequences of impairment or environmental obstacles.

The causes of vocational handicaps are not always obvious, yet they must be determined so that the focus of intervention will be appropriate and effective. Almost by definition, vocational handicaps, and certainly their resolution, involve environmental factors, such as accessibility of the workplace, employer attitudes, and disability insurance provisions.

In recent years, the clinical or medical model of rehabilitation (7) has been increasingly seen as inadequate to address the social disadvantages and barriers that limit the full participation of persons with disability in society. Hahn (2) has identified three competing conceptual models of disability in articulating this issue:

1. the medical model, which defines disability in terms of extent of physical impairment or deviation from normal anatomical function;
2. the economic model, which defines disability in terms of disruption in labor market participation and focuses on the individual's vocational limitations; and
3. the sociopolitical model, which defines disability in terms of a disadvantaged social minority, where disability is the product of environmental response to the social stigma of disability characteristics.

The model of disability adopted in public policy significantly impacts rehabilitation practice. With the passage of the Americans with Disabilities Act in 1990 and the Rehabilitation Act Amendments in 1992, disability and rehabilitation policy has shifted its emphasis from a focus on the individual to a more encompassing view that also addresses individual rights and environmental barriers. Service providers must consider increased expectations and requirements of clients with disabilities for nondiscrimination, self-determination, inclusion, informed choice, and community-based support in the services they receive.

Development and Organization of Vocational Services

Disability can markedly impact upon an individual's opportunity to progress along the usual course of personal development, pursue a desired career, and engage in social and community activities. Society's willingness to attend to the needs of persons with disabilities has been influenced by the perceived cause of the disability and its associated social merit (e.g., war injury) or perceived personal liability (e.g., mental illness), the prevailing economic conditions, sociocultural philosophy, and the existing medical and technological knowledge (6).

While rehabilitation efforts existed in a sporadic fashion prior to the twentieth century in the private and voluntary sectors, the civilian vocational rehabilitation program was only created with the passage of the Smith–Fess Act in 1920. This landmark federal legislation was the first of many such legislative efforts that greatly expanded the public rehabilitation program to address the vocational service needs of individuals with disabilities. Advances in social policy and legislative mandates and changes in the nature of workers' compensation legislation have increasingly broadened the total rehabilitation delivery system to include a wide range of clientele, services, goals, sponsors, and settings. Additionally, these enabling legislative efforts expanded government and other third-party funding for client services and professional rehabilitation education and research, sought to protect the civil rights of consumers, and provided incentives for the employment of individuals with disabilities. Currently, vocational rehabilitation services in this country can be viewed as three distinct efforts: public, private nonprofit, and private for-profit.

PUBLIC SECTOR

Each state has a public rehabilitation program that is funded through both state and federal funds. The Rehabilitation Services Administration (RSA) provides the federal funding for the state/federal program; it is part of the U.S. Department of Education, Office of Special Education and Rehabilitation Services.

These state programs are operated in compliance with federal mandates (RSA). They provide services to individuals with mental or physical impairments that represent substantial vocational handicaps, who have feasible potential for rehabilitation, and who are at least 16 years of age. Typical services provided within state agencies include vocational evaluation, diagnostic evaluation, counseling and guidance, physical and mental restoration, training, job placement, and independent living services. The RSA provides funding to each state on an 80–20 matching basis to facilitate the delivery of these vocational rehabilitation and independent living services. It also provides training funds for rehabilitation professionals and a program for research through the National Institute on Disability and Rehabilitation Research.

PRIVATE NONPROFIT SECTOR

The Vocational Rehabilitation Amendments of 1954 authorized the use of state/federal service dollars to purchase services from private nonprofit facilities. Rehabilitation facilities now number approximately 7,000. They provide individualized vocational rehabilitation services to a wide range of clientele, including vocational assessment, work adjustment, personal adjustment training, vocational skills training, job placement and supported employment, and in some cases sheltered employment.

Clients served within these facilities include individuals sponsored by the state/federal rehabilitation program and the mental health system and, more recently, also industrially injured workers. Each state has an organization of accredited facilities—usually referred to as the Association of Rehabilitation Facilities—where contact can be made regarding the specific types of facilities available for client referral.

PRIVATE FOR–PROFIT SECTOR

For more than 50 years after passage of the Smith–Fess Act, virtually all vocationally related rehabilitation services were provided through public and non-profit agencies. A dramatic and ongoing increase in the private for-profit sector of vocational rehabilitation began in the 1970s due to changes in workers' compensation legislation and the increasingly common provision of rehabilitation benefits by private insurance. Vocational services provided by this sector predominantly focus on return-to-work efforts for employees. This sector—sometimes referred to as "industrial rehabilitation"—is currently the major growth area in rehabilitation.

If an individual becomes disabled in the course of his or her employment, it is generally now viewed as the responsibility of the employer to sponsor the necessary rehabilitation services through workers' compensation insurance. As a result, these services are now provided primarily on a fee-for-service basis by private vocational rehabilitation companies contracted with by the employer or the employer's insurance carrier. Because so many individuals are disabled as a result of occupational injuries or disease, physicians must understand this benefit system in detail. Advocacy by the primary physician for appropriate and timely services is often essential to assure the insurer or employer of their necessity and the benefits of prompt and safe return to work.

The Vocational Rehabilitation Process

The vocational rehabilitation service process can be conceptualized as having four major sequential phases (6). Clients participating in this process usually are of working age and have a physical or mental disability that presents a significant handicap to employment. The extent of vocational handicap that results from disability for any given individual will be influenced by his or her physical capacity, acquired vocational skills and skill-acquisition potential, psychological functioning, and environmental resources.

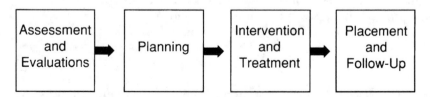

FIGURE 22.1. Vocational rehabilitation process.

ASSESSMENT AND EVALUATION

This initial phase is directed at determining current and potential client function in order to identify appropriate occupations and to develop a plan for effective case management and the provision of rehabilitation services to achieve the identified goal. This process is highly individualized, is comprehensive and systematic in nature, and stresses the active involvement of the client. It should be guided by hypotheses and specific questions generated by interviews with the client and a review of background information. A variety of assessment approaches and instruments are available and should be selected to most appropriately address the hypotheses and questions raised. These include:

1. the counseling interview;
2. tests and inventories, including aptitude, ability, achievement, interests, values, and personality measures;
3. the use of simulated job tasks and real work; and
4. functional assessment and physical capacity evaluation.

The goals of this phase are to:

- describe the individual's functioning level and needs;
- specify the appropriate outcomes to be achieved through the rehabilitation process; and
- identify the interventions or services required to achieve these outcomes (8)

In rehabilitation, special caution must be exercised when utilizing standardized instruments due to the potential confounding effects of disability when such instruments are administered in a nonstandardized fashion (1). Additionally, experiential strategies are preferred to a total reliance on traditional paper-and-pencil tests, especially for individuals who have limited academic backgrounds and work experience.

It is critically important to ascertain the purpose of the proposed vocational assessment, the appropriateness of the selected approach to adequately answer the assessment questions, the professional competence of the evaluation source, and the client's level of understanding and participation in the process. For example, the provision of rehabilitation services in workers' compensation and other insurance-sponsored programs is generally limited to restoring working capacity and facilitating prompt return to employment. The emphasis of evaluation is therefore focused on the identification of transferable skills, residual functional capacities, and essential job requirements in order to make the most efficient match or accommodation of the worker's remaining abilities and work opportunities. Regardless of the purpose for the assessment, the following principles of professional assessment should be followed.

PLANNING

During this phase and after a thorough review of assessment findings and occupational information, the counselor and client decide on appropriate occupational goals and determine what services are required to achieve those outcomes. The planning process is critical to the success of the subsequent intervention and placement stages and must thoroughly identify all interventions and services required and the objectives of each. This plan of service, or an individually written rehabilitation plan, becomes the guide for service for the remainder of the process. Critical to the success of this stage are the counselor's knowledge of available services and community resources and his or her ability to access these services for the client.

INTERVENTION AND TREATMENT

Individual plans of services are implemented in the third phase of the process. Examples of potential interventions include personal adjustment counseling, independent living skills training, physical restoration, adult basic education, work adjustment training, vocational skills training, and rehabilitation engineering. This phase addresses those limitations identified in the assessment phase that are amenable to intervention. The counselor will typically purchase and utilize services from an array of community resources (e.g., hospitals, rehabilitation workshops, vocational training centers) to provide the required service that will prepare the individual for job placement services and independent living.

JOB PLACEMENT

The last phase in the process is that of placement, follow-up, and termination, during which the job-ready client prepares to locate and secure employment. Typical services include job-seeking skills training, individual placement assistance, job and worksite modifications, and employer consultation for reasonable accommodations.

The vocational rehabilitation process described above provides a quick view of the general features involved in most cases. The specific approach, tools, and resources used will vary greatly as a function of (a) impairment–related factors; (b) person–related factors; and (c) system factors (e.g., eligibility and access to benefits and services, labor market opportunities, financial resources, and social support). A few examples may serve to illustrate the range of vocational handicaps, resources, and solutions that come into play as well as why the process must be individualized to reach employment outcomes.

First, consider high-level spinal cord injuries. Most affected individuals are young and have limited education or work experience, and their functional deficits are considerable. Solutions must address equipment needs and environment modifications both for personal independence and community mobility. Individuals usually cannot return to unskilled jobs, and formal training is required to develop specific skills that will utilize intact abilities that relate to local job opportunities. The placement approach is selective, often involving environmental modifications to the worksite and workstation. Long-term involvement and advocacy of a rehabilitation counselor to manage this process is typically required.

On the other hand, consider successfully employed individuals who develop chronic conditions, such as arthritis, or disabilities due to repetitive movements, such as shoulder impingement. In both instances, the vocational rehabilitation goal would be to assist the individual and his or her employer to retain employment in the former job, if possible, or at least in the same company. Through early intervention, the rehabilitation counselor would assist in defining the individual's temporary and long-term functional restrictions and the essential requirements of his or her job; this would be followed by the development of a rehabilitation and return-to-work plan. Timely implementation of this process is essential to its success. Many individuals can resume their former employment in an adapted or in a new capacity using their transferable skills.

The Profession of Rehabilitation Counseling

The field of rehabilitation counseling has developed as the professional discipline that provides vocational services. The rehabilitation counselor is a vocational expert who operates from a psychological base, functions as part of a psychosocial and health-related team, and provides a broad range of services for individuals with disabilities (3). The effective role of the rehabilitation counselor is that of a problem solver who perceives the problems of each individual client as they relate to his or her vocational adjustment within specific environments, and who helps to plan and implement appropriate intervention strategies (5).

Rehabilitation counselors thus play a multifaceted role in providing services to individuals with disabilities. Counselors must be able to assess the functional impact of disability (e.g., psychosocial, vocational aspects) and have the knowledge and skills to utilize all environmental resources available to effect appropriate employment outcomes.

More then 30,000 practicing rehabilitation counselors are employed within the different rehabilitation sectors in the United States, approximately 10,000 of whom are Certified Rehabilitation Counselors (CRC) who have been certified by the Commission on Rehabilitation Counselor Certification as having achieved the minimum standards of practice. It is important that physicians who wish to access vocational services for their clients be aware of the desired credentials, affiliations, and competencies of qualified vocational rehabilitation service providers when making referrals.

Implications for Medical Practice

Physicians occupy a key position in shaping the outcomes of disability and chronic disease. By recognizing the broader implications of health problems on an individual patient's life circumstances and their impact on participation in normal life activities, physicians can help individuals with disabilities to maintain productive activity, with all its economic, psychological, and social benefits. The impact of unemployment and dependency is tremendously negative for individuals in our society. Physicians who are sensitive to these issues and aware of vocational rehabilitation resources and strategies can enhance the quality of life for their patients and achieve accountability in health care.

Conclusions

Some guiding principles that derive from the material presented in this chapter are as follows.

1. Vocational handicaps result from interactions among the impairing condition, personal characteristics, and environmental factors. The needs and solutions necessary to accomplish vocational rehabilitation must therefore be tailored to individual circumstances and address both clinical and environmental barriers

2. The most effective way to prevent unemployment due to disability is to intervene early and to maintain ability to stay in the same job or with the same employer. Early vocational intervention can help prevent the development of psychosocial problems that can interfere with successful outcomes of rehabilitation, maintain motivation for recovery, retain identity as a healthy productive person, guide effective coping and adaptation, reduce needless waiting and frustration with services and benefits, and sustain employer interest in return to work. Communication with the employer or company representative can help to maintain a cooperative, problem-solving atmosphere, and avoid an adversarial process.

3. A knowledge of disability benefit programs and vocational and rehabilitation resources is essential to assisting individuals with disabilities achieve competitive employment and independent living.

4. Patient advocacy and referral often begin with the primary physician. Although most of the vocational rehabilitation processes will occur subsequent to primary care, its continued availability and guidance can facilitate appropriate goal setting, service planning, and the documentation necessary to secure needed benefits and services.

Persons with disabilities insist on equal access to mainstream society and opportunities. Employers insist on reducing unnecessary costs of illness and disability. Demographic changes in our population, public policy goals, and the challenges of international economics require that we protect our human resources and accommodate the limitations resulting from chronic conditions to enable productive contribution. Effective partnerships among physicians, rehabilitation counselors, individuals with disabilities, and employers can significantly address these important needs.

References

Berven NL. Assessment practices in rehabilitation counseling. In Riggar TF, Maki DR, Wolf AW (Eds.), *Applied rehabilitation counseling* (pp. 34–44) New York, Springer, 1986.

Hahn H. The political implications of disability definitions and data. *Journal of Disability Policy Studies* 4(2): 41–52, 1993.

Jacques M. *Rehabilitation counseling: Scope and services.* Boston, Houghton Mifflin, 1970.

Lou Harris & Associates. *The ICD survey of disabled Americans.* New York, 1986.

Maki D, McCracken N, Pape D, Schofield M. The theoretical model of vocational rehabilitation. *Journal of Rehabilitation* 44 (4):26–28, 1978.

Rubin SE, Roessler RT. *Foundations of the vocational rehabilitation process* (3d Ed.). Austin,

TX, Pro-Ed, 1987.

Stubbins J. *The clinical attitude in rehabilitation: A cross cultural view* . Monograph #16. New York, World Rehabilitation Foundation, 1982.

VEWAA Final Report Menomonie, WI: University of Wisconsin–Stout, Materials Development Center, 1975.

Recommended Reading

Isernhagen SJ (Ed.). *Work injury: Management and prevention.* Rockville, MD: Aspen Publishers, 1988.

A comprehensive treatment of physical work injuries, edited by a physical therapist and directed toward all phases of industrial rehabilitation process.

Matkin RE *Insurance rehabilitation,* Austin, TX, Pro-Ed, 1985.

Comprehensive text on insurance rehabilitation and service applications in disability compensation systems.

Rubin SE, Roessler RT *Foundations of the vocational rehabilitation process* (3d ed.). Austin, TX, Pro-Ed, 1987.

The most widely used textbook on the vocational rehabilitation process. Includes chapters on the role of the rehabilitation counselor and the four-stage rehabilitation process.

Resources

Rehabilitation Services Administration (RSA)
U. S. Dept. of Education
Washington, D. C.

National Rehabilitation Association
Alexandria, Virginia

National Council on Rehabilitation Education
Emporia State University
Emporia, KS

American Rehabilitation Counseling Association
Alexandria, VA

Index